PSYCHIATRIC AND BEHAVIORAL DISORDERS IN ISRAEL

PSYCHIATRIC AND BEHAVIORAL DISORDERS IN ISRAEL
From Epidemiology to Mental Health Action

Edited by **Itzhak Levav**

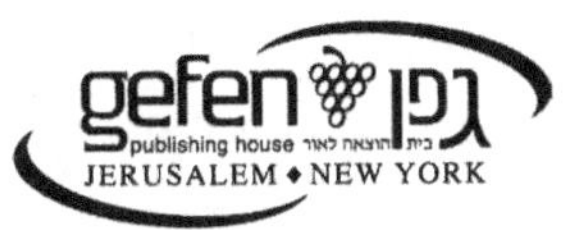

gefen publishing house
JERUSALEM ♦ NEW YORK

Typesetting: KPS, Jerusalem
Cover Design: S. Kim Glassman
Cover Art: S. Levav

ISBN 978-965-229-468-5

Edition 1   3   5   7   9   8   6   4   2

Gefen Publishing House Ltd.
6 Hatzvi Street, Jerusalem 94386, Israel
972-2-538-0247 • orders@gefenpublishing.com

Gefen Books
600 Broadway, Lynbrook, NY 11563, USA
1-800-477-5257 • orders@gefenpublishing.com

www.gefenpublishing.com

Printed in Israel

Send for our free catalogue

Contents

SECTION I: PSYCHIATRIC AND BEHAVIORAL DISORDERS IN POPULATION GROUPS

SECTION II: THE EPIDEMIOLOGY OF PSYCHIATRIC AND BEHAVIORAL DISORDERS

SECTION III: EPIDEMIOLOGY APPLIED TO THE MENTAL HEALTH SERVICES

Authors

Alean Al-Krenawi PhD, Associate Professor, Spitzer Department of Social Work, Ben-Gurion University of the Negev, Beersheba.

Alan Apter MB, Professor, Sackler School of Medicine, Tel Aviv University; and Head, Department of Child and Adolescent Psychiatry, Schneider Children's Medical Center, Petah Tikva.

Orna Baron-Epel PhD MPH, Senior Lecturer, School of Public Health, Faculty of Welfare and Health Studies, University of Haifa, Haifa.

RH Belmaker MD, Hoffer Vickar Chair of Psychiatry, Faculty of Health Sciences, Ben-Gurion University of the Negev, Beersheba.

Cendrine Bursztein Lipsicas MA, Feinberg Child Study Center, Schneider Children's Medical Center, Petah Tikva; and Tel Aviv University, Tel Aviv.

Julie Cwikel PhD, Professor, Spitzer Department of Social Work, Ben-Gurion University of the Negev; and Director, The Ben-Gurion University Center for Women's Health Studies and Promotion, Beersheba.

Richard Ebstein PhD, Professor, Department of Psychology, Hebrew University, Jerusalem; and Head, Scheinfeld Center for Human Genetic Studies in the Social Sciences, Herzog Hospital, Jerusalem.

Ari A. Gershon MD, Department of Psychiatry, Sheba Medical Center, Tel Hashomer.

Galit Geulayov MSc, Researcher, Unit for Mental Health Epidemiology & Psychosocial Aspects of Illness, The Gertner Institute for Epidemiology and Health Policy Research, Sheba Medical Center, Tel Hashomer.

Raz Gross MD MPH, Director, Mental Health Epidemiology, The Gertner Institute for Epidemiology and Health Policy Research, Sheba Medical Center, Tel Hashomer.

Karni Ginzburg PhD, Senior Lecturer, Bob Shappel School of Social Work, Tel Aviv University, Tel Aviv.

Anneke Ifrah MPH, Researcher, Israel Center for Disease Control, Ministry of Health, Tel Hashomer.

Lital Keinan-Boker MD MPH PhD, Lecturer, School of Public Health, Faculty of Welfare and Health Studies, University of Haifa, Haifa; and Israel Center for Disease Control, Ministry of Health, Tel Hashomer.

Ilana Kremer MD, Senior Clinical Lecturer, Faculty of Medicine, Technion, Haifa; and Director, Department of Psychiatry, Emek Medical Center, Afula.

Yaacov Lerner MD, Director, Falk Institute, Ministry of Health, Jerusalem.

Itzhak Levav MD MSc, Adviser in Research, Mental Health Services, Ministry of Health, Jerusalem.

Joseph Levine MD, Associate Professor, Department of Psychiatry, Faculty of Health Sciences, Ben-Gurion University of the Negev, Beersheba.

Daphna Levinson PhD, Director, Research and Development, Mental Health Services, Ministry of Health, Jerusalem.

Joshua D. Lipsitz PhD, Associate Professor, Department of Psychology, Ben-Gurion University of the Negev, Beersheba.

Ivonne Mansbach-Kleinfeld PhD MPH, Researcher, Research and Development, Mental Health Services, Ministry of Health, Jerusalem.

Malka Margalit PhD, Professor, Constantiner School of Education, Tel Aviv University, Tel Aviv.

Anda Massler MD, Schneider Children's Hospital, Petah Tikva; and Tel Aviv University, Tel Aviv.

Julia Mirsky PhD, Associate Professor, Spitzer Department of Social Work, Ben-Gurion University of the Negev, Beersheba.

Hanan Munitz MB BS, Emeritus Professor, Tel Aviv University, Tel Aviv.

Yehuda D. Neumark PhD MPH, Senior Lecturer, Hebrew University-Hadassah Braun School of Public Health and Community Medicine, Jerusalem.

Hadar S. Schwartz BA, Hebrew University-Hadassah Braun School of Public Health and Community Medicine, Jerusalem.

Adi Sharabi PhD, Lecturer, Kibbutzim College of Education Technology and the Arts, Tel Aviv.

Zahava Solomon PhD, Professor, Shappel School of Social Work, Tel Aviv University; and Head, Adler Research Center for Child Welfare and Protection, Tel Aviv University, Tel Aviv.

Mark Weiser MD, Associate Professor, Department of Psychiatry, Sackler School of Medicine, Tel Aviv University, Tel Aviv; and Chief Psychiatrist, Sheba Medical Center, Tel Hashomer.

Perla Werner PhD, Professor and Dean, Faculty of Social Welfare and Health Sciences, University of Haifa, Haifa.

Foreword

Rational decisions require solid data. Cognizant of this, the Ministry of Health established a psychiatric case register (PCR) during the very early years of the state. This move followed a recommendation made by the late American biostatistician Morton Kramer, acting as a World Health Organization consultant.

The Ministry has run the PCR continuously for almost 60 years (1). As needs changed and new services and technologies became available, the system has been expanded and upgraded continuously. Over the years, multiple publications for statistical purposes have been produced (cf. 2, as an example). Also, in recent years it has monitored the process of de-institutionalization (3), changes in the use of services and trends in compulsory hospitalizations (4), as reported in chapter 19.

In addition to the application of psychiatric epidemiology to the planning of services and programs and their evaluation, the PCR has enabled local and foreign investigators to conduct important etiological studies. These have been published in national and international journals with a high-impact factor. The reader will have access to many of these studies since several chapters of this volume illustrate the use of the PCR for etiological research. The reader will thus be able to appreciate the rich contribution of Israeli researchers to the expanding field of psychiatric and behavioral epidemiology, relying on the PCR, other existing data sources as well as ad hoc research strategies.

The Ministry of Health – aware of the PCR's limitations for policy development and program planning (because the data are based mainly on treated prevalence) – joined the World Mental Health Survey initiated and coordinated by the World Health Organization and Harvard University. This study, led by a team of investigators at the ministry, is known as the Israel National Health Survey (INHS) (5). It was funded in collaboration with the Israel National Institute for Health Policy and Health Services Research and the National Insurance Institute (NII). INHS, based on almost 5,000 adult community respondents, has provided true prevalence rates on affective, anxiety and substance abuse disorders and emotional distress. It has also highlighted other important aspects for program planning, such as issues related to treatment gap and delays in seeking help. The database of this large epidemiological study has been made accessible to all researchers, and several chapters in this book present results that originated in this study. In addition, the Ministry of Health, with the support of several local institutions, jointly launched a large epidemiological study on the young, which is reported in chapter 3.

The Ministry of Health firmly believes that all mental health stakeholders need rationally based information to steer their course of action in the field. This book, which takes the reader from research data to intervention, reflects its policy of promoting and circulating knowledge for the widest communities of interested parties (medical and mental health professionals, health insurers and providers, university students, decision makers, service users, families, NGO executives, health journalists and many others) whose purpose is to improve mental health among all sectors of the population. The Ministry of Health and the Israel National Institute for Health Policy and Health Services Research are pleased to offer this publication to local and foreign readers and express their appreciation to the authors, language editors and publisher who collectively made this timely book possible.

Prof. Avi Israeli, *Director-General*
Dr. Boaz Lev, *Associate Director-General*
Dr. Jacob Polakiewicz, *Director, Mental Health Services*
Ministry of Health, Jerusalem
April 2009

❧ References

1. Levav I, Grinshpoon A: Mental health services in Israel. *International Psychiatry* 2004; 4: 10–14.
2. Ministry of Health, Department of Evaluation and Information: *Mental health in Israel. Statistical annual* 2006, Jerusalem, 2006.
3. Levinson D, Lerner Y, Lichtenberg P. Reduction in inpatient length of stay and changes in mental health care in Israel over four decades. *Israel Journal of Psychiatry and Related Sciences* 2003; 40: 240–247.
4. Nahon D, Pugachova I, Yoffe R, *et al.* The impact of human rights advocacy, mental health legislation and psychiatric reform on the epidemiology of involuntary psychiatric hospitalizations. *Medicine and Law* 2006; 25: 283–295.
5. Levinson D, Levav I, Bin Nun G. Special issue. *The Israel Journal of Psychiatry and Related Sciences* 2007; 2.

Preface

It has been often and rightly said that Israel is a population laboratory well suited for epidemiological research. Indeed, it is a small country of 22,072 square kilometers; with slightly over seven million people of diverse origins and from a variety of ethnic communities; comprising secular and religious individuals of different denominations and degrees of observance; where people live in multiple types of social organizations, such as cities, villages, development towns and collective settlements (kibbutzim) and belong to contrasting social classes. In addition, Israel is in a state of continual change, rocked by multiple armed conflicts and attacks and periodically stirred up by small or large waves of immigration. In addition, growing numbers of refugees and foreign workers contribute to enrich this already complex sociodemographic mosaic.

Important for the infrastructure of epidemiological research in this human laboratory is the availability of advanced computerized databases that store easily retrievable records, among those, on the general population, the Israel Defense Forces recruits, the insured in the Health Maintenance Organizations, and persons hospitalized for psychiatric care and in psychosocial rehabilitation services. All these databases operate under laws and regulations that meet ethical concerns. Thus it is no surprise that local epidemiologists have been capitalizing on all of these resources and unique national characteristics to conduct studies that started soon after the state was established in 1948.

Psychiatric epidemiological research in Israel has been thriving over the years. In recent decades it has expanded its concerns from treated populations to community-based studies. An example of the latter is the Israel National Health Survey (INHS), part of the 27-country World Health Survey led by researchers of Harvard University and the World Health Organization. The Israeli component of this cross-national study has yielded many publications; several chapters of this book review various aspects of its findings, together with data collected by other community-based studies.

As attested by this volume, Israeli epidemiological studies cover multiple mental health domains. Thanks to contributions by leading interdisciplinary researchers from academia and the health services, the reader now has at his/her fingertips a full and updated overview of the epidemiology of psychiatric and behavioral disorders in Israel. The information presented is of central relevance for mental health action in the areas of promotion and prevention and, especially, for curative care as well as rehabilitation. Section I of this overview presents epidemiological research conducted on different population groups. It is followed by Section II, which contains a description and analyses of mainly community-based epidemiologic studies of several mental and behavioral disorders. Section III closes the book with epidemiological studies based on the health and mental health services. The reader will note some repetitions; they were unavoidable since each chapter was designed to be self-contained to make it reader friendly.

Epidemiology has three main tasks: the search for causes, the provision of rational bases for planning and the definition of syndromes. Israeli studies have so far mainly addressed the first two tasks. As with all epidemiological research, the ultimate purpose of this book is to provide information that may be applied to prevent the incidence and to reduce the prevalence of disease and disability. This is why most chapters conclude with a discussion entitled "from epidemiology to mental health action."

Epidemiological research aimed at elucidating the causes of mental and behavioral disorders is also well represented in several chapters, including the search for such factors through the use of genetic epidemiology with regard to schizophrenic disorders. Perhaps not all we know about etiology may already be applied to program planning, but the scaffolding under construction will make this possible in the near future as research advances.

The reader will find here a wealth of information impossible to encompass in this introduction, even briefly. It is sufficient to note that the total and specific burden of mental and behavioral disorders in Israel, as highlighted by these 19 chapters, cannot be ignored either by mental health stakeholders or – and most importantly – by decision makers. Attention should also be paid to the fact that this burden falls neither evenly nor randomly: it varies by gender, social class, age, immigrant status, area of residence, ethnic affiliation and past traumatic experiences among civilians and the military. All of these factors must be taken into account by all those advocating for mental health care and those whose task is to formulate mental health policies, and design and lead intervention programs. The findings in this book also address the need to allot commensurate resources, to devise effective planning and deliver appropriately tailored mental health services. Some studies reviewed here present data on the treatment lag and the gaps in mental health care, or stated more simply, their findings revealed that not all those who need care receive it. This untreated prevalence is of particular concern among certain population groups, such as those living in what is commonly known as "the periphery," as noted in the closing chapter of this book.

Another finding emerging from recent epidemiological studies is that disorders come in twos and threes. Comorbidity seems to be not the exception but the rule. Nor is comorbidity limited to mental disorders; it extends to physical disorders as well – a clear indication that the bio-psycho-social constellation is a reality that deserves tangible recognition in both the conceptualization of research, the delivery of care and the training of human resources.

Finally, recognition is due to both the authors who collaborated enthusiastically to make psychiatric epidemiology available to the public and to the institutions that supported their efforts. The Ministry of Health and the Israel National Institute for Health Policy and Health Services Research sponsored and funded the publication of this book, but the sole responsibility for its content rests with the author/s of each chapter.

The authors and the editor are heavily indebted to the following individuals who have made this publication possible: Prof. Alexander Aviram, Prof. Gabi Bin-Nun, Prof. Avi Israeli, Dr. Boaz Lev and Dr. Jacob Polakiewicz. In addition, the authors and the editor acknowledge the editorial assistance of Ms. Judy Siegel-Itzkovich, the graphic design by Shlomit Levav, M.Arch., and the work performed by Gefen Publishing and its helpful staff.

I owe warm personal thanks to the late Prof. Sidney Kark, and Profs J.H. Abramson (in Israel) and B.P. Dohrenwend (in the US). They taught me to appreciate the role of psychiatric epidemiology in advancing the mental health status of the populations.

The authors will feel sufficiently rewarded for their effort if this book is used by teachers, students, researchers, practitioners, service users and families – and by all others within and outside the mental health communities in Israel and abroad.

Itzhak Levav, *Jerusalem*
April 2009

SECTION I

Psychiatric and Behavioral Disorders in Population Groups

Chapter 1

The epidemiology of women's mental health in Israel: A life-course perspective

Julie Cwikel and Anneke Ifrah

This chapter seeks to deconstruct one of the most profound determinants of mental health: the contribution of female sex and gender to patterns of mental and behavioral disorders in general and in Israel in particular. Research has shown that women's mental health is affected by the interaction among biological factors, usually summarized under the term sex (biological classification as either male or female) and gender (self-representation as male or female that is both shaped by exposure to economic, social and cultural factors and reinforced by interaction with the environment) (1–11). The local social reality, shaped by a combination of turbulent historical events and successive waves of immigration, has created a social laboratory for social and psychiatric epidemiology – particularly as it plays out with regard to the gender-based construction of mental health and behavioral disorders.

Over the years, the literature on psychiatric epidemiology has debated the roles of stress, role functions in family, marriage and the workplace and the accumulation of adverse life experiences, particularly child sexual abuse (CSA), as possible determinants for mental health disparities between men and women (5, 12–15). It has been proposed that women's unique experiences over the course of their lives shape the development of mental disorders. The life-course perspective in epidemiology is an interdisciplinary approach that is used to organize diverse findings on the impact of prenatal, childhood and adolescent adverse life exposures and experiences and how these factors interact as determinants of health throughout adulthood (16–21). The basic premise is that various biological, environmental, psychological and social factors affect health and the occurrence of mental health morbidity both independently and interactively. These effects begin at the conception of life and continue in an iterative fashion across the lifespan (16, 17).

Given the importance of gender in framing the differences between women and men in psychiatric and behavioral disorders, we have used an intersection between the life-course perspective and social epidemiological tools to shape the findings presented in this chapter. Social epidemiology looks both at the social determinants of health in general and at the determinants of social conditions such as poverty, violence, stressful life events and mental health conditions

(22, 23). Additionally, social epidemiology seeks to establish evidence-based practice and policy to promote health (22, 24). A further aspect of the field is the integration between qualitative and quantitative research methods and the development of mixed-method research to address challenges in mental health epidemiology (22).

Qualitative methods are important in giving voice to the mental health history of socially excluded groups (25–27). In Israel, a combination of qualitative and quantitative methods is valuable in producing a richer picture – particularly of cross-cultural mental health issues of immigrants and other hard-to-access groups such as the ultra-religious or ethnic minorities. (28–31).

§ Demographic background

Ethnic group, religion and age

Approximately 76% of Israeli women are Jews, 20% are Arabs and about 4% are "others" (non-Arab Christians and those not classified by religion). The main cultural divide in the population is that of Jewish and others on the one hand, 17% of whom are post-1990 immigrants from the former Soviet Union (FSU), and Arabs on the other. The majority (82%) of Arab women in Israel are Muslims, 9% Christians and 9% Druze. The Arab population of Israel is younger than the Jewish population: only 4% of Arab women are aged 65 or over, compared with 13% of Jewish women, and 74% of Arab women are younger than 35, compared with 54% among the Jewish women (32) (see chapter 5).

Fertility

In 2006, the total fertility rate for Israeli women (the average number of expected births in a woman's lifetime) was 2.9, which is higher than the average for Europe (1.5). Total fertility rates are 1.7 times higher among Muslim women (4.0) than Jewish women (2.6). The past decades have seen a decline in total fertility rates, particularly in the Muslim and Druze populations and more moderately in the other groups (32).

Life expectancy at birth

The life expectancy at birth has been increasing steadily over the past three decades for all women. Between 1976 and 2006, it increased by an average of 7.3 years for Jewish women and 5.7 years for Arab women. In 2006, the average life expectancy for Jewish women was 82.7 years and for Arab women, 78.1 (32).

Educational status

The educational status of women, a crucial determinant of physical and mental health, has improved considerably among all Israeli women during the past decade. Between 1993 and 2006, post-secondary education increased by 45% among Jewish women and doubled among Arab women. However, the educational disadvantage of Arab women remains: in 2006, 19% of Arab women, as compared with 46% of Jewish women, had post-secondary education (32).

Health status and social status

The data on morbidity and mortality reflect a poorer health status for Arab than for Jewish women. Among Arab women, mortality rates for heart disease and stroke are higher, and diabetes and obesity are more prevalent (33, 34). The inequalities in health status are related to a complexity of social, demographic and political issues including poverty, lower levels of education, marginal social status and residence in the peripheral areas. Arab women have been termed "a minority within a minority," referring to their ethnic and political status on the one hand and their position as women in a traditional patriarchal society on the other (30) (see chapter 5).

⸹ Depression and its association with women's biology

Mental disorders make a major contribution to the global burden of disease; of them, depression accounts for the largest portion of the mental health burden. In 1990, unipolar major depression was the fourth leading cause of the burden of disease worldwide (as measured by disability-adjusted life years) and by 2020, it is projected to become the second-most-important cause (17, 24, 35). In Israel, unipolar major depression was estimated in 2002 to be the cause of 12.5% of the total burden of disease (35). One of the most commonly reported rates in psychiatric epidemiology is the prevalence rate of depression among women of reproductive age at between 1.5 to three times the rate of men (17, 24, 36–38). An understanding of the determinants of the excess of depression among women could contribute to the lessening of the burden of disease.

Data from the US National Comorbidity Study showed that the increased rate of depression among women first appears at around 10 years of age and disappears when women reach their mid-50s (39). Thus, the time of greatest risk for the development of depressive disorders occurs during women's childbearing years. Studies have shown that a combination of stressful life events, genetic and familial predisposition and neurotic personality style together with hormonal events interact to produce a greater vulnerability to distress and depression (38, 40–44).

Women are more susceptible than men both to stress-induced depression and chronobiological disorders, such as seasonal affective disorder (SAD); more than 80% of those with SAD are women. Women are also susceptible to hormone-related conditions such as premenstrual syndrome, depression in pregnancy and postpartum depression (44, 45). Menstrual hormone fluctuations can result in symptoms that range from mild premenstrual dysphoria to more severe disturbances in work and daily functioning that meet *Diagnostic and Statistical Manual of Mental Disorders – Fourth Edition* (*DSM-IV*) criteria for premenstrual dysphoric disorder. These both occur during the luteal stage when progesterone predominates and disappear during the follicular stage when estrogen increases (46). Interestingly, premenstrual dysphoric disorder occurs in between 2% to 10% of women and among these, comorbid SAD is found in close to half of them (45).

Depression in pregnancy is observed at about 10%, which is a rate comparable to non-pregnant women (44, 47). However, depression during pregnancy predisposes women to postpartum depression (PPD) and difficulties in parenting. PPD is observed in Western countries at a rate of 10% to 15% (46, 48). An Israeli study has estimated the rate of PPD at 23%, however, two-thirds of cases were women already depressed during pregnancy, leaving 7% as incident cases. New immigrant mothers from the former Soviet Union had more than twice the risk for PPD as Israeli-born subjects (49).

Infertility, miscarriage, the use of oral contraceptives and hormone replacement therapy (HRT) have also been observed to produce symptoms of depression (44, 50–52). High rates of dysphoric affect are also observed during menopause (44). Women also have higher rates of eating disorders, somatoform disorders, anxiety disorders including post-traumatic stress disorders (PTSD) and dissociative disorders, while men have higher rates of substance abuse disorders and antisocial personality disorders (12, 17, 53) (table 1).

Table 1. Prevalence rates (%) of mental disorders by gender (53)

Disorders	Rates (%)		Odds ratios
	Women	Men	W/M
Somatization	.4	< .1	7.3
Major depression	5.7	2.7	2.4
Panic disorder	1.8	.8	2.3
Dysthymia	3.9	1.9	2.1
Phobias	18.3	9.5	2.0
Schizophrenia	1.6	1.0	1.5
Obsessive-compulsive disorder	2.4	1.8	1.5
Bipolar disorder	.8	.6	1.3
Drug abuse	3.7	6.2	.6
Antisocial personality	.8	3.7	.2
Alcoholism	4.3	21.2	.1

✿ Distal factors associated with mental health in women

This section addresses the macro or distal factors (as distinct from proximate or micro factors) that affect Israeli women's mental health (22, 36, 54, 55). We outline the general topics that affect women worldwide and discuss the specific Israel-related component. The universal vs. the Israeli nature of macro, societal level factors is illustrated in table 2.

Following an age trajectory, we briefly touch on the salutogenic (health-promoting) factors that affect women's mental health over the course of their lives. These include adequate childhood care and attention during infanthood and childhood, avoidance of child sexual and physical abuse during childhood and adolescence, development of positive self-esteem during the teen years and making good use of opportunities for education to develop social capital (36, 54).

Adequate care in infancy

There is an interaction between parents' psychological resources and their ability to provide adequate care. Mothers who were themselves abused, exposed to stressful life events during pregnancy, lack support or had a difficult delivery are more likely to develop and find caring for an infant difficult (56–59). However, PPD is also associated with infant sleep and feeding problems, parental sleep deprivation and marital stress, making the etiological order of events difficult to tease out (57–61).

Table 2. Examples of distal risk or protective factors over the life course of women by universal vs. local situation-specific factors

	Conception	Birth	Childhood	Adolescence	Adulthood	Old age
Distal universal	Genetic or prenatal nutrition	Access to healthcare and skilled birth attendants, traumatic birth experiences, avoidance of perinatal morbidity.	Development of positive self-esteem, avoidance of sexual violence, access to educational opportunities.	Development of health-promoting coping strategies such as exercise, creative pursuits and avoiding substance abuse and smoking.	Maintenance of adequate friend and family support. Successful choices in work, economic development, partner and family structure. Avoidance of domestic violence and poverty. Successful mothering and caregiving of parents.	Postponing disability, maintaining positive self-esteem, and community involvement. Adequate financial resources in old age.
Distal local-specific	Maternal exposure to Holocaust, war, security-related terrorism, immigration	Crowded hospitals, high birth rate in some areas, lack of cultural-specific attendants for some groups, some interference of security situation in healthcare delivery.	Developing positive self and body image and avoiding eating disorders. Equal access to opportunities in education in some sectors (rural, Arab-speaking, development towns).	High stress during adolescence from security problems, early school dropout and marriage among some groups. Negotiating a positive army service.	Risk of postpartum depression, or fertility-related depression. Balancing between work and family demands. Husbands and children in army. Discrimination for some groups.	Loss of family supports due to immigration, loss of adult children in wars, changing communal structures (e.g., kibbutz).

Social supports

Women are particularly affected by and sensitive to what happens in their social network, which may be both a source of support and a burden on their ability to cope with other stressors (62–64). Women tend to have more social supports to turn to in times of stress and report higher numbers of network connections in comparison with men (63, 65, 66). A comparative study of five European countries found that women report slightly more negative life events than men do, but these are more likely to be associated with events of network members. For both genders, the rate of depression increases as social supports decrease, but at each level of social support the rate of depression among women is higher. For example, even with no negative life events reported, the rate of depression was 7.3% for men and 9.8% for women; with two negative events, it increased to 23.8% for men and 31.2% for women (67).

Poverty

Women living in relative poverty are more than twice as likely to develop psychiatric morbidity, when the lowest socioeconomic groups are compared to the highest, after controlling for age. This finding in psychiatric epidemiology is constant over the decades (24, 54, 68, 69) and is particularly salient with regard to depression (68). Women's greater exposure to poverty, in Israel and worldwide, is due to fewer educational and economic opportunities, lower pay, poorer working conditions, single parenthood, economic dependency on men and a greater portion of their time spent caring for infants, children, disabled persons and the elderly without remuneration (24, 54). Among developing countries with rapid economic growth, the intersection between low income, low levels of education and female gender was strongly associated with increased rates of depression and anxiety (70, 71). Poverty-related food insufficiency and insecurity are also a potent predictor of an increased rate in women's mental disorders (71).

Violence

Although the epidemic of violence against women varies across cultures, it is a consistent and potent factor that adversely affects women's mental health (24, 72). Violence against women includes psychological, physical, sexual and economic violence, each type bringing in its wake an increase in distress and detriments in psychological health. CSA is more common among female than male children but occurs in both sexes and leads to increased mental health morbidity in adulthood (14, 72–75). CSA often interacts with other types of childhood stresses such as chronic mental illness in the family, criminal activity, poverty and substance abuse (76, 77).

The Adverse Childhood Experiences (ACE) Study of 5,060 female members of a managed care organization in the US assessed eight adverse childhood experiences such as abuse, witnessing domestic violence, chronic mental illness or criminal activity of a family member and calculated the ACE score – a measure of cumulative childhood stress. A dose-response relationship was found between ACE score and selected outcomes, as well as with the total number of these outcomes, including smoking, self-rated poor health, many sexual partners, early first-sexual experience, unintended pregnancy, sexually transmitted disease, physical inactivity, substance abuse, severe obesity, chronic illness such as heart disease, cancer, fractures and chronic lung or liver disease (74, 78–83). An Israeli study found that women who had been exposed to CSA had a higher rate of miscarriages than women without this history (an average of 1.3 vs. 1.0) (84). Adverse, intrusive and stressful childhood experiences tend to handicap women in adulthood as they try to establish safe intimate and interpersonal relations, and interfere with the development of health-promoting rather than health-compromising coping behaviors.

The prevalence of intimate partner violence (IPV) among Israeli women has been estimated at 10% to 15% in the general population, with higher rates among some ethnic groups (85–88). A 1998 national survey found that 2.0% reported that they had ever been the victim of rape, 4% reported some other type of sexual violence and 11% reported a lifetime exposure to IPV (89). More recently, in the first national survey of mental health in Israel, 12% of women reported having experienced IPV (163). These findings compare with an IPV prevalence ranging from 15% to 71% in studies conducted around the world (90). This global epidemic has far-reaching health and social effects, including injury, psychological distress, functional impairment in the family and at work, gynecological problems and in some cases, increased mortality through both homicide and suicide (22, 91, 92).

Health-related risk behaviors: smoking

As mentioned above, health behaviors such as smoking are associated with other social conditions that increase risk for both mental and physical morbidity. For example, genetic research with twin pairs has found that mothers who smoked during pregnancy were more likely to be antisocial, had chosen to partner with antisocial men, were bringing up their children in more disadvantaged circumstances and were more likely to have suffered from depression (18, 82, 93). Others have observed strong association between adult smoking and depression, which interferes with women's ability to quit smoking (94–97). Also see chapter 10.

In a survey of the health and welfare of women in the Negev region, it was found that approximately 20% were current smokers and 11% former smokers. Close to 60% of the women started smoking between the ages of 18 to 22, the ages when the majority of women are serving in the army (98). The rate of smoking as reported by other Israeli surveys was found to be highest among the younger age groups (21 to 34, 35 to 44) and is much higher among Jewish than Arab women (20.4% vs. 6.4%) (99). Women in stressful situations are much more likely to smoke, and they may smoke at very high rates, as shown in studies of women with post-traumatic stress symptoms who seek shelter from domestic violence (100) and among women – trafficked and local – who were working in prostitution (101).

❦ Specific sources of stress and distress for Israeli women

Coping under security stress and strain

Since the establishment of the state in 1948, Israeli society has been struggling under the burden of armed conflict and terror. Since the beginning of the *Al-Aqsa Intifada* (insurrection, in Arabic), September 2000, there have been periods when as many as 16 terrorist incidents were perpetrated in a single month (March 2002), with a high proportion of civilian casualties (40% of them women) (102).

Concurrent with this chronic security threat, there has been a serious fraying of the safety net of social programs that used to make up the welfare state, with cuts in income maintenance allowances, unemployment insurance benefits and child allowances, thus creating an additional source of economic distress among the economically disadvantaged. These are disproportionately women and residents of the peripheral areas (103). Thus, many of the macro events, particularly in recent history, have been compounded by socioeconomic stressors.

A major component of psychological and behavioral disorders can be understood as reactions to external events that range from adaptive coping behaviors to severe mental distress. Coping is a multidimensional and dynamic process purported to alter an external event or bring about a solution – or to make tolerable the emotional fallout that stressful situations engender. When a situation cannot be modified by an individual's agency, it becomes a chronic stressor that may affect mental health. Clearly, there are aspects of coping that are universal, such as grief at the loss of a loved one, as well as Israeli-specific aspects of coping.

Early studies differentiated between emotion-focused (expressing the emotions that stress generates) and problem-focused coping (taking concrete actions to alter the situation) (104), with women reporting more frequent use of the former while men use the latter more often (105–107). Later research results were not consistent regarding this gender difference, suggesting that it was both a function of exposure to different types of stressors (e.g., war situations vs. rape) and the gender-based access to power and coping resources (108–110).

Two studies of coping with the *Al-Aqsa Intifada* terrorism among the general population have shown that around 15% of persons were directly exposed to some type of terror attacks and that some 10% showed signs of post-traumatic stress disorder (PTSD)-like symptoms, but there was not a direct relationship between exposure and the development of symptoms (111, 112). Recent analysis showed that women are more vulnerable to the adverse effects of terror attacks than men and more likely to develop post-traumatic stress symptoms in consequence (men, 4.5% and women, 12.7%) (112, 113). This is true among both Arab Israelis and Jews (114). A manifestation of this is the increase during the *Intifada* period in calls made by women in particular for emotional support to a telephone hotline (29).

The interaction between security stress and psychological and physical morbidity

A random telephone survey on the coping of mothers aged 25 to 42 living in the Negev region with chronic security stress associated with the rocket and mortar attacks has shown that security-related stress was associated with health symptoms, particularly gynecological symptoms. Actual personal exposure or knowing someone who had been injured was associated with higher levels of depressive symptoms, as were current domestic violence and a history of sexual abuse as a child (26.4%, 22.0% and 16.7%, respectively, vs. 13.7% depression in the total sample) (115).

As shown in table 2, one of the most persistent and idiosyncratic stressors in Israel is the chronic security situation. This backdrop of pressure and distress interacts with women's decisions and experiences, from decisions on whether to have children, how births and motherhood are experienced, to decisions on family size and spacing (116, 117). This intertwining of the macro political and security events with personal trauma and stressful life events is expressed in the following quote from a 58-year-old mother of four (116, 117):

> *I originally wanted twelve children because I love children, but there is a difference between ideology and reality.... After the first child was born, I was traumatized from the birth itself.... After that first birth I didn't want to have any more children. But the boy was so wonderful that I thought I would try again and this time I made sure not to gain too much weight so that the baby would be small and easy to deliver...But the second birth was complete hell....*
>
> *When my daughter [her second child] was just two weeks old, the Six Day War broke out.... I intended to nurse her, I really wanted to. I started to nurse her, but every evening at 10 there was a siren, and we had to go down to the bomb shelters. My husband was at the front, and there I was by myself.... As you can imagine, my milk dried up.... So I said to myself, "This is it – I am not having any more children." But then my mother died and my husband decided that it would be good for me psychologically to have another baby. A year to the day from when she died my second daughter was born and I named her after my mother.*
>
> *And then after seven years my oldest son got his call-up notice. There was a lot of tension in the country then. I said to myself: "If God forbid, something should happen, I will end up without sons." My husband didn't want another child at age fifty [but we did have]...a beautiful son.*

This quote illustrates how the constant wartime exposure can affect women as they make decisions about family size and how to space their children. The thought of losing a husband or a child in war is an example of a woman's internalization of societal pressures, to have another child so that one does not remain without a son or a child. These macro effects on fertility rate interact with personal stressful life events associated with traumatic pregnancy or birth experiences.

Traumatic birth experiences

Reports of traumatic births are not uncommon. In a study of mothers aged 22 to 45 living in the Negev region (118), 30% reported that they felt fear and anxiety during their first pregnancy (a rate which climbed as the number of children rose to five), and a quarter of the women rated their birth experience as negative or traumatic (119). The rate of caesarean section averaged 9.5% over the first three births. Caesarian section and vacuum delivery were significantly associated with a report of a traumatic experience.

In general, the rate of caesarian section has increased over the years, from 4% to 10% between 1990 and 2000 for low-risk women in Jerusalem (120). Statistics from the Negev show a rate of 10% for low-risk women as well (121). A recent study reported an 18% caesarian rate for women in the central region of Israel (122). Much higher rates were reported among obese women, 28% (121), foreign workers (35%) (122) and women with a pregnancy achieved with *in-vitro* fertilization (IVF) (41%) (123).

Studies from abroad show that both biomedical factors relating to pregnancy and childbirth and pre-existing depression, anxiety and stressful life events adversely affect the experience of childbirth and the likelihood that either childbirth-related PTSD or PPD will develop (42, 43, 124). A prospective study from England reported that 2.8% of women developed PTSD related to childbirth at six weeks postpartum, which decreased to 1.5% at six months postpartum (125). It appears, then, that childbirth experiences, particularly if they are coupled with unpleasant interactions with the healthcare system, can be a potent source of distress among women.

Fertility and psychological distress

There are many macro variables that affect women's fertility. Political and cultural factors relating to the Arab-Israeli conflict are associated with an increase in total fertility rates across all groups (126, 127). For example, religious Jewish women residing in the settlements outside the Green Line were found to have 35% more children than women living within the Green Line. Religious women are also more likely to have more children than secular women, but nationalism interacts synergistically with religious level to accentuate the desire for a large family (126, 128).

Women with fertility problems are under pressure from family, friends and society in general to become mothers (129). In Israel, approximately 12% of couples suffer from infertility (130). Israel is the only country in the world that provides free cycles of assisted reproduction (up to two live births).

Infertility is described as a negative and distressing experience by women from different ethno-cultural backgrounds (131–133). Various studies showed a universal response among all infertile women: an intense emotional reaction regarding their inability to conceive and bring to term a healthy infant (e.g., (132, 134, 135). Among some religious and traditional groups, the social status of the woman is strongly related to her level of fecundity (136, 137).

Fertility treatments, ranging from medical monitoring to hormonal remedies and IVF, are recognized as both a physical and an emotional burden on women and their partners that can cause depression and stress-related somatic symptoms (133, 138). Fertility treatments may also result in lost days of work and income both for the family and the economy (139). In a recent pilot study of a group intervention conducted in a hospital in central Israel on five infertile women who had complete follow-up data, it was found that depression was prominent among women who did not succeed in getting pregnant after years of treatments and that depression lifted only when news came that they had successfully become pregnant (140). Even after succeeding in becoming parents, mothers who have undergone many cycles of IVF treatment have been found to suffer from more parental stress and less secure attachment to their infants, compared to mothers who were treated with fewer cycles (141).

The trauma of women facing army-related stressors

Kessler *et al.* showed that women are more likely to be exposed to sexual violence and men to combat situations, both of which may lead to the development of PTSD (142). This is true also among Israeli populations exposed to stressful life events (143). Thus, most local studies on the impact of the security situation on women have examined the impact of being wives of men who developed PTSD symptoms in war or were prisoners of war, or wives of career officers (e.g., 144–147).

However, for women as well as men the demands of the military framework is often a stressor. A young woman recounted: *"I started to smoke in the army. Why? I started to smoke to relax, and I still smoke today"* (148). A mental health professional who worked in the Israel Defense Forces with both men and women explained that for soldiers who have had traumatic sexual experiences in their childhood or youth, the army framework can aggravate or reactivate psychological scars because it is such an overwhelming and intrusive setting with constant demands and scrutiny (149).

But what happens when women are exposed to both distressing military operations and sexual harassment at the same time? The experience of being part of a combat unit generates both a "tend and befriend response" (63) and a need to be "one of the guys" – not to show distress or react overemotionally to military actions. A study of coping strategies used by women in combat-related roles showed that many felt the need to dress and adopt manly speech and mannerisms to de-emphasize their feminine bodies and to ignore sexual harassment in an effort to demonstrate how they are different from other women (150).

As of now, no study has ever been conducted on PTSD or depressive reactions of Israeli women to their military service. This is so despite a stream of studies on American female combat veterans (151–153). Kang found that both men and women who experienced military sexual trauma and high combat exposure were at a similar level of risk for PTSD (153).

Many Israeli women who volunteered to participate in combat during the War of Independence in 1948 recalled it as an experience that left them permanently scarred (154). Tamar Yarom's film *To See if I'm Smiling* (or *No place for a Lady* in its English title) documented the combat exposures of six women who served in the Israeli-administered territories during the recent *Al-Aksa Intifada*. Moral dilemmas arose in the seams of the friction and harassment of civilians, the handling of cases of civilian casualties and corpses and the interactions with prisoners. These experiences were reviewed retrospectively with pain, doubt and in some cases, post-traumatic symptoms.

One of the women soldiers wrote to her parents: *"One day, I'll tell you everything I went through…."* To this day, she does not wear a watch, read newspapers or listen to the news (155). Incidentally, blocking out news broadcasts was a coping mechanism more commonly used by women than men in managing the stress associated with the *Intifada* (111).

Sexual harassment

A survey of Israeli women found that 9% of working women and 20% in the military reported being sexually harassed each year (156). The attorney who processes sexual harassment cases in the Unit on Women's Status and Advancement in the Civil Service remarked that 25% of the plaintiffs are women soldiers, making the Defense Ministry the source of the highest rate of sexual harassment cases among government agencies (156). It has been commented that sexual harassment is so common in the military that women are expected to "learn to cope" (157). Recent court cases of high-ranking military and government officials suggest that there is less willingness to ignore such harassment, yet the negative media exposure acts as a powerful disincentive to press charges. The introduction of the 1999 Law of Equal Opportunity and the Law for Prevention of Sexual Harassment could help in making a difference (158).

Women working in certain professions are frequently harassed at work. For example, 90% of nurses (80% of whom were women) reported at least one type of sexual harassment at work, and 30% reported four types (159). Over 90% of women working in the police force have also reported sexual harassment on the job (156).

Sexual abuse of women by psychotherapists as well as traditional healers is also of concern in Israel. A recent survey of therapists ($N = 918$) found that close to 30% reported that at least one of their patients had experienced sexual relations with a former therapist (160).

Domestic violence

The prevalence of domestic violence among Israeli women has been estimated at 10% to 15% of the general population, with higher rates among some ethnic groups (86, 87, 161). A survey among women seeking gynecological care showed that 24% reported psychological abuse; 17%, physical attacks; and 6%, sexual coercion. Five percent reported that physical attacks occurred when they were pregnant; no difference in types of abuse was found according to whether they were pregnant or not pregnant (85).

Domestic violence is tolerated by some rabbis, particularly when a woman refuses housework or shows disrespect for her husband's wishes (161, 162). Bedouin women reported threefold rates of domestic abuse compared to Jewish women (30% vs. 10%). These rates decreased if the woman was pregnant (137). This rate is similar to those reported in other Middle Eastern Arab countries. Despite what is generally thought, the Koran does not advocate domestic violence or "honor killings," which are a culturally based way to keep women under control and living in fear (163) (see chapter 5).

Women victims of domestic violence are more likely to show a variety of psychological symptoms. A recent study of 101 women victims of domestic violence who chose to go to battered women's shelters reported that 65% suffered from PTSD; 40%, from major depression; 17%, from dysthymic disorder; 14%, from specific phobias or pain disorders; 11%, from body dysmorphic disorder; 10%, from obsessive compulsive disorder (OCD); and 7%, from binge-eating disorder (100). PTSD and depression were strongly associated, and both were more common among women who grew up in a male-dominated household (100). The strongest predictor of PTSD was exposure to sexual violence.

Discrimination

Israel is a country of immigration and also has significant minority populations. Immigrant status is often associated with socioeconomic stress (see chapter 6), but immigrants may also feel discriminated against and be the victims of the combination of social marginality, meager personal resources and communication difficulties. In another example of how distal and proximate factors interact, a study of self-reported mental health problems (physician-detected depression and sleep disorders, self-reported depressive symptoms, low self-esteem and hopelessness-helplessness) among four different ethnic and immigrant groups showed that immigration interacted with education and income to affect mental health. Immigrants from the FSU were more likely to report mental distress; this was partly explained by higher rates of economic problems, even after education was accounted for (55).

Ethnic group status contributed most strongly to low self-esteem, which suggests an accumulated effect of discrimination (55). Remmenick found that women immigrants from the FSU had often suffered occupational downgrading (164). Another study found that immigrant women from the FSU felt more burdened by family problems, the climate, anxiety about the present and the future and had poorer self-rated health than immigrant men (165).

Discrimination can take other forms too. For example, obese women, as noted earlier, were more likely to have caesarean sections, even without any other risk factors such as hypertension or diabetes. Despite the fact that obesity alone is not associated with any adverse birth outcome, medical teams appear to shortchange obese women of "an adequate trial at vaginal delivery" (121).

Somatic symptoms, especially pain, are the major reason among Bedouin-Israeli women for seeking medical care (166). However, in seeking care, they are more likely than Jewish women to have their symptoms misinterpreted. For example, Bedouin women after birth were assessed by medical teams as suffering from less pain than their Jewish counterparts, despite similar levels of reported discomfort in childbirth. Jewish care providers were not as adept at "reading" pain expression among Bedouin women as they were among Jewish women in Israel (167).

❧ Prevalence of mental disorders: The Israel National Health Survey (INHS)

The INHS, which was carried out in 2003 to 2004 among a representative sample of almost 5,000 community-dwelling adults aged 21 and older, provided estimates of true lifetime and one-year prevalence rates of common mental disorders in Israeli women and men. (This study is reviewed in subsequent chapters as well.)

The survey, which constituted a part of the World Mental Health Survey, was conducted in the respondent's home. The interview schedule included the Composite International Diagnostic Interview (CIDI), which provides diagnoses of disorders according to *ICD-10* and *DSM-IV*. The mental disorders that were assessed were affective disorders (major depressive disorder (MDD), dysthymia, mania, and bipolar disorder); anxiety disorders (generalized anxiety disorder (GAD), agoraphobia, panic disorder, and PTSD); and substance disorders (alcohol abuse, alcohol dependence, drug abuse and drug dependence). Rates are presented in table 3 (168).

The 12-month prevalence and the lifetime prevalence rates of any affective disorder among women were 8.3% and 14.6%, respectively. These rates were, respectively, 1.6 times and 1.5 times higher in women than in men. The most common affective disorder was MDD: 7% of women were diagnosed as having had a MDD during the past 12 months (1.6 times the rate in men) and 12% during their lifetime (1.6 times the rate in men). These rate ratios are similar to the findings from the recent Canadian Community Health Survey (169). As for any anxiety disorder, the 12-month prevalence rate of any anxiety disorder was 1.3 times higher in women than in men, and the lifetime prevalence was 1.6 times higher (table 3). After controlling for sociodemographic correlates (age, income, family status and education), gender differences remained statistically significant for affective disorders but not for anxiety disorders (170).

The 12-month prevalence of PTSD was .6%, with no gender difference in rates. The lifetime prevalence was higher in women, 1.7%, than in men, 1.2%; this difference, however, was of marginal statistical significance (table 3). Women experienced more traumatic events than men (168). Alcohol and substance disorders were more prevalent in men than women. Men compared to women were seven times as likely to meet the criteria for an alcohol disorder (1, 4). The lifetime prevalence of drug abuse was also seven times higher in men than in women (168).

Table 3. Twelve-month and lifetime prevalence rates (%) of mental disorders among Israeli men and women in the INHS, 2003–2004 (168)

Disorders	12-month prevalence rates				Lifetime prevalence rates			
	Men		Women		Men		Women	
	%	SE	%	SE	%	SE	%	SE
Any affective disorder	5.3	(.5)	8.3	(.6)	9.6	(.6)	14.6	(.8)
Major depressive disorder	4.3	(.4)	7.0	(.5)	7.4	(.6)	12.0	(.7)
Minor depressive disorder	.4	(.2)	.8	(.2)	1.1	(.2)	1.8	(.3)
Mania (Bipolar I)	.6	(.2)	.5	(.2)	.9	(.2)	.7	(.2)
Dysthymia	.3	(.1)	.9	(.2)	.6	(.2)	1.3	(.2)
Any anxiety disorder	2.7	(.4)	3.6	(.4)	3.9	(.4)	6.4	(.5)
Generalized anxiety disorder	1.5	(.3)	2.1	(.3)	2.1	(.3)	3.4	(.4)
PTSD	.6	(.2)	.6	(.2)	1.2	(.2)	1.7	(.3)
Panic disorder	.5	(.1)	.6	(.2)	.8	(.2)	1.0	(.2)
Agoraphobia without panic disorder	.2	(.1)	.4	(.1)	.3	(.1)	.8	(.2)
Any substance disorder	2.2	(.3)	.4	(.1)	9.1	(.6)	1.6	(.3)
Alcohol abuse	1.7	(.3)	.3	(.1)	6.9	(.5)	1.1	(.2)
Drug abuse	.4	(.1)	.1	(.1)	2.3	.3	.6	(.2)

Mental disorders among primary care users

In a 2002 study of users of primary care in eight clinics throughout the country, the prevalence of a range of mental health problems was estimated using a variety of methods including the CIDI-short format (SF). Panic attacks, eating disorders and somatization, as well as a global measure of any psychiatric diagnosis, were significantly more prevalent among women than men (table 4) (171).

Table 4. Prevalence rates (%) of psychopathology among primary care patients by gender (171)

Categories of psychopathology	N	Prevalence rates (%)			
		Total N = 976	Men n = 340	Women n = 636	Sig.
Any psychopathology	507	51.2	44.9	54.8	.003
Psychiatric diagnoses	310	31.1	26.0	33.9	.009
Depression	206	20.6	17.4	22.2	.064
General anxiety	111	11.2	10.1	11.9	.373
Panic attack	76	7.4	4.1	9.2	.001
OCD	41	3.9	5.4	3.2	.114
Any anxiety	187	18.7	15.5	20.5	.140
Depression and any anxiety	98	9.8	9.3	10.1	.687
PTSD	28	2.8	3.8	2.2	.183
Hypochondriasis	13	1.3	1.5	1.2	.778
Cognitive impairment	3	.4	0.0	.5	–
Other mental disorders	245	24.3	19.4	27.0	.006
Disordered eating	150	15.0	11.5	17.0	.017
Somatization	123	11.8	9.1	13.2	.041

Rates were weighted for over-sampling of high users. Categories are not mutually exclusive. Sig: significance

Nonspecific psychopathology: Emotional distress and depressive symptoms

In Israel, as in other countries, emotional distress (as assessed by a variety of measures in different populations and settings) has consistently been found to be between 20% to 70% more prevalent among women than men (172–175). In the INHS (176), emotional distress was measured by the 12-item General Health Questionnaire, with scores ranging between 12 and 48, where higher scores indicate greater distress. Women scored higher than men in all age groups, with emotional distress scores increasing steadily with age.

The gender differential was highest among women and men aged 65 and older (figure 1). Mean GHQ scores were approximately 40% higher among Arab-Israeli women and post-1990 immigrant women from the former Soviet Union than among other groups of Jewish-Israeli women.

Figure 1. Mean GHQ-12 scores by age and gender, INHS. Years 2003–2004 (176)

According to the findings of another large national survey, also conducted in 2003–2004, "feeling depressed most or all of the time during the past four weeks" was reported almost twice as frequently by women (5%) than by men (2.9%); rates were higher among Arab than among Jewish Israelis (men and women) and were highest in Arab women (7%) (table 5) (33).

Table 5. Respondents feeling depressed most or all of the time during the preceding four weeks (%) by gender and population group. INHIS. Years 2003–2004 (33)

Gender	Jewish Israelis	Arab Israelis
Men	2.8	3.6
Women	4.7	7.0

Percentages weighted to the age distribution of the Israeli population

Among women, rates followed a J-shaped curve, with slightly elevated rates in the youngest group of women (ages 21–24) followed by a decrease at ages 25 to 34 and thereafter a steady increase with age. Rates were higher among women than men in all age groups (figure 2) (33).

Figure 2. Percent of respondents feeling depressed most or all of the time during the preceding four weeks by gender and age group, INHIS. Years 2003–2004 (33)

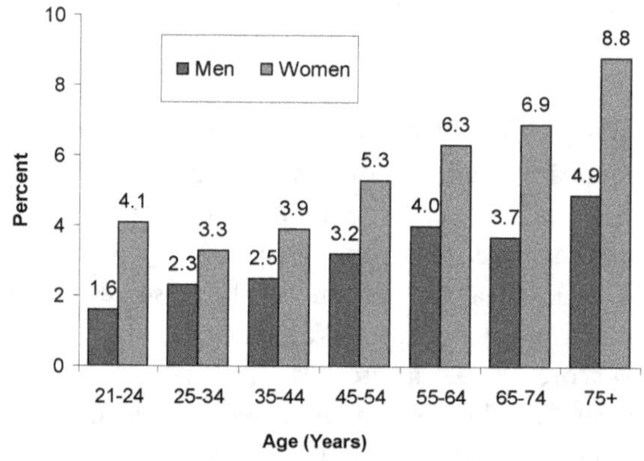

Percentages weighted to the age distribution of the Israeli population

Among women aged 50 and older with at least one chronic illness (hypertension, diabetes, heart disease or arthritis), rates were almost twice as high (6.2%) as among women without chronic diseases (3.2%). The association between feeling depressed and chronic morbidity was also observed among men in this age group, however rates were considerably lower than among women, 3.3%, among men with chronic disease vs. 1.4% of men without chronic disease (37).

Eating disorders

The data generally available on eating disorders (ED) among Israeli women are based mostly on treated populations. A recent study of 698 ED patients found that the profile of clinic patients was typically female, Israeli born, secular, Jewish, urban, of Ashkenazi (Western) origin and with high-level parental education. The percentage of kibbutz patients was high while the Arab-Israeli sector and the Jewish religious sectors were underrepresented (33). In a study of primary clinic attenders, 17% of female patients suffered from eating disorder, as compared with 11.5% of male patients (171).

Data on the incidence and prevalence of ED in the community are scarce. The available data on the prevalence of ED are based on self-reports in health surveys, which almost certainly reflect an underestimate of the true rates due to the stigma associated with such disorders. Of women interviewed in the INHIS, .7% reported that they had at some time been diagnosed with bulimia, anorexia, compulsive eating disorder or other eating disorder (37). More comprehensive population-based data on ED, body image and disordered eating patterns are necessary in order to estimate the extent of these disorders and to explore their correlates.

Suicidal behavior

Suicidal behavior is significantly associated with anxiety, depression, hopelessness and trauma (177–181). While rates of completed suicide are higher among males, attempted suicide is more prevalent among females (182–185).

Epidemiological data on gender differences in attempted suicide in the population have been based mainly on hospital emergency department admissions (186, 187). Community-based data on suicidal behavior have been provided by national surveys on schoolchildren (188). The INHS provided population-based data on suicidal behaviors and tendencies among women and men in the adult population (189).

Many of those with suicidal intentions use the services of ERAN, an NGO which operates a telephone hotline, personal e-mail response and group online support groups (190). A random sample of calls showed that men and women used these services for reporting suicidal threats at approximately the same rate (depending on type of service), but that women used these services at a significantly higher rate than men overall (ranging from 62% to 84% of callers) (see chapter 16).

An analysis of all admissions classified as attempted suicide to the emergency departments of 22 hospitals during the years 1996 to 2002 indicated a significant gender differential in attempted suicide during adolescence and young adulthood (ages 13 to 26). A year-by-year analysis showed that the largest gender difference was at age 14, when the female/male rate ratio reached 8.3 (187). The rate of attempted suicide in females peaked at age 16 to 17, with a rate of 207 per 100,000. The highest rate for males was three years later, at age 19, with a rate of 155 per 100,000. After age 26, rates of attempted suicide were not significantly higher for women than for men.

An inter-ethnic study of adults admitted during a 24-month period to a general hospital in Israel following suicide attempts (N = 175) reported higher rates of self-harm among women. The age patterns of suicide attempts were different in the different population groups: among Jewish-Israeli women rates increased gradually with age, while among Arab-Israeli women there was a peak at ages 20 to 29 followed by a decline at older ages (191).

Suicidal behavior in adolescents

The Health Behaviors in School Children (HBSC) series of studies among school-going youth provided information on suicidal ideation and planning among Jewish-Israeli pupils (188). In the study conducted in 2002, as well as in a similar study conducted in 1998, girls reported higher rates of ideation, planning and attempting suicide (table 6). Boys, however, were more likely to be injured in the course of attempting suicide.

Table 6. Suicide ideation, planning, attempts and injuries (%) during the past 12 months among secular Jewish tenth grade pupils. Year 2002 (188)

Suicidal behavior	Boys (%) n = 510	Girls (%) n = 505	Rate ratios Girls/Boys
Ideation	11.2	15.0	1.3
Planning	8.1	9.1	1.1
Attempt	3.9	7.1	1.8
Injured while attempting	4.0	2.2	.6

Data from the Israel National Health Survey (INHS)

The INHS provided population-based estimates of the prevalence rates of suicidal behaviors in the adult population (189). Gender differences in the prevalence rates of three of the four components of suicidal behaviors (ideation, planning and attempts) are presented in table 7. All outcomes were significantly higher among women than men. The risk of all types of suicidal behavior was greatly increased by the prior presence of mental disorders.

Table 7. Lifetime prevalence rates (%) of suicidal behaviors by gender (N = 4,859), INHS. Years 2003–2004 (189)

	Men		Women	
Ideation	4.8	(.5)	6.2	(.5)
Planning	1.5	(.3)	2.3	(.3)
Attempt	1.0	(.2)	1.7	(.3)

§ Psychiatric hospitalizations

The information presented here was extracted from the National Psychiatric Case Registry, which cumulatively records all admissions and discharges of patients in public and private psychiatric facilities nationwide.

Gender and age differences

Women accounted for about 40% of all psychiatric inpatient admissions in 2005 (192). The hospitalization rates in 2005 were 36% lower among women (2.3 per 1,000 population) than among men (3.6 per 1,000). A similar pattern of gender differences in psychiatric hospitalization rates was evident during the past decade (192). Estimated rates of psychiatric hospitalization in 2007 among ages 15 to 70 were for schizophrenia, delusional disorders and non-affective psychosis, 37 per 10,000 population among men, and 19 per 10,000 among women; for affective disorders, 6 per 10,000 among men, and 16 per 10,000 among women; and for drug and alcohol disorders, 2.7 per 10,000 among men, and .8 per 10,000 among women (193).

Women admitted to psychiatric hospitals were, on average, older than men: in 2005, 15% were aged 65 or older, compared with 10% of men (192). Hospitalization rates were substantially higher among younger and middle-aged men, with the gender differential increasing with age. At ages 65 and older, the trend was reversed, and hospitalization rates were somewhat higher among women (figure 3). Older women were a vulnerable group with regard to psychiatric inpatient admissions: in the 65 and older age group, 50% more women than men were hospitalized in 2005. This may reflect a difference in the availability of mental health support services for older women in the family and in the community.

Figure 3. Psychiatric hospitalization rates (per 100,000 population) by gender and age. Year 2005 (192)

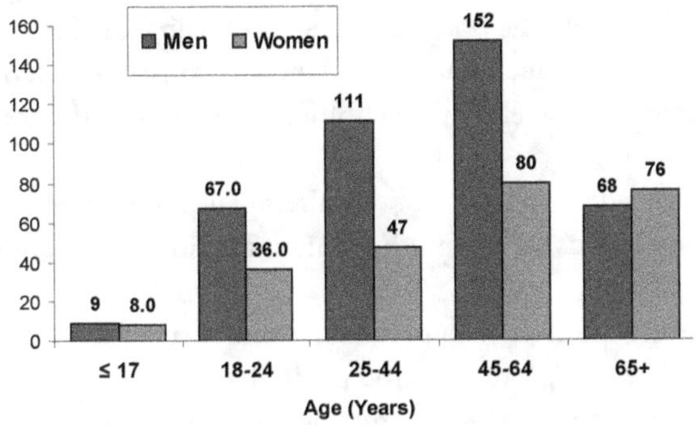

᧬ From epidemiology to mental health action

Effective treatment of women's mental health problems must take into consideration the interaction between difficult life conditions such as poverty and social exclusion, exposure to high levels of stressful life events, and the comorbid nature of somatic difficulties, substance abuse problems, PTSD and depression. Trying to treat one aspect alone is not likely to be effective (194–198). While these studies have been conducted among multiracial groups of women in the US, this social epidemiological approach is relevant to treatment of women's mental health problems in Israel as well.

For example, among women victims of domestic violence, one suggestion is to address the depression and learned helplessness that domestic abuse engenders while addressing the impact of macro issues such as male-dominated upbringing (100). In another study that compared the efficacy of an empowerment model of group therapy with standard group therapy among women seeking treatment for domestic violence, the empowerment model was more effective at reducing symptoms of PTSD, but both types of treatment groups were successful at reducing the extent of partner violence (199). Similarly, findings on female Israeli drug users show that domestic violence and incest are more likely to propel women into drug use, while men are more likely to report that they started substance abuse out of curiosity or because of the influence of friends (200).

A special service, developed at Sheba Medical Center at Tel Hashomer (near Tel Aviv) to address the mental and physical health needs of adolescent girls, showed that while there was an underlying somatic reason for seeking care, one-third of the subjects also mentioned psychosocial problems, and 20% mentioned sexuality-related problems. Curiously, however, they did not state these problems as their reasons for the clinic visits (201, 202). Adolescents especially may feel constrained raising sensitive issues with healthcare providers, who may need additional training to elicit the true reasons for clinic visits.

As we have shown, mental disorders among women of childbearing ages are both prevalent and a considerable public health problem. Although depression affects only 10% of pregnant women, postpartum mental disorders are more common and both are associated with morbidity in affected women and increased morbidity in their children. Despite their prevalence, they are often not recognized by primary-care providers, nor do these problems receive adequate attention among mental health professionals (203). There is a lack of current information and guidelines about how to treat these disorders without causing undue iatrogenic problems to the fetus or the breastfeeding infant. The potential benefits of using antidepressant medications in a pregnant or breastfeeding woman should be balanced against the potential risks to the newborn (47). For this reason, some feel that psychotherapy should be the treatment of choice for mothers with PPD (204).

It has been emphasized as well that psychotherapeutic treatment for depression in the postpartum period should focus on the mother-infant relationship in addition to the mothers' depressive symptoms (205).

Experience in treating mothers with psychiatric disorders (schizophrenia, schizoaffective and mood disorders) in the postpartum period led to the establishment of a Mother and Baby Unit (MBU) in a Jerusalem hospital. This is a treatment possibility for mothers at the severe end of the mental health spectrum, and their infants (206).

❦ Indications for further research

This review has highlighted many of the areas that are associated with women's mental health in Israel. However, there are some areas where current data are lacking. These include sexuality and women's mental health (including the development of sexual identity) and mental health issues of women who are bisexual or lesbian (207). While we reported briefly on issues of ethnic discrimination, more research is needed to explore the mental health consequences of discrimination based on ethnic or religious background, immigration status or skin color.

While research has been conducted on the mental health needs of religious women, more work is needed among this population. For example, some mental health studies have found that PPD and ED are significantly less prevalent among religious women (208, 209), yet other studies have not found such differences (49, 171). Another issue that is currently under-reported in the local literature is the development of empirically based interventions with Israeli women from different cultures (114, 166, 210–215) (see chapters 5 and 6). Clearly, it is difficult to develop evidence-based practice when epidemiological research is lacking; the integration of both the life-course perspective and social epidemiological methods could facilitate this development.

❦ References

1. Tudor W, Tudor JF, Gove WR. The effect of sex role differences on the social control of mental illness. *Journal of Health and Social Behavior* 1977; 18: 98–112.
2. Sen G, George A, Ostlin P. Engendering health equity: a review of research and policy. In: Sen G, George A, Ostlin P, eds. *Engendering international health: the challenge of equity*. Cambridge, MA: Bradford-MIT Press, 2002.
3. Krieger N, Fee E. Man-made medicine and women's health: the biopolitics of sex/gender and race/ethnicity. *International Journal of Health Services* 1994; 24: 265–283.
4. Krieger N. Genders, sexes, and health: what are the connections – and why does it matter? *International Journal of Epidemiology* 2003; 32: 652–657.
5. Fabrega H, Jr., Mezzich J, Ulrich R, *et al*. Females and males in an intake psychiatric setting. *Psychiatry* 1990; 53: 1–16.
6. Doyal L. *What makes women sick: gender and the political economy of health*. New Brunswick, NJ: Rutgers University Press, 1995.
7. Cottingham J, Fonn S, Garcia-Moreno C, *et al*. *Transforming health systems: gender and rights in reproductive health*. Geneva: World Health Organization, 2001.
8. Macintyre S, Hunt K, Sweeting H. Gender differences in health: are things really as simple as they seem? *Social Science and Medicine* 1996; 42: 617–624.
9. Gove WR. Gender differences in mental and physical illness among men and women. *Social Science and Medicine* 1984; 19: 77–91.
10. Wasilow-Mueller S, Erickson CK. Drug abuse and dependency: understanding gender differences in etiology and management. *Journal of the American Pharmaceutical Association* 2001; 41: 78–90.
11. Holden C. Sex and the suffering brain. *Science* 2005; 308: 1574–1577.

12. Gove WR. Gender differences in mental and physical illness: the effects of fixed roles and nurturant roles. *Social Science and Medicine* 1984; 19: 77–91.

13. Gove WR, Tudor JF. Adult sex roles and mental illness. *American Journal of Sociology* 1973; 78: 812–835.

14. Arnow BA. Relationships between childhood maltreatment, adult health and psychiatric outcomes, and medical utilization. *Journal of Clinical Psychiatry* 2004; 65 (Suppl 12): 10–15.

15. Rosenberg SD, Drake RE, Mueser K. New directions for treatment research on sequelae of sexual abuse in persons with severe mental illness. *Community Mental Health Journal* 1996; 32: 387–400.

16. Kuhn D, Hardy R. A life course approach to women's health: does the past predict the present? In: Kuhn D, Hardy R, eds. *A life course approach to women's health*. Oxford: Oxford University Press, 2002.

17. Maughan B. Depression and psychological distress: a life course perspective. In: Kuh D, Hardy R, eds. *A life course approach to women's health*. Oxford: Oxford University Press, 2002.

18. Maughan B, Taylor A, Caspi A, *et al.* Prenatal smoking and early childhood conduct problems: testing genetic and environmental explanations of the association. *Archives of General Psychiatry* 2004; 61: 836–843.

19. Misra DP, Astone N, Lynch CD. Maternal smoking and birth weight: interaction with parity and mother's own in utero exposure to smoking. *Epidemiology* 2005; 16: 288–293.

20. Misra DP, Grason H. Achieving safe motherhood: applying a life course and multiple determinants perinatal health framework in public health. *Women's Health Issues* 2006; 16: 159–175.

21. Misra DP, Guyer B, Allston A. Integrated perinatal health framework: a multiple determinants model with a life span approach. *American Journal of Preventive Medicine* 2003; 25: 65–75.

22. Cwikel JG. *A textbook of social epidemiology: strategies for public health activism.* New York: Columbia University Press, 2006.

23. Kaplan GA. What's wrong with social epidemiology, and how can we make it better? *Epidemiological Review* 2004; 26: 124–135.

24. Cabral M, Astbury J. *Women's mental health: an evidence-based review.* Geneva: Department of Mental Health and Substance Dependence, Mental Health Determinants and Populations Group, World Health Organization, 2000.

25. Lev-Wiesel R, Amir M. Holocaust child survivors and child sexual abuse. *Journal of Child Sexual Abuse* 2005; 14: 69–83.

26. Latzer Y, Ben-Ari A, Galimidi N. Anorexia nervosa and the family: effects on younger sisters to anorexia nervosa patients. *International Journal of Adolescent Medical Health* 2002; 14: 275–281.

27. Luzzatto D, Gvion L. Feminine but not femme: the dual lesbian body. *Journal of Homosexuality* 2004; 48: 43–77.

28. Remennick LI. Immigrants from Chernobyl-affected areas in Israel: the link between health and social adjustment. *Social Science and Medicine* 2002; 54: 309–317.

29. Gilat I, Latzer Y. Characteristics of calls to the Israeli hotline during the *Intifada*. *Community Mental Health Journal* 2007; 43: 401–420.

30. Elnekave E, Gross R. The healthcare experiences of Arab Israeli women in a reformed healthcare system. *Health Policy* 2004; 69: 101–116.

31. Zalcberg S. *The world of Hassidic women "Toldot Aharon": their status as individuals and as a group.* Ramat Gan: Bar-Ilan University, 2005.

32. Central Bureau of Statistics. *Statistical abstract of Israel No. 58.* Jerusalem: Central Bureau of Statistics, 2007.

33. Israel Center for Disease Control. *Israel National Health Interview Survey (INHIS-1) 2003–2004.* European Health Interview Surveys (EUROHIS) project. ICDC Publication No. 249. Tel Aviv: Ministry of Health, 2006.

34. Ifrah A. Women's health in Israel: progress and gaps. *bridges, Israeli-Palestinian Health Magazine* 2005; 1: 8–12.

35. Murray JL, Lopez AD. *The global burden of disease: a comprehensive assessment of mortality and disability from diseases, injuries and risk factors in 1990 and projected to 2020. Summary.* Boston: Harvard School of Public Health and the World Health Organization, 1996.

36. Piccinelli M, Wilkinson G. Gender differences in depression. Critical review. *British Journal of Psychiatry* 2000; 177: 486–492.

37. Gofin R, Palti H, Mandel M. Fighting among Jerusalem adolescents: personal and school-related factors. *Journal of Adolescent Health* 2000; 27: 218–223.

38. Kessler RC. Gender and mood disorders. In: Goldman MB, Hatch MC, eds. *Women & health.* San Diego: Academic Press, 2000.

39. Kessler RC, McGonagle KA, Swartz M, *et al.* Sex and depression in the National Comorbidity Survey. 1: Lifetime prevalence, chronicity and recurrence. *Journal of Affective Disorders* 1993; 29: 85–96.

40. Kendler KS, Kessler RC, Neale MC, *et al.* The prediction of major depression in women: toward an integrated etiologic model. *American Journal of Psychiatry* 1993; 150: 1139–1148.

41. Kendler KS, Neale MC, Kessler RC, *et al.* A longitudinal twin study of personality and major depression in women. *Archives of General Psychiatry* 1993; 50: 853–862.

42. Verkerk GJ, Denollet J, Van Heck GL, *et al.* Personality factors as determinants of depression in postpartum women: a prospective 1-year follow-up study. *Psychosomatic Medicine* 2005; 67: 632–637.

43. Verkerk GJ, Pop VJ, Van Son MJ, *et al.* Prediction of depression in the postpartum period: a longitudinal follow-up study in high-risk and low-risk women. *Journal of Affective Disorders* 2003; 77: 159–166.

44. Noble RE. Depression in women. *Metabolism.* 2005; 54 (Suppl 1): 49–52.

45. Alexander JL, Dennerstein L, Kotz K, *et al.* Women, anxiety and mood: a review of nomenclature, comorbidity and epidemiology. *Expert Review of Neurotherapeutics* 2007; 7 (Suppl 11): S45–58.

46. Gorman LL, O'Hara MW, Figueiredo B, *et al.* Adaptation of the structured clinical interview for DSM-IV disorders for assessing depression in women during pregnancy and post-partum across countries and cultures. *British Journal of Psychiatry* 2004; 46: Suppl. s17–23.

47. Gorman JM. Gender differences in depression and response to psychotropic medication. *Gender Medicine* 2006; 3: 93–109.

48. O'Hara M, Swain AM. Rates and risks of postpartum depression: a meta-analysis. *International Review of Psychiatry* 1996; 8: 37–54.

49. Glasser S, Barell v, Shoham A, *et al.* Prospective study of postpartum depression in an Israeli cohort: prevalence, incidence and demographic risk factors. *Journal of Psychosomatic Obstetrics and Gynaecology* 1998; 19: 155–164.

50. Mindes EJ, Ingram KM, Kliewer W, *et al.* Longitudinal analyses of the relationship between unsupportive social interactions and psychological adjustment among women with fertility problems *Social Science and Medicine* 2003; 56: 2165–2180.

51. Cwikel J, Gidron Y, Sheiner E. Psychological interactions with infertility among women. *European Journal of Obstetric and Gynecological Reproductive Biology* 2004; 117: 126–131.

52. Broen AN, Moum T, Bodtker AS, *et al.* The course of mental health after miscarriage and induced abortion: a longitudinal, five-year follow-up study. *BMC Medicine* 2005; 3: 18.

53. Weissman MM, Bruce M, Leaf PJ, *et al.* Affective disorders. In: Robins LW, Regier DA, eds. *Psychiatric disorders in America*. New York: Free Press, 1991.

54. Astbury J. The state of the evidence – Gender disparities in mental health. In: Cabral de Mello M, Borneman T, Levav I, eds. *A call for action by world health ministers*. Geneva: World Health Organization, 2001.

55. Cwikel J, Segal-Engelchin D. Implications of ethnic group origin for Israeli women's mental health. *Journal of Immigrant Health* 2005; 7: 133–143.

56. Bloch M, Rotenberg N, Koren D, *et al.* Risk factors associated with the development of postpartum mood disorders. *Journal of Affective Disorders* 2005; 88: 9–18.

57. Zelkowitz P, Milet TH. The course of postpartum psychiatric disorders in women and their partners. *Journal of Nervous Mental Disease* 2001; 189: 575–582.

58. Astbury J, Brown S, Lumley J, *et al.* Birth events, birth experiences and social differences in postnatal depression. *Australian Journal of Public Health* 1994; 18: 176–184.

59. Atkinson L, Paglia A, Coolbear J, Niccols A, *et al.* Attachment security: a meta-analysis of maternal mental health correlates. *Clinical Psychology Review* 2000; 20: 1019–1040.

60. Hiscock H, Wake M. Infant sleep problems and postnatal depression: a community-based study. *Pediatrics* 2001; 107: 1317–1322.

61. Zelkowitz P, Milet TH. Postpartum psychiatric disorders: their relationship to psychological adjustment and marital satisfaction in the spouses. *Journal of Abnormal Psychology* 1996; 105: 281–285.

62. Belle D. The stress of caring: women as providers of social support. In: Breznitz LGS, ed. *Handbook of stress: theoretical and clinical aspects*. New York: Free Press, 1982.

63. Taylor SE, Klein LC, Lewis BP, *et al.* Biobehavioral responses to stress in females: tend-and-befriend, not fight-or-flight. *Psychological Review* 2000; 107: 411–429.

64. Carver CS, Scheier M, Weintraub F, *et al.* Assessing coping strategies: a theoretically based approach. *Journal of Personality and Social Psychology* 1989; 56: 267–283.

65. Ptacek JT, Smith RE, Zanas J. Gender, appraisal, and coping: a longitudinal analysis. *Journal of Personality* 1992; 60: 747–770.

66. Rosario M, Shinn M, March H, *et al.* Gender differences in coping and social supports: testing socialization and role constraint theories. *Journal of Community Psychology* 1988; 16: 555–569.

67. Dalgard OS, Dowrick C, Lehtinen v, *et al.* Negative life events, social support and gender difference in depression: a multinational community survey with data from the ODIN study. *Social Psychiatry and Psychiatric Epidemiology* 2006; 41: 444–451.

68. Belle D. Poverty and women's mental health. *American Psychologist* 1990; 45: 385–389.

69. Paltiel FL. Is being poor a mental health hazard? *Women's Health* 1987; 12: 189–211.

70. Patel V, Araya R, de Lima M, *et al.* Women, poverty and common mental disorders in four restructuring societies. *Social Science and Medicine* 1999; 49: 1461–1471.

71. Heflin CM, Siefert K, Williams DR. Food insufficiency and women's mental health: findings from a 3-year panel of welfare recipients. *Social Science Medicine* 2005; 61: 1971–1982.

72. Watts C, Zimmerman C. Violence against women: global scope and magnitude. *The Lancet* 2002; 359: 1232–1237.

73. Bohn DK, Holz KA. Sequelae of abuse. Health effects of childhood sexual abuse, domestic battering, and rape. *Journal of Nurse Midwifery* 1996; 41: 442–456.

74. Dube SR, Anda RF, Whitfield CL, *et al.* Long-term consequences of childhood sexual abuse by gender of victim. *American Journal of Preventive Medicine* 2005; 28: 430–438.

75. Chapman DP, Whitfield CL, Felitti VJ, *et al.* Adverse childhood experiences and the risk of depressive disorders in adulthood. *Journal of Affective Disorders* 2004; 82: 217–225.

76. Horwitz AV, Widom CS, McLaughlin J, *et al.* The impact of childhood abuse and neglect on adult mental health: a prospective study. *Journal of Health and Social Behavior* 2001; 42: 184–201.

77. Dong M, Anda RF, Felitti VJ, *et al.* The interrelatedness of multiple forms of childhood abuse, neglect, and household dysfunction. *Child Abuse and Neglect* 2004; 28: 771–784.

78. Felitti VJ, Anda RF, Nordenberg D, *et al.* Relationship of childhood abuse and household dysfunction to many of the leading causes of death in adults. The Adverse Childhood Experiences (ACE) Study. *American Journal of Preventive Medicine* 1998; 14: 245–258.

79. Dube SR, Miller JW, Brown DW, *et al.* Adverse childhood experiences and the association with ever using alcohol and initiating alcohol use during adolescence. *Journal of Adolescent Health* 2006; 38: 444 e1–10.

80. Dube SR, Anda RF, Felitti VJ, *et al.* Childhood abuse, household dysfunction, and the risk of attempted suicide throughout the life span: findings from the Adverse Childhood Experiences Study. *Journal of the American Medical Association* 2001; 286: 3089–3096.

81. Hillis SD, Anda RF, Felitti VJ, *et al.* Adverse childhood experiences and sexual risk behaviors in women: a retrospective cohort study. *Family Planning Perspective* 2001; 33: 206–211.

82. Anda RF, Croft JB, Felitti VJ, *et al.* Adverse childhood experiences and smoking during adolescence and adulthood. *Journal of the American Medical Association* 1999; 282: 1652–1658.

83. Dietz PM, Spitz AM, Anda RF, *et al.* Unintended pregnancy among adult women exposed to abuse or household dysfunction during their childhood. *Journal of the American Medical Association* 1999; 282: 1359–1364.

84. Lev-Weisel R, Daphna-Tekoa S. Prenatal posttraumatic stress symptomology in pregnant survivors of childhood sexual abuse: a brief report. *Journal of Trauma and Loss* 2007; 12: 145–153.

85. Fisher M, Yassour-Borochowitz D, Neter E. Domestic abuse in pregnancy: results from a phone survey in northern Israel. *Israel Medical Association Journal* 2003; 5: 35–39.

86. Rabin B, Markus E, Voghera N. A comparative study of Jewish and Arab battered women presenting in the emergency room of a general hospital. *Social Work in Health Care* 1999; 29: 69–84.

87. Eisikovits Z, Fishman G, Mesch G, *et al. The prevalence and correlates of domestic violence in the Israeli population.* Haifa: Minerva Center for the Study of Society, 2002 (Hebrew).

88. Cwikel J, Lev-Weisel R, Al-Krenawi A. The physical and psychosocial health of Bedouin Arab women in the Negev area of Israel – the impact of high fertility and pervasive domestic violence. *Violence against Women* 2003; 9: 240–257.

89. Gross R, Brammli-Greenberg S. *The health and welfare of women in Israel: findings from a national survey.* RR-361-00. Jerusalem: JDC-Brookdale Institute, 2000.

90. Garcia-Moreno C, Jansen HA, Ellsberg M, *et al.* Prevalence of intimate partner violence: findings from the WHO multi-country study on women's health and domestic violence. *The Lancet.* 2006; 368: 1260–1239.

91. Mahoney P, Williams LM, West CM. Violence against women by intimate relationship partners. In: Renzetti CM, Edleson JL, Kennedy Bergen R, eds. *Sourcebook on violence against women.* Thousand Oaks, CA: Sage, 2001.

92. Raphael J. Domestic violence as a welfare-to-work barrier. In: Renzetti CM, Edleson JL, Kennedy Bergen R, eds. *Sourcebook on violence against women* Thousand Oaks, CA: Sage, 2001.

93. Kendler KS, Neale MC, MacLean CJ, *et al.* Smoking and major depression. A causal analysis. *Archives of General Psychiatry* 1993; 50: 36–43.

94. Tsoh JY, Humfleet GL, Muñoz RF, *et al.* Development of major depression after treatment for smoking cessation. *American Journal of Psychiatry* 2000; 157: 368–374.

95. Murphy JM, Horton NJ, Monson RR, *et al.* Cigarette smoking in relation to depression: historical trends from the Stirling County Study. *American Journal of Psychiatry* 2003; 160: 1663–1669.

96. Covey LS, Glassman AH, Stetner F. Cigarette smoking and major depression. *Journal of Addictive Disorders* 1998; 17: 35–46.

97. Borrelli B, Bock B, King T, *et al.* The impact of depression on smoking cessation in women. *American Journal of Preventive Medicine* 1996; 12: 378–387.

98. Cwikel J, Barak N. *The health and welfare of Israeli women in the Negev.* Beersheba: The Center of Women's Health Studies and Promotion, Ben-Gurion University of the Negev, 2003.

99. Garti N, Ifrah A, Blau S. *European Health Interview Surveys (EUORHIS) – Women's health. Report No. 237,* Tel Aviv: Israel Center for Disease Control, 2004.

100. Bargai N, Ben-Shakhar G, *et al.* Posttraumatic stress disorder and depression in battered women: the mediating role of learned helplessness. *Journal of Family Violence* 2007; 22: 267–272.

101. Chudakov B, Ilan K, Belmaker RH, *et al.* The motivation and mental health of sex workers. *Journal of Sex and Marital Therapy* 2002; 28: 305–315.

102. Radlauer D. Statistical analysis of casualties in the Palestinian-Israeli conflict. International Policy Institute for Counterterrorism, 2005.

103. Achdut L, Cohen R, Endwald M. Trends of development in poverty and income inequality. Jerusalem: The National Insurance Institute, 2004 (Hebrew).

104. Lazarus RS, Folkman S. *Stress, appraisal, and coping.* New York: Springer, 1984.

105. Billings AG, Moos RH. The role of coping responses and social resources in attenuating the stress of life events. *Journal of Behavioral Medicine* 1981; 4: 139–157.

106. Vingerhoets AJJM, Van Heck G. Gender, coping and psychosomatic symptoms. *Psychological Medicine* 1990; 20: 125–135.

107. Heiman T. Examination of the salutogenic model, support resources, coping style, and stressors among Israeli university students. *Journal of Psychology* 2004; 138: 505–520.

108. Bekker MHJ, Nijssen A, Hens G. Stress prevention training: sex differences in types of stressors, coping, and training effects. *Stress and Health* 2001; 17: 207–218.

109. Davis MC, Matthews KA, Twamley EW. Is life more difficult on Mars or Venus? A meta-analytic review of sex differences in major and minor life events. *Annals of Behavioral Medicine* 1999; 21: 83–97.

110. Lengua LJ, Stormshak EA. Gender, gender roles, and personality: gender differences in the prediction of coping and psychological symptoms. *Sex Roles* 2000; 43: 787–820.

111. Gidron Y, Kaplan Y, Velt A, *et al.* Prevalence and moderators of terror-related post-traumatic stress disorder symptoms in Israeli citizens. *Israel Medical Association Journal* 2004; 6: 387–391.

112. Bleich A, Gelkopf M, Solomon Z. Exposure to terrorism, stress-related mental health symptoms, and coping behaviors among a nationally representative sample in Israel. *Journal of the American Medical Association* 2003; 290: 612–620.

113. Bleich A, Gelkopf M, Melamed Y, *et al.* Emotional impact of exposure to terrorism among young-old and old-old Israeli citizens. *American Journal of Geriatric Psychiatry* 2005; 13: 705–712.

114. Al-Krenawi A, Lev-Wiesel R, Sehwail MA. Psychological symptomatology among Palestinian male and female adolescents living under political violence 2004–2005. *Community Mental Health Journal* 2007; 43: 49–56.

115. Cwikel JG, Segal-Engelchin D, *et al.* Developing resilience – the structure of mothers' coping strategies under chronic security threats in Israel. Paper presented as the International Society for Traumatic Stress Studies, Hollywood CA, 2006.

116. Cwikel J, Mendlinger S. Origins of and influences on women's health behaviors: examining intergenerational and multi-cultural effects. Grant from the Ministry of Science, Culture and Sport 83667101–301. Beersheba: Ben-Gurion University Center for Women's Health Studies and Promotion, 2003.

117. Mendlinger S, Cwikel J. Spiraling between qualitative and quantitative data on women's health behaviors: a double helix model for mixed methods. *Qualitative Health Research* 2008; 18: 280–293.

118. Amir LH, Cwikel J. Why do women stop breastfeeding? A closer look at 'not enough milk' among Israeli women in the Negev Region. *Breastfeed Review* 2005; 13: 7–13.

119. Cwikel J, Segal-Engelchin D, *et al. Women's perceptions of pregnancy and childbirth among mothers in the Negev.* Beersheba: The Center for Women's Health Studies and Promotion, 2007.

120. Cohain JS, Yoselis A. Caesareans and low-risk women in Israel. *Practical Midwifery* 2004; 7: 28–31.

121. Sheiner E, Levy A, Menes TS, *et al.* Maternal obesity as an independent risk factor for caesarean delivery. *Paediatric and Perinatal Epidemiology* 2004; 18: 196–201.

122. Maslovitz S, Kupferminc MJ, Lessing JB, *et al.* Perinatal outcome among non-residents in Israel. *Israel Medical Association Journal* 2005; 7: 315–319.

123. Friedler S, Mashiach S, Laufer N. Births in Israel resulting from in-vitro fertilization/embryo transfer, 1982–1989. *Human Reproduction* 1992; 7: 1159–1163.

124. Gupton A, Heaman M, Cheung LW. Complicated and uncomplicated pregnancies: women's perception of risk. *Journal of Obstetric and Gynecological Neonatal Nursing* 2001; 30: 192–201.

125. Ayers S, Pickering AD. Do women get posttraumatic stress disorder as a result of childbirth? A prospective study of incidence. *Birth* 2001; 28: 111–118.

126. Fargues P. Protracted national conflict and fertility change: Palestinians and Israelis in the twentieth century *Population and Development Review* 2000; 26: 441–482.

127. Stypińska J. Jewish majority and Arab minority in Israel-demographic struggle *Polish Sociological Review* 2007; 157: 105–120.

128. Anson J, Meir A. Religiosity, nationalism and fertility in Israel. *European Journal of Population* 1996; 12: 1–25.

129. Shalev C, Gooldin S. The uses and misuses of *in vitro* fertilization in Israel: some sociological and ethical considerations. *Nashim* 2006; 12: 151–176 (Hebrew).

130. Lunenfeld B, Insler V. Human gonadotropins. In: Zacur HA, ed. *Reproductive medicine and surgery* St. Louis, MO: Mosby, 1995.

131. Benyamini Y, Gozlan M, Kokia E. Variability in the difficulties experienced by women undergoing infertility treatments. *Fertility and Sterility* 2005; 83: 275–283.

132. Nasseri M. Cultural similarities in psychological reactions to infertility. *Psychological Report* 2000; 86: 375–378.

133. Schmidt L. Psychosocial burden of infertility and assisted reproduction. *The Lancet* 2006; 367: 379–380.

134. Franco JG, Jr., Razera Baruffi RL, Mauri AL, *et al.* Psychological evaluation test after the use of assisted reproduction techniques. *Journal of Assisted Reproduction Genetics* 2002; 19: 274–278.

135. Matsubayashi H, Hosaka T, Izumi S, *et al.* Increased depression and anxiety in infertile Japanese women resulting from lack of husband's support and feelings of stress. *General Hospital Psychiatry* 2004; 26: 398–404.

136. Cwikel J, Barak N. *The health and welfare of Bedouin Arab women in the Negev.* Beersheba: The Center of Women's Health Studies and Promotion, Ben-Gurion University of the Negev, 2002.

137. Cwikel J, Lev-Weisel R, Al-Krenawi A. The physical and psychosocial health of Bedouin-Arab women of the Negev area of Israel: the impact of high fertility and pervasive domestic violence. *Violence against Women* 2003; 9: 240–257.

138. Cwikel J, Gidron Y, Sheiner E. Psychological interactions with infertility among women: a review. *European Journal of Obstetrics & Gynecology and Reproductive Biology* 2004; 117: 126–131.

139. Van Balen F. The psychologization of infertility. In: Inhorn MC, Van Balen F, eds. *Infertility around the globe.* Berkeley: University of California Press, 2002.

140. Sarid O, Cwikel J, Bloch M. If I had a child – Voices of Israeli women in treatment for infertility. *Society and Welfare* (In press) (Hebrew).

141. Peleg-Lazar G. The relationship between parental stress, parental attitudes and security of attachment among mothers and their IVF children. [Ph.D.thesis]. Tel Aviv: Tel Aviv University, 2001.

142. Kessler RC, Sonnega A, Bromet E, *et al.* Posttraumatic stress disorder in the National Comorbidity Survey. *Archives of General Psychiatry* 1995; 52: 1048–1060.

143. Amir M, Sol O. Psychological impact and prevalence of traumatic events in a student sample in Israel: the effect of multiple traumatic events and physical injury. *Journal of Traumatic Stress* 1999; 12: 139–154.

144. Anson O, Rosenzweig A, Shwarzmann P. The health of women married to men in regular army service: women who cannot afford to be ill. *Women's Health* 1993; 20: 33–45.

145. Ben Arzi N, Solomon Z, Dekel R. Secondary traumatization among wives of PTSD and post-concussion casualties: distress, caregiver burden and psychological separation. *Brain Injury* 2000; 14: 725–736.

146. Solomon Z, Waysman M, Levy G, *et al.* From front line to home front: a study of secondary traumatization. *Family Process* 1992; 31: 289–302.

147. Dekel R, Solomon Z. Marital relations among former prisoners of war: contribution of posttraumatic stress disorder, aggression, and sexual satisfaction. *Journal of Family Psychology* 2006; 20: 709–712.

148. Mendlinger S, Cwikel J. Health behaviors over the life cycle among mothers and daughters from Ethiopia. *Nashim* 2006; 12: 57–94 (Hebrew).

149. Ifergan A. personal communication. 2008.

150. Sasson-Levy O. Feminism and military gender practices: Israeli women soldiers in "masculine" roles. *Sociological Inquiry* 2003; 73: 440–465.

151. Zinzow HM, Grubaugh AL, Monnier J, *et al.* Trauma among female veterans: a critical review. *Trauma and Violence Abuse* 2007; 8: 384–400.

152. Turner JB, Turse NA, Dohrenwend BP. Circumstances of service and gender differences in war-related PTSD: findings from the National Vietnam Veteran Readjustment Study. *Journal of Traumatic Stress* 2007; 20: 643–649.

153. Kang H, Dalager N, Mahan C, *et al.* The role of sexual assault on the risk of PTSD among Gulf War veterans. *Annals of Epidemiology* 2005; 15: 191–195.

154. Shiloh D. A rite of passage: women in the Israeli Army. WIN: *Women's International Network* 1998; 10B.

155. Karpel D. My God, what did we do? A new film reveals the trauma of the female soldiers of the *Intifada. Haaretz Magazine* 2007; Sect. 14–7 (Hebrew).

156. Mazali R. And what about the girls? What a culture of war genders out of view. *Nashim* 2003; 6: 39–50.

157. Sered S. What makes women sick? *Maternity, modesty and militarism in Israeli society.* Hanover and London: University Press of New England/Brandeis University Press, 2000.

158. Tabak N, Livneh A. Sexual harassment – abuse or flirtation. *Medicine and Law* 2005; 24: 479–488.

159. Bronner G, Peretz C, Ehrenfeld M. Sexual harassment of nurses and nursing students. *Journal of Advance Nursing* 2003; 42: 637–644.

160. Aviv A, Levine J, Shelef A, *et al.* Therapist-patient sexual relations: results of a national survey in Israel. *Israel Journal of Psychiatry and Related Sciences* 2006; 43: 119–125.

161. Anson O, Sagy S. Marital violence: comparing women in violent and nonviolent unions. *Human Relations* 1995; 48: 285–305.

162. Graetz N. *Silence is deadly: Judaism confronts wifebeating.* Northvale, NJ and Jerusalem: Jason Aronson, 1998.

163. Douki S, Nacef F, Belhadj A, *et al.* Violence against women in Arab and Islamic countries. *Archives of Women's Mental Health* 2003; 6: 165–171.

164. Remennick L. Immigration, gender and psychosocial adjustment: a study of 150 immigrant couples in Israel. *Sex Roles* 2005; 53: 847–863.

165. Ritsner M, Ponizovsky A, Nechamkin Y, *et al.* Gender differences in psychosocial risk factors for psychological distress among immigrants. *Comprehensive Psychiatry* 2001; 42: 151–160.

166. Al-Krenawi A, Graham JR. Gender and biomedical/traditional mental health utilization among the Bedouin-Arabs of the Negev. *Culture, Medicine and Psychiatry* 1999; 23: 219–243.

167. Sheiner EK, Sheiner E, Shoham-Vardi I, *et al.* Ethnic differences influence care giver's estimates of pain during labour. *Pain* 1999; 81: 299–305.

168. Levinson D. Unpublished data from the Israel National Health Survey, 2003–2004.

169. Romans SE, Tyas J, Cohen MM, *et al.* Gender differences in the symptoms of major depressive disorder. *Journal of Nervous and Mental Disease* 2007; 195: 905–911.

170. Levinson D, Zilber N, Lerner Y, *et al.* Prevalence of mood and anxiety disorders in the community: results from the Israel National Health Survey. *Israel Journal of Psychiatry and Related Sciences* 2007; 44: 94–103.

171. Cwikel J, Zilber N, Feinson M, *et al.* Prevalence and risk factors of threshold and sub-threshold psychiatric disorders in primary care. *Social Psychiatry and Psychiatric Epidemiology* 2008; 43:184–191.

172. Gross R, Feldman D, Rabinowitz Y, *et al.* Characteristics of adults with emotional distress, and patterns of mental health services use. *Harefuah* 1998; 134: 341–348 (Hebrew).

173. Levav I, Abramson JH. A community study of emotional distress in Jerusalem. *Israel Journal of Psychiatry and Related Sciences* 1984; 21: 19–45.

174. Levav I, Gilboa S, Ruiz F. Demoralization and gender differences in a kibbutz. *Psychological Medicine* 1991; 21: 1019–1028.

175. Merom D. *A national survey of women's health.* Tel Aviv: Israel Center for Disease Control (ICDC), Ministry of Health, 1998.

176. Ifrah A. Gender differences in mental health and mental disorders in Israel: findings from National Mental Health Survey. Paper presented at the Meeting of the Israel Psychiatric Association, Tel Aviv, 2006.

177. Goldney RD, Wilson D, Dal Grande E, *et al.* Suicidal ideation in a random community sample: attributable risk due to depression and psychosocial and traumatic events. *Australia and New Zealand Journal of Psychiatry* 2000; 34:98–106.

178. Lester D, Walker R. Hopelessness, helplessness, and haplessness as predictors of suicidal ideation. *Omega* 2007; 55: 321–334.

179. Sareen J, Cox BJ, Afifi TO, *et al.* Anxiety disorders and risk for suicidal ideation and suicide attempts: a population-based longitudinal study of adults. *Archives of General Psychiatry* 2005; 62: 1249–1255.

180. Suominen K, Isometsä E, Suokas J, *et al.* Completed suicide after a suicide attempt: a 37-year follow-up study. *American Journal of Psychiatry* 2004; 161: 562–563.

181. Jenkins GR, Hale R, Papanastassiou M, *et al.* Suicide rate 22 years after parasuicide: cohort study. *British Medical Journal* 2002; 325: 1155.

182. Knox KL, Caine ED. Establishing priorities for reducing suicide and its antecedents in the United States. *American Journal of Public Health* 2005; 95: 1893–1903.

183. Lewinsohn PM, Rohde P, Seeley JR, *et al.* Gender differences in suicide attempts from adolescence to young adulthood. *Journal of the American Academy of Child and Adolescent Psychiatry* 2001; 40: 427–434.

184. Lubin G, Glasser S, Boyko v, *et al.* Epidemiology of suicide in Israel: a nationwide population study. *Social Psychiatry and Psychiatric Epidemiology* 2001; 36: 123–127.

185. Prosser JM, Perrone J, Pines JM. The epidemiology of intentional non-fatal self-harm poisoning in the United States: 2001–2004. *Journal of Medical Toxicology* 2007; 3: 20–24.

186. Information and Computerization Services, Information Section, Ministry of Health. *Suicidality in Israel.* Jerusalem: Information and Computerization Services, Information Section, Ministry of Health, 2005 (Hebrew).

187. Levinson D, Haklai Z, Stein N, *et al.* Suicide attempts in Israel: age by gender analysis of a national emergency departments database. *Suicide & Life Threatening Behavior* 2006; 36: 97–102.

188. Harel Y, Molchl M, Tillinger E. *Youth in Israel: health, well being and risk behavior: summary of findings from the third national study (2002) and trend analysis (1994–2002).* Ramat Gan: Bar-Ilan University, 2003 (Hebrew).

189. Levinson D, Haklai Z, Stein N, *et al.* Suicide ideation, planning and attempts: results from the Israel National Health Survey. *Israel Journal of Psychiatry and Related Sciences* 2007; 44: 136–143.

190. Gilat I, Shahar G. Emotional first aid for a suicide crisis: comparison between telephonic hotline and Internet. *Psychiatry* 2007; 70: 12–18.

191. Ashkar K, Giloni C, Grinshpoon A, *et al.* Suicidal attempts admitted to a general hospital in the Western Galilee: an inter-ethnic comparison study. *Israel Journal of Psychiatry and Related Sciences* 2006; 43: 137–145.

192. Department of Information and Evaluation, Mental Health Services. Ministry of Health. *Mental health in Israel. Statistical annual, 2006.* Jerusalem: Department of Information and Evaluation, Mental Health Services. Ministry of Health, 2007 (Hebrew).

193. Personal communication. Mental Health Services. Jerusalem: Department of Information and Evaluation, Ministry of Health, 2008.

194. Amaro H, Raj A, Vega RR, *et al.* Racial/ethnic disparities in the HIV and substance abuse epidemics: communities responding to the need. *Public Health Report* 2001; 116: 434–448.

195. Amaro H, Hardy-Fanta C. Gender relations in addiction and recovery. *Journal of Psychoactive Drugs* 1995; 27: 325–337.

196. Arevalo S, Prado G, Amaro H. Spirituality, sense of coherence, and coping responses in women receiving treatment for alcohol and drug addiction. *Evaluation and Program Planning* 2008; 31: 113–123.

197. Amaro H, Dai J, Arevalo S, Acevedo A, *et al.* Effects of integrated trauma treatment on outcomes in a racially/ethnically diverse sample of women in urban community-based substance abuse treatment. *Journal of Urban Health* 2007; 84: 508–522.

198. Morrissey JP, Jackson EW, Ellis AR, *et al.* Twelve-month outcomes of trauma-informed interventions for women with co-occurring disorders. *Psychiatric Services* 2005; 56: 1213–1222.

199. Aronson EA, Cwikel JG. *Group treatment of battered women as an empowerment tool for violence prevention: a randomized controlled trial.* Ben-Gurion Center for Women's Health Studies and Promotion. Beersheba, 2007.

200. Lev-Wiesel R, Shuval R. Perceived causal and treatment factors related to substance abuse: gender differences. *European Addiction Research* 2006; 12: 109–112.

201. Wilf-Miron R, Glasser S, Sikron F, *et al.* Using a health concerns checklist as a bridge from reason for encounter to diagnosis of girls attending an adolescent health service. *Pediatrics* 2000; 106: 1065–1069.

202. Wilf-Miron R, Sikron F, Glasser S, *et al.* Community-based adolescent health services in Israel: from theory to practice. *International Journal of Adolescent Medical Health* 2002; 14: 139–144.

203. Stuart S, O'Hara MW, Blehar MC. Mental disorders associated with childbearing. Report of the Biennial Meeting of the Marce Society. *Psychopharmacological Bulletin* 1998; 34: 333–338.

204. Stuart S, O'Hara MW, Gorman LL. The prevention and psychotherapeutic treatment of postpartum depression. *Archives of Women's Mental Health* 2003; 6 Suppl 2: S57–69.

205. Forman DR, O'Hara MW, Stuart S, *et al.* Effective treatment for postpartum depression is not sufficient to improve the developing mother-child relationship. *Developmental Psychopathology* 2007; 19: 585–602.

206. Maizel S, Kandel Katzenelson S, Fainstein V. The Jerusalem psychiatric mother-baby unit. *Archives of Women's Mental Health* 2005; 8: 200–202.

207. Rabinerson D, Ninio A, Greenblat BZ, *et al.* Kos and lesbos or the physician and the lesbian patient. *Harefuah* 2005; 144:554–557 (Hebrew).

208. Dankner R, Goldberg RP, Fisch RZ, *et al.* Cultural elements of postpartum depression. A study of 327 Jewish Jerusalem women. *Journal of Reproductive Medicine* 2000; 45: 97–104.

209. Latzer Y, Vander S, Gilat I. Socio-demographic characteristics of eating disorder patients in an outpatient clinic: a descriptive epidemiological study. *European Eating Disorders Review* 2008; 16:139–46.

210. Abu-Baker K. Arab women, sex and sexuality: the presence of Arab society and culture in individual and marital therapy among Palestinian women. *Hamizrah Hahadash* 2002; MG: 229–245 (Hebrew).

211. Al-Krenawi A, Graham JR, Ophir M, *et al.* Ethnic and gender differences in mental health utilization: the case of Muslim Jordanian and Moroccan Jewish Israeli out-patient psychiatric patients. *International Journal of Social Psychiatry* 2001; 47: 42–54.

212. Al-Krenawi A, Slonim-Nevo V. A comparative study of polygamous and monogamous marriages as they affect Bedouin-Arab women. In: Lev-Weisel R, Cwikel J, Barak N, eds. *Shimri nafshech ("Guard your soul"): mental health among women in Israel.* Jerusalem: JDC-Brookdale Institute, The Center for Women's Health Studies and Promotion and the Spitzer Department of Social Work, Ben-Gurion University of the Negev, 2005.

213. Hundt GL, Chatty D, Thabet AA, *et al.* Advocating multi-disciplinarity in studying complex emergencies: the limitations of a psychological approach to understanding how young people cope with prolonged conflict in Gaza. *Journal of Biosocial Sciences* 2004; 36: 417–431.

214. Savaya R. Associations among economic need, self-esteem, and Israeli Arab women's attitudes toward and use of professional services. *Social Work* 1998; 43: 445–454.

215. Shemesh AA, Kohn R, Blumstein T, *et al.* A community study on emotional distress among Arab and Jewish Israelis over the age of 60. *International Journal of Geriatric Psychiatry* 2006; 21: 64–76.

Chapter 2

THE EPIDEMIOLOGY OF MENTAL HEALTH PROBLEMS IN ISRAELI YOUTH

Ivonne Mansbach-Kleinfeld, Anda Massler and Alan Apter

§ Socioeconomic and demographic characteristics

By the end of 2006, the number of Israeli children and adolescents below the age of 18 totaled 2,365,800 (1). Of these, 69.1% were Jews; 24% Muslims; 1.9% Christians; 2% Druze; and 3% did not have a registered religion. Although more children are born every year, their proportion in the general population has been decreasing: in 1970 this group comprised 39.2% of the population while by the end of 2006 they were 33.2% of the total population. Such a decrease has occurred among all religious groups, including Muslim Israelis, among whom the proportion of children and youth decreased from 58.7% in 1970 to 48.7% in 2006.

In 2006, 9% of the young lived in single-parent families. This trend seems to be on the rise, even when controlling for population growth; while in 2000 there were 170,874 children living with a single parent, in 2006 there were 201,649. Among new immigrants, there were almost three times as many one-parent families compared to veteran Israeli families, 27.4% vs. 10.2%. The percentage of children without citizenship rights in 2007 was 6.8% (N = 160,120); 71% of them were residents of east Jerusalem and the rest were born to migrant workers, new immigrants with undetermined status or in mixed marriages without reunification rights (an Arab Israeli married to a Palestinian). About 54,000 children, mainly Bedouin, lived in unrecognized villages, where they comprise 61% of the population.

Poverty and mental health

There is extensive inequality in healthcare delivery, health status and health outcomes resulting from marked disparities in income, housing, education and employment (2). In 2004, the top 20% of the population held 44% of the total wealth, while the lower 20% received only 6% (3). Differences in income by gender and ethnicity are particularly worrisome, due to the percentage of children living with a single mother. In 2004, women's monthly wages were, on average, 63% of those earned by men and women's average hourly wages were 84% those of men. As for ethnicity, Israeli adults of Asian or African origin earned less than those born to European or American fathers, while Arab Israelis earned less than any of them (3). Accordingly, in 2007,

50% of Arab children were poor. Importantly, not only the number of poor families in a community affects its health status but also the size of the gap between the richest and the poorest sectors – "countries with a wide distribution of income have poorer health status, even after adjusting for the overall wealth of each country" (4).

In the past two decades, the percentage of children living in poverty has increased. In 1980, 8.1% of children lived below the poverty line, while in 2006, the percentage increased to 35.8%. Poverty, however, is not distributed equally among all population groups – about 24.3% of Jewish children and 67% of Muslim and Christian Arabs, Druze and Bedouin in Israel lived in poverty in 2007 (5). Among immigrant children, 27.1% lived in poverty. The percentage of poor families in which there were four or more children increased from 54.7% in 2004 to 60% in 2006 (1). This increase reflects changes in governmental policies that have reduced child subsidies and the number of recipients of unemployment benefits (1).

The proportion of children in urban areas is inversely proportional to the socioeconomic status of the residents: while in the poorest localities they include 57.2% of the population, in the richest localities they represent 25%.

The percentage of pupils who received a matriculation certificate in 2004 was 47.8%, but their distribution varied by sector: among Jews, 58.7%; 35.7%, in the Arab sector; 44%, in the Druze sector; and 27.9%, among Bedouins (1). This variation was directly related to the socio-economic status of their locality.

In sum, the government trend that began two decades ago of massive cuts in the different subsidies and benefits for families in need, coupled with the reduction of welfare services, is leading to an increase in poverty and inequality with its subsequent adverse results.

❧ Major mental and behavioral disorders of children and adolescents

There are five major groups of child psychiatric disorders: the first includes developmental disorders, which reflect pathology in psychological development from an early age. These disorders may involve the entire range of mental and emotional functioning – e.g., pervasive developmental disorders that include the autistic spectrum, early-onset schizophrenia and infantile dementias such as Heller's disease – or specific disorders of development in which only specific areas of mental and emotional functioning are affected. These include learning or developmental language disorders (see chapter 3).

The second group includes disorders that mainly affect emotions and are often termed "internalizing disorders." The major conditions under this heading are depression and anxiety, which are probably the most common chronically disabling medical disorders of childhood. They are usually underdiagnosed.

A third group includes the disruptive behavior disorders of childhood. These are also termed externalizing disorders, since their problems are obvious to the observer. Attention-deficit hyperactivity disorder (ADHD), conduct disorder and oppositional defiant disorder are the major representatives of this class of problems.

The fourth group includes disorders expressed by physical symptoms, such as eating disorders (anorexia, bulimia and obesity); tic and Tourette's syndromes; enuresis and encopresis; sleep disorders and body dysmorphobia.

The final subdivision refers to children who suffer from intellectual disability.

⸹ The epidemiology of mental and behavioral disorders

The literature on the epidemiology of mental health among Israeli youth is slowly developing. A relatively large number of studies addressing different topics have been conducted at Israel Defense Forces (IDF) induction centers where most youth are assessed prior to military service (6–8). At the national level, rates of disabilities and special needs among children have been determined (9), and more localized studies have dealt with issues such as eating disorders and suicide attempts (10–13). In addition, a nationwide community-based study of psychiatric disorders in younger populations, the Israel Survey of Mental Health among Adolescents (ISMEHA) was carried out in 2004–2005 (14). However, this survey is limited by its restricted age range and by the inclusion of only selected psychiatric conditions.

The following is a summary of some key epidemiological studies.

Pervasive Developmental Disorders

There are no systematic studies of these conditions in Israel. Davidovitch *et al.* (15) reported an incidence rate of autism of one per 1,000 children born between the years 1989 and 1993 in the Haifa area and a male/female ratio of 4.2:1.0. Conceivably, although there are no hard data, the diagnosis of autism seems to be made more commonly than in previous decades, as is the case in other Western countries.

Studies have looked for an association between autism and neonatal problems. Stein *et al.* (16) investigated birth complications in probands with autism born in the Tel Aviv area between 1970 and 1998 (75% of all probands diagnosed with autism during that period). They compared their mothers with those of healthy controls using a structured tool assessing prenatal, perinatal and neonatal complications. No differences in prenatal complications were found, although the controls had a somewhat elevated perinatal sub-optimal score, and the autistic probands had a significantly greater neonatal sub-optimal score. These differences in obstetric sub-optimality remained after controlling for confounders (sex of the probands and mothers' years of schooling). The findings suggested that the presence of nonspecific neonatal factors, rather than the specific influence of individual severe insults, may account for the elevated neonatal sub-optimality found in probands diagnosed with autism compared with healthy controls.

A combined Israeli-American research team investigated autistic spectrum disorder (ASD) using the IDF data on draftees (17). This data set has proven invaluable for a number of studies. Kolevzon *et al.* (17) examined the association between month and season of birth and risk for autism spectrum disorders. The cohort included all local-born Jewish Israelis over five consecutive years (n=311,169), assessed at age 17 as part of the eligibility examination for military service. Autism spectrum disorders were ascertained from the IDF Draft Board, which contains clinical information about medical and psychiatric disorders for this population. The findings from this cohort study did not support an association between season of birth and ASD.

The same research group used similar data to look at paternal age and autism (18). Also in this study, ASD cases were identified from the registry. The study included Jewish recruits born in Israel during six consecutive years. Almost all men and about three-quarters of women in this cohort underwent Draft Board assessment at age 17. Paternal age at birth was obtained for most of the cohort; maternal age was obtained for a smaller subset. The authors used the smaller subset (n=132,271) with data on both paternal and maternal age for the primary analysis and the larger subset (n=318,506), with data on paternal but not maternal age for sensitivity analyses. The registry identified 110 individuals diagnosed with ASD according to the *International Classification of Diseases – Tenth Edition (ICD-10)* (19) (incidence rate, 8.3 per 10,000 persons), mainly autism, in the smaller subset with complete parental age data. There was a significant monotonic association between advancing paternal age and risk of ASD. Offspring of men 40 years or older were 5.8 times (95% CI 2.7–12.5) more likely to have ASD compared with offspring of fathers younger than 30 years, after controlling for year of birth, socioeconomic status and maternal age. The children of relatively older mothers were at no higher risk of ASD after adjusting for paternal age. Sensitivity analyses indicated that these findings were not the result of bias due to missing data on maternal age. Thus, advanced paternal age was associated with increased risk of ASD (see chapter 14).

Schizophrenia

The same Israeli-American team also used the IDF draft data to seek evidence for cognitive difficulties in adolescence that predict later onset of psychosis (20). Indeed, subtle behavioral and intellectual abnormalities were often present in apparently healthy adolescents who later developed schizophrenia. The authors investigated whether these abnormalities can predict vulnerability for schizophrenia before the first psychotic manifestation. The study consisted of linking the IDF Draft Board Registry, which has measures of intelligence, social functioning, organizational ability, interest in physical activity and individual autonomy, with the nation-wide Psychiatric Case Registry (PCR). Patients (N = 509) were compared to non-patients, i.e., adolescents not appearing in the registry (N = 9,215), matched by age, gender and school attended at time of testing. Healthy male adolescents who were later hospitalized for schizophrenia had significantly lower test scores on all measures than adolescents not included in the PCR. The strongest predictors for schizophrenia were deficits in social functioning, organizational ability and intellectual functioning. When patients were compared to matched non-patients, the prediction model had 75% sensitivity, 100% specificity, a positive predictive value of 72% and an overall rate of correct classification of 87.5%. Applied to the IDF Draft Board, the model yielded a sensitivity of 74.7%, a specificity of 99.7%, and a positive predictive value of 42.7%. This study would demonstrate that simple assessment tools can predict predisposition to schizophrenia in healthy male adolescents. The predictive ability of the model did not change as a function of the time elapsed between testing and first psychiatric hospitalization.

Another study (21) merged data on measures of intellectual, language and behavioral functioning for the unselected population of 16- to 17-year-olds obtained from the IDF Draft Board with the PCR. The database was used to identify adolescents with no evidence of illness during assessment who were later hospitalized for bipolar disorder (N = 68), schizoaffective disorder (N = 31) or schizophrenia (N = 536). The pre-morbid functioning of these subjects was compared to that of non-hospitalized controls matched for age, gender and school attended at the time of assessment. The diagnostic groups of hospitalized subjects were also compared. Relative to the controls, subjects with schizophrenia showed significant pre-morbid deficits on all intellectual and behavioral measures. Repeated analyses indicated that future patients with schizophrenia were significantly impaired on reading and reading comprehension tests relative to the comparison subjects, but performed better than the comparison subjects on the writing test. The interaction of language measures and gender was the result of significantly larger differences between female future patients and their comparison subjects than between male future patients and their comparison subjects on the reading and reading comprehension tests.

The direct comparison of pre-morbid intellectual performance indicated significant main effects of diagnosis and intellectual measures and a significant interaction of intellectual measures and gender. No other significant main effects or interactions were found. Bivariate analyses showed that both future schizophrenia and schizoaffective disorder patients had significantly lower (worse) Raven's Progressive Matrices-R, Otis-R and Arithmetic-R scores than future non-psychotic bipolar disorder patients. In addition, future schizophrenia patients had significantly lower Similarities-R scores, compared to future non-psychotic bipolar disorder patients. The effect sizes were small to medium (effect size = .43–.66) for the group with schizophrenia and medium to large (effect size = .50–.85) for the group with schizoaffective disorder. Descriptive analysis also showed that the interaction between intellectual measures and gender was accounted by lower scores of female patients on the Arithmetic-R (21).

Weiser *et al.* (22), also using IDF data, looked at body mass index (BMI) as an adolescent predictor of future schizophrenia. Compared with the general population, individuals suffering from schizophrenia are more likely to be overweight, a finding attributed to the effect of antipsychotic medications, poor nutrition and sedentary lifestyle. As evidence accumulates indicating that some aspects of the illness manifest themselves before the onset of psychosis and the established diagnosis, it has been suggested that increased weight, like other metabolic dysfunctions, might precede active illness. Data were analyzed on height and weight of 203,257 male adolescents assessed by the IDF and followed for two to six years for later hospitalization for schizophrenia using the PCR. From the entire cohort, 309 persons, .15%, were later hospitalized for schizophrenia (ICD-10). After removing adolescents with evidence of disorder before or within one year of the IDF assessment, 204 future patients with schizophrenia were available for analysis. Compared with the rest of the cohort, future schizophrenia patients had lower body mass indexes (21.24 +/- 3.3 kg/m2 vs. 21.77 +/- 3.5 kg/m2; $F = 4.682$, df = 1, $p = .03$) and weighed slightly but significantly less (64.2 +/- 11.6 kg vs. 66.3 +/- 12.0 kg; $F = 6.615$, df = 1, $p = .01$). The mean height of the future patients did not differ significantly from the mean height of the remaining cohort (173.63 +/- 6.7 cm vs. 174.40 +/- 6.9 cm; $F = 2.520$, df = 1, $p = .112$). Reanalysis of the data, controlling for physical activity and socioeconomic status, showed that the differences between the groups remained significant. Thus, before the onset of the disorder, those individuals who would develop schizophrenia were not found heavier compared with their peers. This would suggest that the increased weight of patients with schizophrenia is related to illness effects, including the effects of antipsychotic medication.

Specific Developmental Disorders
Brook and Boaz (23) studied 543 high schools pupils in the city of Holon. They found that the prevalence rate of ADHD according to the *Diagnostic and Statistical Manual of Mental Disorders – Fourth Edition* (DSM-IV) among pupils was 15.2% and, of them, 9.7% had ADHD inattentive; 1% had ADHD hyperactivity-impulsivity (HI); and 4.5% had combined ADHD. The prevalence rate of learning disability (LD) was 17.6%. The gender ratio in both groups (ADHD and LD) was equal. These pupils had lower academic achievements and lower marks.

Gross-Zur *et al.* (24) selected 140 11-year-olds with development dyscalculia from a cohort of 3,029 fourth graders from Jerusalem to determine demographic features and prevalence of this primary cognitive disorder. They were evaluated for gender, IQ, linguistic and perceptual skills, symptoms of ADHD, socioeconomic status and associated learned disabilities. The IQs of the 140 children (75 girls and 65 boys) ranged from 80 to 129 ($M = 98.2$, $SD = 9.9$); 26% of them had symptoms of ADHD, and 17% had dyslexia. Their socioeconomic status was significantly lower than of the rest of the cohort; 42% had first-degree relatives with learning disabilities. The prevalence of dyscalculia in the original cohort was 6.5%, similar to that of dyslexia and ADHD. However, unlike other learning disabilities, dyscalculia affected the two sexes in about the same proportions.

It is beyond the scope of this chapter to review the educational literature on learning disabilities, which is done fully in chapter 3. Suffice to note here that the IDF data have been used to look at this issue also in relation to psychopathology (25). Research indicates that persons with learning disorders often suffer from psychopathology. Current and future psychopathology in male adolescents with discrete impairments in reading comprehension (IRC) or arithmetic abilities (IAA), but with average or above-average general intellectual abilities were assessed. The subjects included a population-based cohort of 174,994 male adolescents screened by the IDF with average or above-average intellectual abilities but with low scores (eighth and tenth lowest percentile respectively) on reading or arithmetic tests. They were compared with a group of adolescents who scored in the tenth percentile and above on these tests. Relative to the comparison group, male adolescents with IRC, IAA, or IRC and IAA had poorer scores on most behavioral assessments and higher prevalence of current psychopathology: 4.2% (comparison group), 8.0% (IRC), 7.0% (IAA), and 9.8% (IRC and IAA). Adolescents with IRC were also at increased risk for later hospitalization for schizophrenia (hazard ratios = 1.8, 95% CI = 1.3–2.6). Male adolescents with average and above-average general intellectual abilities but with IRC or IAA were more likely to have current and future psychopathology. Impairments in intellectual functioning and abnormal behaviors leading to mental illnesses may share common neurobiological substrates.

Weiser *et al.* (26) also investigated cognitive performance on a large population-based sample of individuals. They compared unaffected individuals with a sibling who at the time of testing was affected by either a non-psychotic or a psychotic disorder. Subjects were taken from a population-based cohort of 523,375, 16- to 17-year-old male adolescents who had been assessed by the IDF. Cognitive test scores were examined in sib-pairs discordant for non-psychotic (N = 19,489) and psychotic (N = 888) disorders and compared with 224,082 individuals from sibships with no evidence of mental illness. There appears to be a gradient in cognitive performance (worst to best) from individuals currently affected by psychotic disorders (*Cohen's d* = -.82), followed by individuals currently affected by non-psychotic disorders (*Cohen's d* = -.58), unaffected siblings of individuals affected by psychotic disorders (*Cohen's d* = -.37), unaffected siblings of individuals affected by non-psychotic disorders (*Cohen's d* = -.27) and members of sibships with no evidence of mental disorders. Unaffected siblings of both psychotic and non-psychotic individuals from multiple affected sibships (more than one affected sibling) had worse cognitive test scores compared with unaffected siblings from simplex sibships (only one affected sibling).

Suicidal behavior

The IDF database has also been used for psychological autopsy studies of young soldiers who committed suicide (see chapter 16). Apter *et al.* (7) studied 43 consecutive male suicides, 18 to 21 years of age that occurred during compulsory military service, using pre-induction assessment data, service records and postmortem interviews with family and peers. At pre-induction, subjects were above average in intelligence, physical fitness and measures predictive of successful adaptation to military service. Active duty performance was generally satisfactory.

Ascertained postmortem, 53.5% met formal criteria for major depressive disorder; most cases, however, appeared recent and reactive. Narcissistic and/or schizoid traits were common. Substance abuse was absent, and antisocial personality disorder was rare, 4.7%. Furthermore, in eight soldiers, 18.6%, no Axis I diagnosis could be made; half of these also lacked any significant Axis II pathology. These findings, at partial variance with US studies (27), suggest a complex relationship between suicide and mental disorder. The striking failure of intensive screening and other measures to prevent these suicides highlights unresolved questions of etiology and intervention.

In this same study, Apter *et al.* (7) examined similarities and differences between adolescent suicide completers, adolescents with non-fatal suicidal behaviors and non-suicidal psychiatric controls. The 43 consecutive completed suicides were compared with 171 consecutive psychiatric clinic outpatients presenting near-fatal suicide attempts, serious suicide attempts, parasuicidal gestures, threats, ideation or other non-suicidal complaints. Systematic pre-induction and service data were available for all subjects, with detailed postmortem inquest data for suicides. Systematic clinical data, including the Kiddie-Schedule for Affective Disorders and Schizophrenia (K-SADS), Hamilton Depression Scale, and Eysenck Personality Inventory were obtained on all clinic subjects. For completers, instrument evaluation was based on informant interviews. The following factors did not differentiate between any of the groups: immigrant status or parental country of birth; number of recorded disciplinary infractions; parental marital status and age of death; subject's degree of religious observance; and urban versus rural residence. None of the subjects in any of the groups abused alcohol or other substances. The subjects who made serious or near-fatal attempts or actually committed suicide were older and had served longer in the military than the other subjects. There was a significant linear trend across the groups of increasing age ($F(1,206) = 44.47$, $p < .001$) and longer duration of service ($F(1,206) = 105.26$, $p < .001$) with greater seriousness of suicidality.

The groups differed significantly by type of military assignment, with the most serious attempters and those who had committed suicide being predominantly in combat units, while those from the other five groups were predominantly in basic training, support, administrative, technical or transitional units ($X^2 = 41.76$, df$= 25$, $p < .02$). The combat suitability ratings of those who committed suicide or made near-fatal attempts significantly exceeded those of all five other groups. At pre-induction assessment, significantly fewer completed suicides and near-fatal suicides – 25% – had been given a psychiatric diagnosis, compared to 45% among inductees in the other groups ($X^2 = 26.32$, df$= 6$, $p < .001$). In addition, completed suicides had received significantly higher ($F(6,206) = 13.02$, $p < .001$) pre-induction Physician's Global Assessment ratings than the subjects with no suicidal behavior and those with serious, but not near-fatal, attempts. There was a significant linear trend across the groups with higher physical fitness ratings associated with greater severity of suicidality ($F(1,206) = 78.5$, $p < .001$). The suicide completers' ratings were very high ($M = 86.3$ of a possible 97), well above the demanding minimum requirement for combat troops (e.g., the minimum required for paratroopers is 72). Thus at pre-induction assessment, the soldiers who subsequently committed suicide or made near-fatal attempts showed relatively fewer physical and mental symptoms. Similarly, the completed and near-fatal suicide groups had Cognitive Indices (a measure of intelligence used by the IDF) significantly higher ($F(6,206)=21.77$, $p < .0001$) than those of all the other groups. A significant linear trend across the groups was found of increasing intelligence with increasing seriousness of suicidality ($F(1,206)=78.5$, $p <. 001$). Eleven, 25.6%, of the subjects who completed suicide and two (25%) of the near-fatal suicide attempters had the highest possible Cognitive Index score of 90, corresponding to an IQ of 135 (28). In contrast, those making suicidal gestures scored below the national mean on this index.

Interestingly, prior to induction, the subjects who subsequently made non-lethal suicidal gestures received significantly higher scores on the sociability subscale of the IDF Pre-induction Interview Schedule than did the non-suicidal psychiatric controls or subjects who only had suicidal ideation. Thus, at the time of induction, most soldiers who were later to commit suicide or make near-fatal suicide attempts appeared highly qualified on screening instruments that were generally reliable and valid for predicting overall functioning in the face of service-related stress. Clinical assessment data at time of index suicidal or psychiatric event, in contrast with the relative pre-induction appearances of the groups, showed a very different picture. Major depressive disorder (MDD) was diagnosed in half of those completing suicide, making near-lethal attempts, or having suicidal ideation while schizophrenia was diagnosed in four subjects of these groups. In the other clinical groups, i.e., soldiers with low lethal types of suicidal behaviors, MDD was absent and adjustment disorder was the commonest diagnosis.

HAM-D depression scores showed a significant ($F(1,164)=30.62$, $p < .001$) linear trend across the groups with increasing depression associated with increasing severity of suicidal symptoms, with the exception of suicidal ideators, who had scores comparable to the serious and near-fatal attempters. Compared to subjects with less severe attempts, gestures, or threats, near-fatal attempters had significantly lower scores ($F(5,164)=8.23$, $p < .01$) on the Psychoticism or AP Scale of the Eysenck Personality Inventory (29), a factor usually taken to relate to suspicion and emotional isolation. Extroversion did not differentiate between the groups, except for the ideators, who had significantly lower scores than did the non-suicidal controls ($F(5,164)=5.70$, $p < .001$). The retrospectively reported data on prior suicidal behavior for each group showed an almost linear trend of increasing numbers of prior suicidal threats and gestures with increasing severity of the index suicidal event. The frequency with which suicide letters were left at the time of the index suicidal episode also increased with the seriousness of the episode. Such letters were left by 10% of serious attempters, by 12.5% of the near-fatal attempters, and by 37% of the completers; no letters were left by subjects of the other groups.

Finzi *et al.* (30) conducted the main study of childhood that assessed depressive symptoms and suicidality in 114 children aged six to 12 years, of whom 41 had been physically abused (group 1); 38, neglected (group 2); and 35, neither abused nor neglected (group 3). Six months after legal intervention for their protection commenced, children were recruited for participation in the study through welfare department records and various child protection officer registrations in the Tel Aviv area. The officers were asked to locate physically abused children who had not been neglected and neglected children who had not been physically abused. Subsequently, they obtained the parents' approval to being approached for consent by the research project team. Sexually abused children were excluded from the study, as were those who suffered both abuse and neglect (including two abused children who were also neglected and one child that might have suffered from neglect). Beyond the legal definitions of abuse or neglect, which necessitated legal intervention of Welfare Department officers, all the children met the criteria described in the literature: physical abuse was defined by the National Center on Child Abuse and Neglect (31) as "acts of commission that involve either demonstrable harm or endangerment to the child." Current parental abuse was reported verbally by children in the physically abused group, although five reported that the abuse had recently been reduced by the intervention of child protection officers (evidence of burn, bruises and fractures from being kicked or hit very badly – sometimes with solid objects – were observed). Neglect was defined as "acts of omission, implying lack of proper parental control or guardianship" (32). Specific elements of neglect included lack of adequate food, clothing, shelter, supervision, necessary medical care and adequate schooling, in addition to acts of abandonment and an immoral environment. Children reported that current neglect was expressed in lack of parental concern to maintain adequate physical, health and educational conditions.

In the study, one-way ANOVA revealed significant differences in total Children Depression Inventory (CDI) scores among the three groups. The lowest level was observed in group 3 (the non-abused children), and the highest in group 1 (the physically abused children). When the CDI items were divided into factors, one-way MANOVA showed that scores in the physically abused group on the behavioral and social domains and on the domain of depression were significantly higher than those of the neglected group. Scores for the neglected group – group 2 – and on the neither abused nor neglected group 3 were similar to each other in the emotional, social and behavioral domains, but were significantly higher for group 2 than for group 3 in the vegetative and cognitive domains. Suicidal behavior was noted in 22 of the children from group 1, compared to two from each of the other groups. Of these 22, seven, 17.1%, reported suicidal ideation; nine, 22%, suicide threats; five, 12.2%, a minor suicidal attempt (e.g., slight cutting of the hand joints or jumping from a high point); and one, 2.4%, a major suicide attempt (he was run down intentionally by a car and injured. In an interview following rehabilitation he said "only in heaven will I have peace without suffering from my father").

Suicidal expression was found in 23 of the children from the physically abused children of group 1, compared to two from groups 2 and 3. Among these 23 children from group 1, 12 (29.3%) thought about jumping from a high place or being hit by a moving car and two (4.9%) did so; five (12.2%), thought about taking an overdose of pills and one (2.4%) did so; seven (17.1%), considered initiating a fatal traffic accident and two (4.9%) had done so; three (7.3%) of the five (12.2%) children who threatened self-infliction of stab wounds attempted it. Risk-taking behavior was observed in 31 children from group 1, compared to two and three children from groups 2 and 3, respectively. These 31 children described such behavior as running into the road without caution, climbing tall trees or buildings, and ingesting poisonous substances. No significant gender differences were found on any of the suicidal variables.

Aggression was measured on a spectrum of assaultive and destructive types of behavior; aggression; antisocial behavior; and impulsiveness. Pearson's correlations were calculated to examine links among scores on CDI domains, suicidality and the aggression variables. Significant correlations were found in the range of $r = .18$ to $.62$. Correlations between the vegetative domain of depression and aggression characteristics were not significant (this domain was most characteristic of the neglected group, which exhibited a low aggression level).

❧ Externalizing disorders

Obsessive Compulsive Disorder

The IDF data set has also been used to study obsessive compulsive disorder (OCD) (33). During pre-induction military screening, 861 16-year-old adolescents completed a questionnaire regarding the lifetime presence of eight obsessive-compulsive (OC) symptoms (disturbing thoughts, intrusive images, repetitive actions, urge to repeat, ritualized routines, extreme neatness, orderliness and hoarding), and three severity measures (time occupied with the endorsed symptoms, the perceived senselessness of the symptoms and the amount of distress caused by these symptoms). The presence or absence of OCD or subclinical OCD was ascertained by structured interviews administered by experienced child psychiatric clinicians who were blind to self-report. Although only 8.0% and 6.3% of respondents reported disturbing and intrusive thoughts, respectively, 27% to 72% of subjects endorsed the six remaining OCD symptoms. Twenty percent of subjects regarded the symptoms they endorsed as senseless and 3.5% found them disturbing; 8.0% reported spending more than an hour daily on symptoms. OCD and subclinical cases differed significantly from non-OCD cases, but not from each other in distress and mean number of symptoms. Although the distribution of nine of the items differed for non-cases, compared with OCD and subclinical OCD cases, the distributions for all items overlapped markedly across the three groups. Thus, OC phenomena appear to be on a continuum with few symptoms and minimal severity at one end and many symptoms and severe impairment on the other. Defining optimal cutoff points for distinguishing between psychiatric disorder and OC phenomena that are common in the general population remains an open question.

King *et al.* (34) studied trichotillomania among Jewish adolescents before military service at the IDF induction center. The 794 17-year-olds were screened for current and past hair pulling and comorbid psychopathology, using a questionnaire consisting of 11 OCD screening items plus one trichotillomania screening question: "Have you ever or do you now pull out hair from your scalp, eyebrows or elsewhere?" Eight current or past hair pullers (five males and three females) were identified, yielding a lifetime prevalence rate of hair pulling of 1%. Four subjects reported current hair pulling (point prevalence rate of .5%). None of these reported alopecia, distress or tension before pulling; only two reported relief after pulling. Thus, none met the full *DSM-III-R* criteria for trichotillomania. The authors found that only two of the eight subjects reported bare spots, and none admitted to rising tension and subsequent relief. Compared with non hairpullers, the prevalence of OC symptoms or disorder (other than hair pulling) was significantly elevated in the hair pulling subjects. Hair pullers did not differ significantly from non hairpullers in IQ, physical fitness, overall competence or prevalence of other comorbid disorders.

A random sample of 16- to 17-year-old consecutive inductees into the IDF, 562 of their cohort, were screened for OCD, Tourette's syndrome, transient tics (TT), chronic multiple tics (CMT), and ADHD (35). Two child psychiatrists interviewed the subjects, using screening items from structured interviews that generate *DSM-III-R* diagnostic criteria. For OCD, a point prevalence rate of 3.6% was found; 3.9% for ADHD; 1.8% for CMT; and 1.6% for TT. There was a higher prevalence of ADHD, TT and CMT, but not of OCD among male inductees than among female inductees. Among the OCD individuals, there was an elevation of TT, CMT and Tourette's syndrome relative to the population rates.

Apter *et al.* (8) used the IDF inductees's database to estimate the lifetime prevalence of Tourette's syndrome (GTS) in adolescents aged 16 to 17 years. This study included 18,364 males and

9,673 females. Of the 28,037 individuals screened, 12 met diagnostic criteria for GTS. The point prevalence rate in this population was 4.3, SE = 1.2 per 10,000. The rate was higher for males. The rate of OCD was significantly elevated among the subjects with GTS, 41.7%, compared with the population point prevalence of OCD, 3.4%, in those without GTS. The rate of attention deficit hyperactivity disorder was 8.3% compared with the population point prevalence rate of 3.9% in individuals without GTS. The prevalence estimates from this population-based study were in agreement with previous results based on surveys of younger children.

Zohar *et al.* (8) studied subtypes of OCD in adolescents in the IDF Draft Board sample. Forty individuals with obsessive-compulsive spectrum disorders were ascertained in a sample of 861 adolescents. Child and adolescent psychiatrists used semi-structured diagnostic interviews that included the clinician-rated Yale-Brown Obsessive Compulsive Scale (36). This scale is a reliable and valid instrument for estimating total scores of obsessive-compulsive symptom severity in children and adolescents with OCD. Reliability and validity appeared to be influenced by age of the child and the hazards associated with integrating data from parental and patient sources (37). Discriminant function analysis was performed to compare the scores on the Yale-Brown scale of groups with and without comorbid tics and to compare boys and girls. Adolescents with tics were more prone to aggressive and sexual images and obsessions than were adolescents without tics; these differences could not be wholly attributed to gender differences. The subtypes among un-referred adolescents were similar to those of adult patients with obsessive-compulsive disorder with and without Tourette's syndrome.

Disruptive Behavior Disorders

There has not been a systematic epidemiological investigation of disruptive behavior disorders in Israel, but some surveys do indicate that these conditions are probably quite common. Molcho *et al.* (38) examined the comorbidity of substance use and violence among a representative sample of 8,394 pupils from sixth to tenth grade. Measures included smoking, alcohol consumption and illicit drug use, predicting involvement in bullying, injury during a fight and weapon carrying in the past 30 days. They found across all grades, genders and ethnicities that daily smoking, use of hard drugs, history of drunkenness and binge drinking were the best predictors of violent behavior. Although girls were less often involved in substance use, girls who did were at much higher risk of involvement in youth violence than boys.

In addition, Smith-Khuri *et al.* (39) compared frequencies of adolescent violence-related behaviors in cross-sectional, school-based, nationally representative surveys that included 22,139 pupils aged 11.5, 13.5 and 15.5 years from five countries (Ireland, Israel, Portugal, Sweden and the US). The study examined associations between violence-related behaviors and potential explanatory characteristics. Most countries had lower percentages of male respondents, with the greatest discrepancy in Portugal, where 20.4% fewer boys than girls responded. A difference in age distribution was notable in the Israeli data due to an oversampling of 11-year-olds, so a weighting scheme was developed. A weighting scheme was also used for the intentionally oversampled Arab-Israeli population. The researchers looked at frequency of physical fighting, bullying, weapon carrying and fighting injuries in relation to other risk behaviors and characteristics in home and school settings. Fighting frequency among youth was similar in all five countries (nonfighters: M frequency of five countries = 60.2%), as were the frequencies of weapon carrying (noncarriers: M frequency of five countries = 89.6%), and fighting injury (noninjured: M frequency of five countries = 84.6%). Bullying frequency varied widely cross nationally (nonbullies: from 57.0% for Israel to 85.2% for Sweden). Fighting was most highly associated with smoking, drinking, feeling irritable or bad-tempered and having been bullied. Adolescents in the five countries behaved similarly in their expression of violence-related behaviors. Occasional fighting and bullying were common, whereas frequent fighting, frequent bullying, any weapon carrying or any fighting injury were infrequent behaviors. These findings were consistent across countries, with little cross-national variation except for bullying rates. Traditional risk-taking behaviors (smoking and drinking) and being bullied were highly associated with the expression of violence-related behavior.

Shoval *et al.* (40) looked at illicit substance use and common comorbidity in adolescent-onset schizophrenia/schizoaffective patients. A total of 188 adolescents, consecutively admitted to psychiatric inpatient units between 1994 and 2004, were compared to a representative sample of 26,543 controls screened for substance use by the Anti-Drug Authority during the same time period. All illicit substances, except for opiates, were used in significantly higher rates by the inpatient sample (28.2% of inpatients vs. 10% of controls).

§ Psychiatric illnesses with physical symptoms

Eating attitudes have been surveyed in Israeli adolescents. Apter *et al.* (11) assessed eating attitudes and body image on a sample of 850 adolescents using the Eating Attitudes Test-26 (EAT) (41, 42), a measure originally developed to identify people at risk of any eating disorder, and a 17-item bodyimage scale that dealt with the way the subjects viewed their body. As indicated by the control group, the higher the scores on the tests, the more likely the subjects had an eating disorder. The study was conducted among Jewish female high school populations in five distinct residential settings (kibbutz – at the time, mostly collective settlements; moshav – private, mostly agricultural villages; city; and two different types of boarding schools); in five ethnically distinct Arab-Israeli female high school populations (Muslim, Christian, Druze, Bedouin and Circassian); and in a mixed group of hospitalized adolescent girls with anorexia nervosa. The authors hypothesized that the attitudes of the adolescent females most exposed to Western body shape ideals, and simultaneously undergoing role conflict between traditional and modern images of the female role would most resemble attitudes of individuals with anorexia. This was partly supported by the findings. Circassian adolescents had the lowest scores for total eating pathology and most subscales of the EAT-26, whereas the Bedouin adolescents had the higher scores: Bedouins, 19.4%; Muslims, 18.6%; Christians, 15.4%; Druze, 14.3%; and Circassians, 8%.

Ethnic differences also emerged in attitude towards food. All the Arab-Israeli populations, except the Circassian, showed strong Western influences in their attitudes toward eating and body image, and thus may be at higher risk for epidemics of anorexia and similar eating disorders. Kibbutz adolescent females had the highest positive scores on the EAT-26 for the total and for most subscales; thus, they were most similar to the anorectic group.

Scheinberg *et al.* (43) administered the EAT to 1,112 female soldiers at the beginning of their military service and determined weight and height for each one. Those with high EAT scores or low weights were subsequently interviewed by the study psychiatrist. Two of them, .2%, were diagnosed with anorexia nervosa. Both were identified by their low weights, but their EAT scores were both normal. Twenty-seven females, 2.4%, were diagnosed as having a partial eating disorder syndrome, and it was severe in a third. The youngsters with severe cases of the disorder were also identified by their weights and not by EAT scores. In addition, four (.5%) had bulimia nervosa, all of whom were identified from their EAT scores. These findings were similar to some of the most recent studies in the field (44, 45). Because of its relatively low positive predictive value as well as the apparent reluctance of many subjects to answer reliably, the scale is not effective by itself for screening purposes. As was shown in this study, additional measures of weight and height considerably improved accuracy of diagnosis.

Stein *et al.* (12) administered questionnaires on eating behaviors, depression, obsessionality and impulsivity to 534 female high school pupils. A diagnosis of partial eating disorder was made on the basis of the combination of a pathological EAT score (22 points) and the relevant criteria of the DSM-III-R (46). EAT scores revealed maladaptive behavior in 18% of the subjects. The combination of the EAT and DSM-III-R criteria identified 20.8% of the subjects as having partial anorexia nervosa and 11.3% as having partial bulimia nervosa. Both definitions were significantly associated with risk factors known to predict anorexia nervosa or bulimia nervosa in female adolescents: relatively higher mean weight and BMI, smaller ratio between desired and mean BMI, greater weight fluctuations, dieting, menstrual disturbances and higher rates of depression, obsessionality and preoccupation with food, weight and dieting in the family (47, 48). Partial bulimics fared worse on most of these parameters when compared to normal students and to students with partial anorexia. Adolescents with partial anorexia were not more psychologically distressed than normal subjects.

✎ Intellectual disability

To the best of our knowledge, only one study of dual diagnosis in children with intellectual disability (ID) has been carried out in Israel. Gothelf *et al.* (49) evaluated the prevalence of DSM-IV-TR-defined psychiatric disorders in adolescents with ID, focusing on OCD. Eighty-seven adolescents with mild to moderate ID attending the special education system in the Central Region of Israel, were screened for psychiatric disorders in general and OC symptoms in particular. Sixty-one percent had at least one psychiatric disorder. Of the 13 participants receiving antipsychotic medication, none had an underlying psychotic disorder and most had anxiety or depressive disorders. OCD was detected in 11% of participants and was characterized by high rates of psychiatric comorbidities. The severity of autistic symptoms predicted 39% of the variance in the severity of OCD symptoms. Adolescents with mild to moderate ID have high rates of psychiatric comorbidities that are often inappropriately treated. Autism scores were significantly higher in individuals with OCD than in those without ($M = 15.7$, $SD = 7.2$ vs. $M = 10.0$, $SD = 7.0$, $z = 2.8$, $p = .01$). Further studies are required in adolescents with mental retardation to better delineate psychiatric morbidities and their appropriate treatment in this at-risk population.

✎ The Israel Survey of Mental Health among Adolescents (ISMEHA)

This is the first countrywide epidemiological study of mental health carried out in a representative sample of adolescents (14, 50, 51). It aimed to determine: (a) the prevalence rates of mental disorders among adolescents and their association with risk and protective factors, (b) mothers' and adolescents' use of services for the adolescent's mental and behavioral problems and (c) the gap existing between needs and use of services (treatment gap). The sampling frame used was the Population Register of the Interior Ministry, updated to August 2002. Fourteen hundred adolescents between 14 and 17 years of age were selected, with a response rate of 68.3%.

The final sample included 957 adolescents and their mothers, who were independently interviewed at home.

The interview schedule comprised of the Development and Well-Being Assessment (DAWBA) (52), the Strengths and Difficulties Questionnaire-Hebrew version (SDQ-H) (53), a services utilization questionnaire, and questions tapping health status and sociodemographic characteristics of the population. The DAWBA provides period and point prevalence rates of psychiatric disorders in children and adolescents according to DSM-IV and ICD-10 criteria. This measure uses a mixture of closed and open questions about child psychiatric symptoms and their resultant impairment and impact on those surrounding him/her. The SDQ (54) is a brief screening questionnaire for 3- to 16-year-olds. It includes 25 attributes related to five areas: emotional symptoms, conduct problems, hyperactivity/inattention, peer- related problems and pro-social behavior. A total difficulties score is generated based on 20 attributes, excluding the prosocial behavior items. The SDQ includes an impact supplement, as well as questions about chronicity, distress, social impairment and burden to others (53).

A questionnaire was administered by lay interviewers to the young respondents, their parents and, in an abbreviated form, to teachers. The interviewers also recorded verbatim their accounts of reported symptoms but did not rate them. Experienced clinicians subsequently reviewed these accounts and the computerized diagnosis based on the answers to the structured questions. The questions in the structured section are closely related to the diagnostic items of the ICD-10 and DSM-IV and focus on current rather than lifetime problems. They provide prevalence estimates relevant to service planning.

Selected characteristics of the study population

There were slightly more boys than girls in the sample, 40% of the mothers had a post-high school education and 80% of the adolescents lived in a Jewish or mixed Jewish/Arab town or city, and 20% in Arab towns. One-quarter of the fathers were unemployed. Unemployment was higher in the Arab than in the Jewish sector. The characteristics of this sample reflected a socioeconomically polarized population, one group was highly educated and a large minority was unemployed and had a relative low educational level.

Prevalence rates of mental disorders

The overall prevalence rates of mental disorders were 11.7%; 8.1% of the adolescents had an internalizing disorder and 4.8% had an externalizing disorder. The following groups had higher rates of any mental disorder: girls more than boys (13.9% vs. 9.7%, $p = .06$); adolescents whose parents were single or divorced more than those whose parents were married (22.9% vs. 10.1%, $p < .001$); and adolescents whose families were on welfare more than those whose families were not (23.4% vs. 10.1%, $p < .001$). No differences in prevalence rates of mental disorders were found by parental educational level and employment status, family size or type of locality of residence. More adolescents who were either a single child or had only one sibling than those belonging to large families had an externalizing disorder. As well, more adolescents living in a Jewish or mixed Jewish-Arab location than adolescents living in exclusively Arab locations had an externalizing disorder.

Depression was the most prevalent disorder, about 3.3% of the adolescents, followed by ADHD (3.0%) and specific phobia (2.5%). Less than 1% of the population had PTSD.

Comorbidity

The study found mental disorders to be associated with learning disabilities and with physical complaints of the adolescents. Among adolescents with a diagnosed mental disorder, 45% had a learning disability. Regarding physical symptoms, it was found that many more complained of headache, stomach pains, decreased appetite, dizziness and sleep problems among those with any disorder than among those with no mental disorder. A relationship was also found with diagnosed chronic diseases: among those with any mental disorder 33% had a chronic health condition, compared with 20% among those who had no mental disorder ($p = .01$).

Mothers' and adolescents' use of services

About 11% of mothers consulted professional or paraprofessional agents regarding the emotional or behavioral problems of their adolescent son or daughter. Consultation rates differed according to locality of residence and mother's marital status. More mothers who lived in Jewish or mixed Jewish/Arab localities consulted when they felt concerned about their offspring's emotional or behavioral problems, compared to mothers who lived in all-Arab localities (13.0% vs. 1.0%, $p < .0001$). Also, more single or divorced mothers than married mothers consulted (22.0% vs. 9%, $p < .0001$).

About 22.0% of adolescents consulted someone at school for emotional problems not related to their studies. Different consultation rates were found according to gender and mother's marital status. More girls than boys (26.0% vs. 19.0%, $p = .01$), and more adolescents living with a single or divorced parent than with married parents consulted someone in school (33% vs. 20%, $p = .002$).

Treatment gap

Among mothers whose child had any mental disorder (N = 112), about 40% (95% CI 24.4%–49.0%) consulted any agent in the past year. More than half of the mothers whose child had an externalizing disorder and about one third of those whose child had an internalizing disorder consulted someone. The treatment gap was larger for adolescents living in all-Arab localities compared with those living in all-Jewish or mixed Jewish/Arab localities. More than 90% of mothers of adolescents diagnosed with any disorder and living in all-Arab localities (N = 20) did not consult anyone in the past year, compared with about 50% of mothers living in an all-Jewish or mixed localities ($p < .001$).

The adolescents themselves consulted in school when they felt the need: 33% among those with any disorder and over 40% among those with an internalizing disorder sought help. Among adolescents living in all-Arab localities over 50% of those with any disorder consulted someone in school.

❧ Lessons learned from the ISMEHA with regard to cultural considerations and inclusion strategies in community studies conducted in multicultural societies

Studying mental disorders of adolescents living in multicultural societies such as Israel's demands focusing attention on some basic assumptions and methodological issues. First, the assumption of universality of psychiatric disorders or symptoms is controversial. These may differ in their core definitions and in the constellation of symptoms, depending on cultural or contextual factors (55). The social and developmental context in which behavior occurs distinguishes normal from disordered behavior since this distinction is ultimately a "social judgment that may differ across cultures" (55). Relativists claim that culture can shape not only the manifestation and content of symptoms but the development of the syndrome and symptom cluster per se, while universalists claim that the role of culture is merely in shaping the expression of the symptom and the magnitude and intensity of psychosocial risks and protective factors. Fabrega *et al.* (56) claimed that the nosological criteria should be developed on the basis of culture-specific information to avoid misclassification. Otherwise, there is the danger of missing the existence of symptoms that are not listed in the DSM-IV (55).

Added to the question of cultural differences, there is the methodological question of differences in the classificatory systems and in iterations of the same classification. Canino and Alegria (55) claimed that the different instruments, methods and classifications used among studies may account for the different rates obtained among different population groups.

The ISMEHA used a single instrument, translated and adapted to the languages used by the population groups (i.e., Hebrew, Arabic and Russian), under the assumption that psychiatric disorders and syndromes have core symptoms that cluster into universal syndromal patterns. Although efforts were made to adapt the instruments to the cultural subgroups by employing culturally-trained professionals who carried out the interview and the clinical diagnoses, the question of cross-cultural comparability remains open.

Another issue to consider when carrying out epidemiological studies in nationwide community samples is the inclusion of non-mainstream subcultures to assure the representation of the findings. The following is an example of the ISMEHA, where two subpopulation groups could not be included in the study due to cultural and sociopolitical sensitivities.

The case of the ultra-Orthodox Jewish population

This population sector follows the most theologically conservative form of Orthodox Judaism and comprises 17.8% of the population among adolescents between 14 and 17 years of age. They attend schools where girls and boys learn separately and live in more or less segregated neighborhoods in several cities. Children are not allowed to watch TV or films, read secular newspapers or use the Internet – thus enabling parents and teachers to control the information to which children are exposed. To conduct a survey that includes the ultra-Orthodox community has to be conceived and planned in agreement with its religious leaders.

The case of Palestinian residents of East Jerusalem

This population group has a complex relation with the Israeli authorities, so requests coming from the latter risk meeting with mistrust or evoking outright refusal, either because of compromised confidentiality or misuse of the information. This population group perceives extensive surveillance of their daily life.

These issues were taken into consideration when planning the ISMEHA, and those population groups were not included. This limitation should be addressed in future studies. A national survey that attempts to include all groups, including others not cited here such as children of migrant workers or residing in unrecognized settlements, might consider a basis of common core questions and additional differential supplements for the different cultural groups and close collaboration with the community leaders.

§ ISMEHA: From epidemiology to mental health action

A review (57) of mental health services for children and adolescents worldwide stated that the priority is to develop and implement evidence-based interventions, modern training programs and effective policies. The ISMEHA responded to this call by providing the evidence that can be used to design interventions, training programs, and the formulation and development of effective policies for Israeli adolescents.

This study has shown that psychopathology with functional impact is found in about 12% of adolescents. The study did not find significant differences in prevalence of mental disorders between Jewish-Israeli and Arab-Israeli adolescents.

In this study, only a small number of mothers of adolescents sought consultation. As in other studies (58, 59), the authors found differential treatment gaps according to type of mental disorder: mothers of adolescents with an internalizing disorder consulted less often than mothers of adolescents with an externalizing disorder.

The groups especially at risk of greater treatment gaps are mothers of adolescents living in Arab localities and peripheral areas in Israel and those belonging to low socioeconomic groups. Geraisy (51, 60) has attributed the low consultation rates of Arab Israelis to the following factors – some of them are common to the Jewish-Israeli majority as well:

(a) Lack of accessibility and availability: few services are available in the Arab-Israeli localities, and seeking services in the neighboring Jewish or mixed Jewish/Arab localities demands confronting language barriers and transportation costs. Therefore, families may consult only as a last resource (see chapter 5);

(b) Fear of stigma: adolescents approaching marriageable age are at special risk to be stigmatized if they seek help for psychiatric problems. Therefore, families postpone or refuse consultation. Education of the population is thus needed to overcome stigma (61, 62);

(c) Lack of awareness of the Arab-Israeli population regarding possibilities of treatment of mental disorders: young people may be more aware than their parents of the need for and the possibilities of treating mental disorders, but the attitudes of the latter prevail; and

(d) School staff remains almost the only source available to Arab-Israeli adolescents who need to consult regarding mental health concerns: the school staff responds to language needs, the school is a non-stigmatic setting and teachers are seen as an authority on many subjects.

ISMEHA showed that more adolescents than their mothers consulted someone at school when they felt the need for it, 22% vs. 11%, but among those with an internalizing disorder the percentage that consulted was over 40%. This indicates the need to improve the on-site school-based interventions and the linkage between the mental health and the educational systems.

Several tasks confront the adolescent mental health specialists working with different population groups. One is creating awareness of the need to identify and treat mental disorders. Primary care and school staff are the professionals of choice to identify and refer adolescents in need of specialized help. Schools are the ideal site to provide awareness and primary prevention programs if the staff receives the appropriate training, and primary care practitioners should also be recruited for the task of identifying and treating some students with mental health problems. It has been estimated that between 15% and 25% of the adolescents who visit a primary health practitioner annually for nonrelated problems have a mental disorder that requires treatment

(63–65). Lastly, both parents and professional organizations should advocate for the development of additional preventive and curative services for adolescents.

But not only services are needed. This chapter briefly reviewed the association between poverty and mental health, and the ISMEHA has shown that more adolescents whose parents who were divorced and presumably poorer than families with two breadwinners – as well as more adolescents who lived in families that were cared for by the welfare agencies than those who were not – have a mental disorder. The salutogenic effect of emerging from poverty has been shown by Costello *et al.*, who noted that while "adversity and stress associated with low social status" (66) are associated with psychiatric disorders among children, in families emerging from poverty conduct and oppositional disorders decreased (although no changes were noted in the children's mood and anxiety level). Dunn (4) stated that even when a large proportion of the population has a low income, universal access to free health and mental health care, a progressive taxation system and universal public services that redistribute non-cash benefits, such as free high-level and quality "public goods" (healthcare, education, safe streets, good municipal infrastructure, public recreation, etc.) will reduce the gap between the have and the have not. In a country where over one-third of minors live under the poverty line, government measures to remedy this situation should be a national priority as a first mental health preventive measure.

❧ References

1. Zionit Y, Kamhi M, Ben-Arieh A, eds. *Children in Israel 2007-Statistical yearbook.* Jerusalem: National Council for the Child (NCC), Research and Development Center, 2007.

2. Epstein L, Goldweg R, Ismail S, *et al.* Reducing health inequality and health inequity in Israel: toward a national policy and action program. Executive Summary-R 76–06. Jerusalem: Myers-JDC-Brookdale Institute, 2006.

3. Swirski S, Konor-Attias E. Workers, employers and the distribution of Israel's national income-Labor report: 2005. Tel Aviv: ADVA Center, 2006.

4. Dunn, JR. Housing and inequalities in health: a study of socioeconomic dimensions of housing and self reported health from a survey of Vancouver residents. *Journal of Epidemiology and Commmunity Health* 2002; 56: 671–681.

5. National Council for the Child. Executive Summary. *Statistical yearbook on children in Israel-2007* (Hebrew). [Cited September 10, 2008.] Available from URL: http://yeled.zahav.net.il.

6. Apter A, Bleich A, King RA, *et al.* Death without warning? A clinical postmortem study of suicide in 43 Israeli adolescent males. *Archives of General Psychiatry* 1993; 50: 138–142.

7. Apter A, Pauls D, Bleich A, *et al.* An epidemiologic study of Gilles de la Tourette's syndrome in Israel. *Archives of General Psychiatry* 1993; 50: 734–738.

8. Zohar AH, Pauls DL, Ratzoni G, *et al.* Obsessive-compulsive disorder with and without tics in an epidemiological sample of adolescents. *American Journal of Psychiatry* 1997; 154: 274–276.

9. Naon D, Morginstin B, Schimmel M, *et al.* Children with special needs: an assessment of needs and coverage by services. Report No. 335-00. Jerusalem: Meyers-JDC-Brookdale Institute, National Insurance Institute, 2000 (Hebrew).

10. Apter A, Abu Shah M, Iancu I, *et al.* Cultural effects on eating attitudes in Israeli subpopulations and hospitalized anorectics. *Genetic, Social, and General Psychology Monographs* 1994; 120: 83–99.

11. Horesh N, Apter A, Ishai J, *et al.* Abnormal psychosocial situations and eating disorders in adolescence. *Journal of the American Academy of Child and Adolescent Psychiatry* 1996; 35: 921–927.

12. Stein D, Meged S, Bar-Hanin T, *et al.* Partial eating disorders in a community sample of female adolescents. *Journal of the American Academy of Child and Adolescent Psychiatry* 1997; 36: 1116–1123.

13. Ponizovsky A M, Ritsner MS, Modai I. Suicidal ideation and suicide attempts among immigrant adolescents from the former Soviet Union to Israel. *Journal of the American Academy of Child and Adolescent Psychiatry* 1999; 38: 1433–1441.

14. Mansbach-Kleinfeld I, Levinson D, Farbstein I, *et al.* The Israel Survey of mental health among adolescents: aims, methods, strengths and limitations. *Israel Journal of Psychiatry and Related Sciences* (In press).

15. Davidovitch M, Holtzman G, Tirosh E Autism in the Haifa area: an epidemiological perspective. *Israel Medical Association Journal* 2001; 3: 188–189.

16. Stein D, Weizman A, Ring A, *et al.* Obstetric complications in individuals diagnosed with autism and in healthy controls. *Comprehensive Psychiatry* 2006; 47: 69–75.

17. Kolevzon A, Weiser M, Gross R, *et al.* Effects of season of birth on autism spectrum disorders: fact or fiction? *American Journal of Psychiatry* 2006; 163: 1288–1290.

18. Reichenberg A, Gross R, Weiser M, *et al.* Advancing paternal age and autism. *Archives of General Psychiatry* 2006; 63: 1026–1032.

19. World Health Organization. *The ICD-10 classification of mental and behavioral disorders. Diagnostic criteria for research*. Geneva: World Health Organization, 1993.

20. Davidson M, Reichenberg A, Rabinowitz J, *et al*. Behavioral and intellectual markers for schizophrenia in apparently healthy male adolescents. *American Journal of Psychiatry* 1999; 156: 1328–1335.

21. Reichenberg A, Weiser M, Rabinowitz J, *et al*. A population-based cohort study of pre-morbid intellectual, language and behavioral functioning in patients with schizophrenia, schizoaffective disorder, and non-psychotic bipolar disorder. *American Journal of Psychiatry* 2002; 159: 2027–2035.

22. Weiser M, Knobler H, Lubin G, *et al*. Body mass index and future schizophrenia in Israeli male adolescents. *Journal of Clinical Psychiatry* 2004; 65: 1546–1549.

23. Brook U, Boaz M. Attention deficit and learning disabilities (ADHD/LD) among high school pupils in Holon (Israel). *Patient Educational Counseling* 2005; 58: 164–167.

24. Gross-Tsur v, Manor O, Shalev RS. Developmental dyscalculia: prevalence and demographic features. *Developmental Medicine and Child Neurology* 1996; 38: 25–33.

25. Weiser M, Reichenberg A, Rabinowitz J, *et al*. Impaired reading comprehension and mathematical abilities in male adolescents with average or above general intellectual abilities are associated with comorbid and future psychopathology. *Journal of Nervous and Mental Disease* 2007; 195: 883–890.

26. Weiser M, Reichenberg A, Rabinowitz J, *et al*. Cognitive performance of male adolescents is lower than controls across psychiatric disorders: a population-based study. *Acta Psychiatrica Scandinavica* 2004; 110: 471–475.

27. Holinger PC, Barter JT, Bell CC. *Suicide and homicide among adolescents*. New York: Guildford Press, 1994.

28. Gal R. *The selection, classification and placement process: a portrait of the Israeli soldier*. Westport, CT: Greenwood Press, 1986.

29. Eysenck HJ. The classification of depressive illnesses. *British Journal of Psychiatry* 1970; 117: 241–250.

30. Finzi R, Ram A, Shnit D, *et al*. Depressive symptoms and suicidality in physically abused children. *American Journal of Orthopsychiatry* 2001; 71: 98–107.

31. National Center on Child Abuse and Neglect. *Caregiving of young children: preventing and responding to child maltreatment*. Washington, DC: Department of Health and Human Services,1992.

32. Paget K, Philp JD, Abramczyk LW. Perspective on child neglect. *Advances in Clinical Child Psychology* 1993; 15: 121–173.

33. Apter A, Fallon TJ Jr, King RA, *et al*. Obsessive-compulsive characteristics: from symptoms to syndrome. *Journal of the American Academy of Child and Adolescent Psychiatry* 1996; 35: 907–912.

34. King RA, Zohar A, Ratzoni G, *et al*. An epidemiological study of trichotillomania in Israeli adolescents. *Journal of the American Academy of Child and Adolescent Psychiatry* 1995; 34: 1212–1215.

35. Zohar AH, Ratzoni G, Pauls D., *et al*. An epidemiological study of obsessive-compulsive disorder and related disorders in Israeli adolescents. *Journal of the American Academy of Child and Adolescent Psychiatry* 1992; 31: 1057–1061.

36. Storch EA, Purphy TK, Adkins JW, *et al*. The Children's Yale-Brown Obsessive-Compulsive Scale: psychometric properties of child and parent report formats. *Journal of Anxiety Disorders* 2006; 20: 1055–1070.

37. Scahill L, Riddle MA, McSwiggin-Hardin M, *et al*. Children's Yale-Brown Obsessive Compulsive Scale: Reliability and validity. *Journal of the American Academy of Child and Adolescent Psychiatry* 1997; 36: 844–852.

38. Molcho M, Harel Y, Dina LO. Substance use and youth violence: a study among sixth to tenth grade Israeli school children. *International Journal of Adolescent Medical Health* 2004; 16: 239–251.

39. Smith-Khuri E, Iachan R, Scheidt PC, *et al*. A cross-national study of violence-related behaviors in adolescents. *Archives of Pediatric and Adolescent Medicine* 2004; 158: 539–544.

40. Shoval G, Zalsman G, Nahshoni E, *et al*. The use of illicit substances in adolescent schizophrenia inpatients. *International Journal of Adolescent Medicine and Health* 2006; 18: 643–648.

41. Garner DM, Garfinkel PE. The Eating Attitudes Test: an index of the symptoms of anorexia nervosa. *Psychological Medicine* 1979; 9: 273–279.

42. Garner DM, Olmsted MP, Bohr Y, *et al*. The eating attitudes test: psychometric features and clinical correlates. *Psychological Medicine* 1982; 12: 871–878.

43. Scheinberg Z, Bleich A, Koslovsky M, *et al*. Prevalence of eating disorders among female Israel Defence Force recruits. *Harefuah* 1992; 123: 73–78 (Hebrew).

44. Patton GC, Coffey C, Carlin JB, *et al*. Prognosis of adolescent partial syndromes of eating disorder. *British Journal of Psychiatry* 2008; 192: 294–299.

45. Steinhausen HC, Winkler C, Meier M. Eating disorders in adolescence in a Swiss epidemiological study. *International Journal of Eating Disorders* 1997; 22: 147–151.

46. American Psychiatric Association. *Diagnostic and statistical manual of mental disorders. Third edition-revised*. Washington, DC: American Psychiatric Association, 1987.

47. Bruch H. Thin fat people. *Journal of the American Medical Women's Association* 1973; 28: 187–188.

48. Dancyger I F, Garfinkel PE. The relationship of partial syndrome eating disorders to anorexia nervosa and bulimia nervosa. *Psychological Medicine* 1995; 25: 1019–1025.

49. Gothelf D, Goraly O, Avni S, *et al*. Psychiatric morbidity with focus on obsessive-compulsive disorder in an Israeli cohort of adolescents with mild to moderate mental retardation. *Journal of Neural Transmission* 2008; 115: 929–936.

50. Farbstein I, Mansbach-Kleinfeld I, Levinson D, *et al*. Prevalence rates and correlates of mental disorders in adolescents: results from the Israeli Survey on Mental Health among Adolescents (ISMEHA). (Manuscript available from senior author).

51. Mansbach-Kleinfeld I, Farbstein I, Levinson D, *et al*. Use of services for mental disorders and treatment gap: results from the Israel Survey on Mental Health among Adolescents (ISMEHA). (Manuscript available from senior author).

52. Goodman R, Ford T, Richards H, *et al.* The Development and Well-Being Assessment: description and initial validation of an integrated assessment of child and adolescent psychopathology. *Journal of Child Psychology and Psychiatry* 2000; 41: 645–655.
53. Goodman R. The extended version of the Strengths and Difficulties Questionnaire as a guide to child psychiatric cases and consequent burden. *Journal of Child Psychology and Psychiatry* 1999; 40: 791–799.
54. Goodman R. The Strengths and Difficulties Questionnaire: a research note. *Journal of Child Psychology and Psychiatry* 1997; 38: 581–586.
55. Canino G, Alegria M. Psychiatric diagnosis – is it universal or relative to culture? *Journal of Child Psychology and Psychiatry* 2008; 49: 237–250.
56. Fabrega H. Hispanic mental health research: a case for cultural psychiatry. *Hispanic Journal of Behavioral Sciences* 1990; 12: 339–365.
57. Remschmidt H, Belfer M. Mental health care for children and adolescents worldwide: a review. *World Psychiatry* 2005; 4: 147–153.
58. Verhulst FC, Ende VJ. Factors associated with child mental health service use in the community. *Journal of the American Academy of Child and Adolescent Psychiatry* 1997; 36: 901–909.
59. Wu P, Hoven CW, Cohen P, *et al.* Factors associated with use of mental health services for depression by children and adolescents. *Psychiatric Services* 2001; 52: 189–195.
60. Mansbach-Kleinfeld I, Farbstein I, Levinson D, *et al.* Met and unmet needs: results from the Israeli survey of mental health among adolescents in the community. Workshop presented at the World Congress of the International Association for Child and Adolescent Psychiatry and Allied Professions (IACAPAP), Istanbul, 2008.
61. Al-Krenawi A. Mental health service utilization among the Arabs in Israel. *Social Work in Health Care* 2002; 35: 577–589.
62. Al-Krenawi A, Graham JR, Dean YZ, *et al.* Cross-national study of attitudes towards seeking professional help: Jordan, United Arab Emirates and Arabs in Israel. *International Journal of Social Psychiatry* 2004; 50: 102–114.
63. Williams J, Linepeter K, Palmes G, *et al.* Diagnosis and treatment of behavioral health disorders in pediatric practice. *Pediatrics* 2004; 114: 601–606.
64. Kramer T, Garralda ME. Psychiatric disorders in adolescents in primary care. *British Journal of Psychiatry* 1998; 173: 508–513.
65. Leaf PJ, Owens PL, Leventhal JM, *et al.* Pediatricians' training and identification and management of psychosocial problems. *Clinical Pediatrics* 2004; 43: 355–365.
66. Costello EJ, Compton SN, Keeler G, *et al.* Relationships between poverty and psychopathology: a natural experiment. *Journal of the American Medical Association* 2003; 290: 2023–2029.

Chapter 3

LEARNING DISABILITIES AMONG THE YOUNG IN ISRAEL:
FROM THEORY TO RESEARCH TO INTERVENTION

Adi Sharabi and Malka Margalit

৯ Definitions and diagnosis

Definitions are essential to explore the epidemiology of any disorder; learning disorders (LD) are no exception. Therefore, this chapter starts with a discussion on the complex definition of these disorders both in the US and in Israel. Importantly, these definitions have had an effect on the development of educational conceptualizations in many countries.

৯ US definitions

The current Individuals with Disabilities Education Act (1) in the US accepted the earlier general definitions of learning disabilities. Since 1977, a significant discrepancy between academic achievement and intellectual abilities (IQ) is required to characterize LD – which is defined as "a disorder in one or more of the basic psychological processes involved in understanding or in using written or spoken language. This disorder may manifest itself in the imperfect ability to listen, think, speak, read, write, spell or perform mathematical calculations."

This definition includes conditions such as perceptual disabilities, brain injury, minimal brain dysfunction, dyslexia and developmental aphasia. It does not include learning problems that are primarily the result of visual, hearing or motor disabilities, intellectual disability, emotional disorders or environmental, cultural or economic disadvantage.

Response to intervention (RTI)

Starting in October 2006, changes in US educational regulations were introduced, such as eliminating the requirement for LD diagnosis of pupils to show a "severe discrepancy" between intellectual abilities and academic achievements. This "discrepancy requirement" was at first internationally accepted, but later it became the target of criticism due to the growing number of pupils with heterogeneous characteristics that were identified with the disorder. In addition, schools and families opposed the requirement of waiting until significant discrepancies were established, as it became clear that the delayed delivery of needed services has undesired outcomes, both academic and emotional. Under the new regulations, schools could intervene earlier.

The diagnosis of LD includes measures of abilities (frequently IQ) and achievements. Currently, US regulations expect schools to use assessment approaches that are more relevant to the pupils' instruction and learning. Accordingly, school districts are asked to assess the pupil's ability to respond to a research-based intervention (Response to Intervention or RTI). This recommendation is based on the assumption that early and intensive intervention for children and their families is necessary to prevent more severe problems (2).

In addition, pupils who show signs of learning difficulties are provided with individualized instructional or behavioral interventions – designed and delivered by general education staff, in collaboration with experts such as special education personnel and school psychologists. These scientifically based intervention procedures must include systematic monitoring activities to examine the child's progress. Those who do not show meaningful improvement (responsiveness) to these interventions are considered to be at risk for LD.

As expected, a reduction in the prevalence rates of LD resulted from the application of the RTI diagnostic approach. This also reduced the over-representation of minorities in special education classes and institutions. However, these procedures aroused many objections on the grounds of ethics and validation. Treatment fidelity appears to be one of the greatest threats to the validity of RTI assessments, because there is no commonly agreed list of research-based remedial interventions appropriate for diverse academic domains and ethnic groups. There is also uncertainty regarding appropriate procedures to determine whether the pupil's failure may be considered within the category of "nonresponse to intervention" that warrants formal referral for evaluation of special education eligibility (3).

The impact of LD on the individual's education and daily life can range from mild to severe, with academic underachievement or failure being the most common outcome in specific domains. LD is considered a neurological deficit that interferes with a person's ability to store and process or produce information, causing discontinuity between his or her ability and performance. This results in significant academic and social difficulties (4).

Importantly, previous efforts had focused on isolating a single underlying cause of LD, while today the heterogeneous nature of LD has been acknowledged. Accordingly, current research is focusing on attempting to solve the difficulties in identifying multiple interactive factors (5).

Determining whether a person has LD cannot be based on any single criterion such as a single test, assessment, observation or report. Indeed, LD requires a variety of assessment tools, including inputs from teachers and parents, RTI results, observations of pupils' academic performance and classroom behavior. Comparison of these approaches with Israeli definitions and diagnostic procedures clarifies the complexity of the disorder within different contextual conditions, at-risk populations and prevalence rates.

❧ Israel-based definitions of LD and assessment procedures

This definition is based on both the Interagency Committee on Learning Disabilities definition (6) and the current *Diagnostic and Statistical Manual of Mental Disorders – Fourth Edition (DSM-IV)* (7): "Learning disability is defined when there is a significant discrepancy between the individual achievement in standard tests of reading, mathematics or writing. Those tests results are significantly lower than expected by the predicted achievements according to his/her age, intellectual abilities and educational history. LD interferes severely with academic functioning or activities that require reading, writing or mathematics abilities." (www.education.gov.il/mankal/indux/sd4bk4_3_25.htm).

The procedures for identifying children with LD were based on the discrepancy model. Recently, however, there has been growing interest in introducing the RTI model for the identification of LD (8).

According to the discrepancy model (9), LD assessment includes the evaluation of cognitive abilities and difficulties and standardized achievement testing of reading, math and written language. Neurological evaluation may be requested, usually upon identification of attention deficits and other specific difficulties. Some educators and other practitioners disagree over the choice of assessment tools as well as the necessary qualifications of professionals for diagnosing LD.

The following summary of the current main diagnostic approaches illustrates this debate:

(a) Didactic assessments were adopted to evaluate the pupils' academic difficulties and abilities, as well as their basic learning skills. The identification of pupils' learning strategies must be performed by qualified educational diagnosticians;

(b) Psychological assessments were adopted to evaluate children's psychological profiles, including cognitive, emotional and behavioral functioning. These assessments must be performed by qualified psychologists; and

(c) Comprehensive assessments – consisting of psychological and didactic assessments – were adopted to provide a comprehensive profile of pupils with severe learning difficulties.

§ The epidemiology of learning disabilities

Prevalence rates in international studies

Epidemiologic studies of LD address issues related to prevalence rates, distributions and determinants. Learning disability constitutes the largest diagnostic group in special education. Since its recognition in 1968 as a federally designated condition of disability, about half of all pupils receiving special education services in the US have been diagnosed with LD (10). In other countries, the number of diagnosed children continues to grow, even in educational systems that in the past did not recognize LD as a disability (e.g., Australia), and in countries that adopted different terminologies, such as the United Kingdom (i.e., LD is referred to as mental retardation, Down syndrome and developmental disabilities). Children with average intellectual functioning and specific LD are recognized as having learning difficulties (11).

In the US, 2.8 million pupils – or about 1 in 10 children – were identified with LD (12). In addition, the number of identifications has also increased across grades, from .5% of children in kindergarten to 6.5% of fifth graders. More boys than girls were identified (13). These children experience higher rates of health risks than children with typical development (14). The 2003 US National Survey of Children's Health found 9.0% and 14.4% among children without and with asthma, respectively. Similarly, the prevalence rates of LD among children without and with diabetes were 9.7% and 18.3%, respectively. These results remained stable in the adjusted logistic regression models (14).

Due to their academic difficulties, these children often experience social and emotional problems, such as low self-esteem and loneliness. They often struggle with interpersonal relations, such as initiating and maintaining friendships (15). As they move into adolescence, they often exhibit more pronounced adjustment challenges, such as learned helplessness, decreased confidence in their ability to learn or succeed at school, low academic motivation, attention deficits and maladaptive behavior (16). However, within every group of individuals with LD, a subgroup is successful and resilient. This suggests the need to move from deficit-based models to one exploring risk and protective factors for understanding these children's development and wellbeing regardless of their disabilities.

Prevalence rates in Israel

LD was recognized relatively late in Israel. Today, the prevalence rates of pupils with LD are growing faster than the international average. The State Comptroller reported in 2002 that the percentage of high school pupils aged 16–18 who received LD testing accommodations for their matriculation examinations was 15.5%. This figure, considerably higher than the less than 10 percent rate in countries such as US and Canada, is a source of concern for policymakers and educational administrators. One way to explain the difference stems from differences in the reported age groups. The Israeli report dealt with high school students, while in other countries most statistics include a wide range of age groups. In addition, the reported proportions referred to different levels of severity, such as pupils who need extensive help with reading and writing and those with very mild LD who need only more time to take exams.

Rates of identified LD distribution in the US and Israel according to socioeconomic status (SES) differ; they are higher among American children in the lower SES (17), while in Israel, the higher the SES, the higher the rates. Historical reasons may explain this difference. In the 1970s, LD was rarely diagnosed in the US, and LD served for parents and children as a preferable explanation for the pupils' difficulties in school. The collective pressure of relatively privileged parents was critical in getting schools to recognize and accommodate those pupils (18). In Israel, LD diagnosis is still in its early stages, requiring parental initiative and the investment of resources. Thus, more learning disabilities are identified in the privileged population – but currently efforts are being made to identify children in a range of economic and cultural contexts (19).

What follows is a multidimensional developmental construct of LD for exploring interactions between risk and protective factors, predicting resilience and reporting current trends in international and Israeli research on intervention and future research trends.

❧ Etiology and subtypes of learning disabilities

Israeli researchers have helped enlarge the pool of information available on the etiology and subtypes of LD. This section reports both local and international contributions.

Epidemiology has identified genetic and neuro-developmental factors in LD, particularly with regard to reading and mathematical disabilities (5). The genetic basis of LD has been a focus of interest (20) because of the family history of LD such as dyslexia (21, 22) and dyscalculia (23), which showed an increased risk for developing learning, reading and mathematical problems in several families (24). Twin-based studies further demonstrated the contribution of genetic factors (22). However, genetic research has not been able to identify a single LD gene (25); several genes may be responsible for the high heritability of LD. For example, a specific gene was reported to be associated with dyslexia (26). Subsequent studies, however, have yielded different results: three different genes that have deviant forms among dyslectic individuals were identified. Molecular genetic studies focused on multiple genes (27), implicating five chromosomal regions (1p, 2p, 6p, 15q and 18p) and provided more modest evidence for supporting the assumption related to 6q, 3p, 11p and Xq (22).

Findings from the current explosion in neuro-scientific knowledge seem confusing, yet they have important implications for understanding the disability. In addition, the new knowledge contributes to the emergence of a new discipline of "pedagogical neuroscience" designed to combine psychological, medical and educational perspectives (4). Studies have identified specific cortical malformations involving neuronal migration and axon growth as being involved with a number of different reading-related processes. Those malformations can also affect the sensory-motor, perceptual and cognitive processes considered to be critical for effective learning. Brain plasticity related to initial cortical developmental events, triggered by the aberrant gene function, may vary with respect to age and sex, resulting in differences in the behavioral phenotype (27).

Evaluations of children with LD showed significantly more neuro-developmental deficits or delays across domains (e.g., language, motor, attention and social behavior) than are found in children with typical development (28). A number of anatomical brain correlates have been studied, including cerebral lateralization abnormalities, cerebral asymmetry, minor cortical malformations, immune disturbances and genetics (5). A report by the US-based National Committee on Learning Disabilities in 2002 concluded that experts do not yet know the exact causes of LD, and factors such as heredity, problems during pregnancy or childbirth and postpartum incidents such as poisoning and head injury may be considered risk factors (5).

In addition, current neuro-developmental approaches have extended their research interests to the interactions between genetic predisposition and contextual/environmental impacts. Thus the impact of heritability may not be considered unchangeable, since the proportions of the total variance attributable to genes are partly dependent on the variance in exposure to the relevant – but sometimes unknown –environmental risk factors and on the characteristics of the population studied (22).

Cognitive basis for LD

Decades of Israeli and foreign research in cognitive neuroscience and genetics have suggested several possible causes of LD and recognized their heterogeneous nature. Various cognitive difficulties such as slow temporal processing, deficient phonological processing, difficulties in visual attention span and memory difficulties (including short-term memory and working memory and strategic deficiency in learning skills) were examined (29–34). The specific domains of LD involved different phenotypic characteristics and intervention needs, and in many individuals, LD is comorbid with other impairments (9).

Commenting on the heterogeneity of the learning difficulties and accompanying adjustment problems, Margalit and Tur-Kaspa (35) suggested moving from the pathogenic approach that examined children's difficulties in depth to the risk and protective multidimensional model. They suggested taking into consideration both individual and environmental characteristics to explain profiles of individual differences in learning, performance and coping. In addition, they focused on the interacting roles of additional specific disabilities as risk factors. For example, dyslexia may appear together with dyscalculia or with attention-deficit hyperactivity disorder (ADHD), and their interactions may contribute to a more severe dysfunctional performance than the impact of each one of these difficulties separately.

According to this paradigm, LD represents a heterogeneous group of learners with a wide range of abilities. LD children approach learning challenges in a variety of ways and respond differently to interventions. Separate descriptions of several subgroups of LD are presented in the next section. Of particular interest are two subtypes: dyslexia as basic phonological-processing disabilities (BPPD), and dyscalculia as a nonverbal learning disability (NLD).

Dyslexia

Developmental dyslexia is the most common form and most researched subtype of LD (2).

Developmental dyslexia is a specific reading disability defined as an unexpected, specific and persistent failure to acquire efficient reading skills despite conventional instruction, adequate intelligence and sociocultural opportunities. This exclusionary definition was adopted by DSM-IV (7) and by the *International Classification of Diseases – Tenth Edition (ICD-10)* (36). The prevalence rate of dyslexia in school populations of developed countries is around 5%. It has a clear, wide-ranging impact, not only on the development of literacy skills, but also throughout life (4). In a review of dyslexia, Demonet *et al.* (37) identified three major deficits: (a) phonological deficits; (b) sensory deficits; and (c) cerebellar deficits.

(a) The phonological model proposes that affected individuals have impaired reading ability due to a deficit in phonological processing. Listening to and understanding speech requires the identification of individual sounds that make up words. The processes identifying those sounds (phonemes) and, subsequently, enabling them to be combined into words is known as phonological processing. This process takes place automatically at a preconscious level in spoken language. According to this model, individuals with dyslexia have difficulties with written language because of their impaired ability to deconstruct written words into phonemes, thus preventing word identification. This low-level phonological deficit prevents words from reaching high-level linguistic processing, which would allow the reader to understand the meaning of the text;

(b) The sensory deficit framework considers impairment of the visual or audition pathways as the source of dyslexia. The visual demands of reading require age-appropriate capabilities in the visual magnocellular system, and any weakness can lead to visual confusion of letter order and poor visual memory for the written word; and

(c) The cerebellar deficit framework proposed that the cerebellum is a key structure in skill automatization and that dyslexia is related to difficulties in acquiring automatization in reading. Today, no conclusions have been reached regarding subtypes' differentiation, since perceptual attention difficulties and visual processing deficits tend to occur together with phonological disorders. Similarly, the cerebellar theory of dyslexia proposes that problems in motor control affecting speech articulation and automation may result in poor phonological skills.

Dyslexia in Israel

Hebrew presents unique challenges to Israeli researchers, as their studies only partially support international findings. Several studies examined speed and accuracy in processing of words (30). Oren and Breznitz (38) used behavioral and electrophysiological measures to examine differences in the processing of reading material in Hebrew and English among regular and bilingual readers with dyslexia. Their studies found that affected individuals read significantly slower and less accurately than regular readers in Hebrew and English. Other researchers examined ongoing arguments regarding the existence of different dyslexia subtypes. Their results supported the move from general conceptualization of heterogenic nonspecified dyslexia to identifying unique subtypes such as neglect dyslexia and letter-position dyslexia.

Neglect dyslexia (neglexia) involves difficulty in directing attention to letters that are located at the initial or final position of the word, in most cases on the left side (the final position in Hebrew). In letter-position dyslexia (LPD), the letters are well recognized, but their position in the word is wrong. Studies of these two dyslexia subtypes must consider the unique characteristics of Hebrew orthography. Hebrew has 22 letters, five of which appear in two different forms – one used for the word's initial and medial positions and the other only for the final position. Additionally, Hebrew is read from right to left.

Friedmann and Givon (39) investigated the blocking effect of the final letter form on the addition of letters to the end of the word. They also examined whether omissions of letters after letters in the nonfinal form are avoided in both acquired and developmental neglexia and LPD. The participants included both acquired and developmental neglexia and LPD. The first group included seven Hebrew-speaking and Hebrew-reading adults aged 43 to 79 with acquired word-based neglexia. They all had brain lesions following a cerebrovascular accident (stroke) in the right hemisphere that caused neglect dyslexia.

The nine participants in the second group were aged 9 and 10 to 12 with developmental left word-based neglect dyslexia. Their results indicated a strong effect of final-letter form, which almost completely prevented form-changing errors in acquired neglexia and in acquired and developmental LPD, but not in developmental neglexia. Words that end in final-form letters were more impaired than other words in developmental neglexia. The researchers argued that final-form letters appear only on the neglected side of the word for Hebrew-reading children with left developmental neglexia. Research in Hebrew opens new theoretical explorations with clear educational implications (39).

The importance of phonological awareness for promoting the acquisition of reading (40) was demonstrated through effective intervention approaches that targeted reading of words and their segmentation, without neglecting awareness of reading comprehension. Surprisingly, Hebrew readers with dyslexia, in contrast to their counterparts, did not show morphological priming – awareness of the linguistic form and of its morpheme component. This research called attention to unique morphological processing as an additional source of dyslexia and to the need for focused remedial training (33).

Reading and writing are important skills that affect every academic task. Pupils who do not develop age-appropriate reading and writing skills will face increased difficulty in meeting varied and more complex academic demands at different age levels (2).

Nonverbal learning disabilities (NLD) and dyscalculia

NLD were described as a part of the clinical characteristics of the Developmental Right-Hemisphere Syndrome (41). Rourke (42) described NLD by characterizing a specific pattern of relative assets and deficits in several main categories, such as a deficit in academic functioning that included "a well-developed single-word reading relative to severe difficulties in arithmetic" and a deficit in social domains. In different age groups, children demonstrated their problems not only in mathematical difficulties, but also in their behavior patterns. For example, at preschool level, many children with NLD were considered "hyperactive" and "inattentive." In later childhood and early adolescence, their typical behavior also included withdrawal, anxiety, depression and social-skill deficits.

In the absence of community-based data, Gross-Tsur *et al.*'s hospital-based study (41) becomes relevant. They examined clinical aspects of 20 children (nine girls and 11 boys) aged six to 17 years (mean age, 9.5 years), who were referred to the neuro-pediatric unit at Jerusalem's Shaare Zedek Medical Center. The diagnostic criteria for this study included emotional and interpersonal behavioral disorders; paralinguistic communication problems; verbal IQ higher than performance IQ (a score higher than 85); dyscalculia and soft neurological signs on the left side of the body. The results were that the participants reported emotional and interpersonal problems, social incompetence, withdrawal and social isolation. These youngsters had difficulty maintaining friendships and understanding social rules. Most of them were very shy, and half of them found it hard to maintain eye contact. All participants had inadequate paralinguistic communicative abilities.

Developmental dyscalculia (DC) is defined as a specific learning difficulty with mathematics, expressed by the failure to achieve satisfactory proficiency in arithmetic despite normal intelligence, scholastic opportunity, emotional stability and sufficient motivation (7). Pupils with dyscalculia have difficulty learning basic number facts (43). Relatively few pupils have been diagnosed with pure dyscalculia (44). More often, this difficulty has been related to pervasive underachievement and reading difficulties (45).

Children with dyscalculia are often slow at counting and calculating; have difficulties in retrieving number facts; fail to learn multiplication and division tables; use learning strategies for calculations similarly to younger children and are error-prone; and monitor their counting and detect computational errors poorly (46).

Research studies distinguished two subtypes of mathematical difficulties – those that originated from a nonverbal system (thought to be controlled by right-hemisphere processes) and those related to the verbal number system (controlled by the left hemisphere). Thus, several children experienced difficulties in learning mathematical concepts, while others showed deficits of the calculation systems (36, 47). Their research also regards working memory difficulties as related to arithmetic problems, since numbers have to be stored in short-term memory during the process of mental calculations, and the memory of the problem's spatial representation may support and facilitate effective problem solving. Verbal short-term memory difficulties, as well as a wide range of mental control processes, were also involved in selecting appropriate solutions and monitoring performance; for example, checking that the solution to a problem is within the estimated range (47).

Another group of studies focused on long-term memory processes and considered children's difficulties in retrieving information as the major explanation for problems such as remembering basic number facts. Additional sources of disabilities were attributed to difficulties in subtraction, computing long division and solving word problems (48).

Dyscalculia in Israel

Children with developmental dyscalculia fail in many numerical tasks. They have difficulties performing arithmetic operations, solving problems and using numerical reasoning (47). In addition, they have problems automatically associating numerals with magnitudes even though no problems were found in associating letters with phonemes (47).

The familial perspectives of dyscalculia (DC) have been examined by Shalev *et al.* (23). Their studies included 39 children from elementary and middle school diagnosed with DC, and 21 of their mothers, 22 fathers, 90 siblings, and 16 second-degree relatives. The researchers showed that 66% of mothers, 40% of fathers, 53%, of siblings and 44% of second-degree relatives had DC. In another longitudinal study, Shalev *et al.* (32) showed that severity of the dyscalculia, lower IQ, inattention and writing problems were related to the chronic and persistent nature of the disorder.

In conclusion, cognitive difficulties with familial sources play an important role in predicting the performance of children with LD, both with reading as well as with mathematical difficulties. However, there is a growing recognition that several studies identified children who were able to cope successfully with their deficits, overcoming their reading and mathematical difficulties. This calls for special attention to predictors of resilience.

⑂ LD and positive psychology perspectives

Resilience conceptualization

As a result of positive views among psychologists in the field of LD (49), attention has extended to children's struggles with their difficulties, including the identification of the sources of pupils' resilience with regard to their academic achievements, well-being and social adjustment (50). This novel paradigm involves the study of interactions between risk and protective factors, searching for inner energy resources and external energizing factors that may increase probabilities for effort investment and successful outcomes (51).

Hope theory and LD

The change in Israeli LD research – from identifying stable and deficient cognitive-based traits to exploring dynamic processing sequences – was exemplified by studies of "hope theory" (52). Snyder (53) defines "hope" as a set of beliefs that involves two relatively distinct ways of thinking about future goals – agentic thinking and pathways thinking. Agentic thinking refers to thoughts related to success in reaching one's goals, while pathways thinking refers to thoughts about one's effectiveness when pursuing different means to attain goals. In addition, hope is related to a belief in the ability to pursue goals and envision desirable future goals (54). Reciprocal relations were found between hopeful thinking and achievements, thus adolescents with LD reported lower levels of hope (52).

Hope may be nurtured in different social contexts, such as schools and/or families, which, according to their nature, may be conceptualized as protective or risk factors. In a study that compared self-efficacy, mood, effort and hope in 123 Israeli adolescents with LD and a group of 123 non-LD peers matched for their level of academic performance and gender, the results showed that those with LD reported lower academic and social self-efficacy. They also rated their mood as more negative and reported lower levels of hope and less investment of effort in their academic work. In addition, among high school pupils with LD who were successful in their studies, a subgroup continued to report low levels of hope expectations (52). These results demonstrated that, even when the academic performance of pupils with LD is similar to their non-LD peers, their specific and global self-perceptions continue to reflect their ongoing emotional distress.

❧ Contextual factors

Risk and protective factors

Children and adolescents with LD are exposed to challenges in similar ways as their classmates who developed normally. However, their adjustment during different developmental stages reflects the outcomes of interactions between personal and contextual risk and protective factors. Many children with LD function well in society, indicating their resilience (55, 56), but the combination of LD and pressures in the family, school and community may put them at greater risk than others, leading to negative emotional and social outcomes. For example, Israeli children with LD who were exposed to terror attacks experienced more post-traumatic stress disorder (PTSD) reactions. They were found more vulnerable to stress situations, expressing higher levels of anxiety than their normally developed peers who experienced the same terror attacks (57).

Considering the importance of the risk and protective paradigm and the consistent challenges that individuals with LD are experiencing, research has been devoted to children's emotional distress, their self-perception, self-efficacy, self-determination and experiences of loneliness (15). In a recent study (58), adolescents with LD (as a group), showed lower levels of achievement, academic self-efficacy, belief in themselves and effort investment. They also experienced lower positive mood and less hope.

Social difficulties and loneliness

Studies of children and adolescents with LD showed that they were rejected by peers and that their personal characteristics predicted their loneliness experience, thus making it more difficult to cope with these aversive feelings (59). Studies carried out in different countries and cultures showed that pupils with LD often experienced higher levels of loneliness (60). This experience has often been a true reflection of realistic social difficulties related to their poor social network, lower social status and peer rejection (61). Yet, it was also closely linked to their self-perceptions, expectations from classmates, distress and frustrations.

In conclusion, research has consistently showed that children and adolescents with LD are at a greater risk for experiencing loneliness and related interpersonal difficulties along with their academic difficulties and cognitive disabilities. However, previous studies focused attention on groups of individuals with LD who were resilient and did not experience more loneliness or lower self-perception than their peers. The study emphasized the need to move beyond academic and cognitive dysfunction to a more comprehensive conceptualization of LD – with clear educational and interventional implications – and sensitize teachers and parents to the emotional cost of the children's distress from LD, their effort investment and frustrations resulting in increased loneliness experience.

Research also highlighted the important protective role of environmental factors in promoting resilience. In addition, the growing knowledge in genetic studies paradoxically enhanced the understanding of dynamic interactions with environmental factors and contextual conditions (62). Individuals with different genetically-based traits will react differently (either feeling vulnerable or resilient) to different processes in their environment.

❧ Protective factors

Family Support

Supporting families and empowering teachers are two major protective factors. Their role in predicting resilience among pupils with LD was demonstrated in several studies (56, 63, 64). Research has indicated that parents of children with LD are more likely to experience greater stress, anxiety, depressive moods and parent-child conflicts than parents of those without disabilities (65). Experiencing higher levels of stress and anxiety may decrease their ability to provide meaningful support to their children (66). Attachment processes with their LD children will predict supportive parenting and better adjustment (63). Parents' expectations for partnership with schools and teachers' perceptions were often the source of misunderstandings, frustrations, conflicts and mistrust that contributed to increased parental distress (67).

Teacher's support

Teachers have a critical role in promoting well-being among all pupils and their families, but the LD groups are more vulnerable to teachers' perceptions and support. Most children and adolescents with LD are in inclusive classes, together with average-achievement pupils. Only a few with severe disabilities attend special educational classes or institutions. Intervention programs were developed to meet their unique individualized academic needs. In Israel, teachers provide remedial teaching to develop the children's basic skills and learning strategies, adapted to various age groups, e.g., programs for preschool children and for elementary and middle-school pupils. This material can be accessed at: http://cms.education.gov.il/EducationCMS/Units/Shefi/gapim/likuylemida/Shutafut.htm.

However, current limited resources in the educational system are slowing the implementation of these school-based services. Nevertheless, different programs do continue with support from municipalities, foundations, parents' organizations and special projects of the Ministry of Education.

ẞ Testing accommodations

Following identification and diagnosis, accommodations (adjustment) of testing conditions are granted in Israeli schools to enable students with LD to demonstrate their knowledge. The ministry of Education developed detailed regulations to accommodate pupils with LD across grades and in different cultural groups. Their regulation consists of processes for identifying proposed steps of intervention and support suggestions within a developmental continuum. See http://cms.education.gov.il/EducationCMS/Units/Shefi/gapim/likuy_lemida/RatzyonalHitarvut.htm.

The accommodations are divided according to three levels of severity from mild changes (such as time extension – for pupils with LD who are slow in reading and writing) to major changes in testing formats (such as oral answers instead of written ones for children with more severe writing difficulties). The Ministry has reported a yearly increase in the proportion of high school pupils with LD who are entitled to accommodations; by 2006, the total percentage for final exams reached 21.1% (68). This is a much higher percentage than reported in most Western countries. The most prevalent accommodation was time extension. It was also noted that in contrast to the high proportions of pupils with LD in the high school age-group, only a few pupils were identified in elementary schools.

As mentioned above, the current situation in Israel reflects increased awareness with regard to LD among parents with higher education. Thus, the difficulties of adolescents with LD in economically challenged environments emerge not only from their disabilities, but also from prolonged neglect and delayed identification. To help rectify this situation, the ministry's department of welfare educational services, together with the LD department, is attempting to identify and develop better ways to support LD pupils from disadvantaged homes. Obviously, the identification and diagnosis of LD does not solve the children's other difficulties. Accordingly, the next section addresses intervention approaches and accommodation alternatives.

❧ From epidemiology to mental health action

The goals of intervention are to enable LD children at various age levels to experience high-quality educational opportunities and to enhance their opportunities for future academic success. Early indicators that a child may be at risk for developing LD include delays in speech and language development as well as motor coordination and perception difficulties. These indicators may occur concomitantly with problems in self-regulation, attention and/or social interaction (12). Early intervention requires children with developmental delays to be exposed to high-quality learning opportunities even before they start kindergarten.

Different age groups present different developmental, educational challenges and interventional needs. No single instructional-remedial model is expected to provide effective help to all children, considering the heterogeneity of LD pupils and their disabilities. Research identified several instructional components that can be generalized as "effective intervention approaches" in designing remediation programs for many pupils with various learning disabilities (69), pinpointing attention to strategic learning, modeling of performance and repeated training.

The support provided through remedial approaches may focus on children's needs and/ or would target school-based comprehensive systemic changes – as presented by the learning skills centers at Israel's ORT educational networks. It is beyond the goals of this chapter to provide a detailed survey of the existing intervention approaches.

Currently, there is no comprehensive roster of research-based and effective intervention programs, needed for the Reaction to Intervention approach. However, meta-analysis of studies that examined the effectiveness of various academic intervention programs for pupils with LD at schools (69) identified two major effective approaches: (a) direct teaching and (b) strategy teaching. Each one consists of several elements such as explicit direct instruction (including sequencing and segmentation of the tasks); explicit strategy training (including teachers' explaining and modeling effective learning strategies); systemic monitoring of pupils' learning and performance; individualized remedial training in small interactive groups; and technology-mediated instruction. The combination of direct teaching and strategy instruction within small-group training procedures may provide a valid model for improving outcomes for LD pupils across a broad array of samples, age groups, settings and dependent measures (69).

Socioemotional interventions

Several interventional approaches target the socioemotional needs of LD pupils, challenging their deficits in social skills, need for personal empowerment, hopeful thinking and self-advocacy. Interventions were performed in small groups using different therapeutic approaches. Research revealed that changes were achieved through the promotion of self-monitoring, self-evaluation, self-reinforcement and self-instruction.

Studies also showed the positive outcomes of humanistic therapeutic approaches (70, 71). The heterogeneous needs of children with LD preclude debates among different intervention approaches such as strategy training versus humanistic approaches; a focus on children versus a focus on parents; and small-group instruction versus individualized tutoring.

Technology and socioemotional aspects of LD

Progress in technology may help pupils with LD in various ways. Computers may support several academic activities such as typing school projects or using the Internet as a source of information. Assistive technology has a potential for improving their educational performance, achievements and quality of life (72). For example, the Internet was used to promote motivation and writing performance among children with LD (73). The Internet was also supportive in a self-advocacy program for LD children developed by Israel's Center for Educational Technology (CET), which taught them to present and express their needs. An evaluation of this program showed that children with LD identified individual paths in developing advocacy skills (70), and the significant role of promoting hopeful thinking in predicting children's competence was demonstrated.

Internet and social connections

Internet has become part of the youth culture, providing leisure-time activities and opportunities for communication with peers (74). The needs and difficulties of children with LD were expressed in SparkTop (a special discussion group for pupils with LD), with regard to their social adversity and academic challenges (75). In another discussion group for parents of children with LD, mothers wrote about their frustrations and struggles with the educational institutions and described their children's coping with social rejection (67).

To examine the impact of children's virtual relationships and how they dealt with alienation, a recent study (76) examined the association between Internet use for interpersonal communication and loneliness among adolescents with and without LD. It showed a unique gender difference in the group of pupils with LD. Girls who experienced relatively high levels of virtual friendships reported higher levels of loneliness than those without virtual friendships. Structural equation modeling analysis differentiated between the use of the Internet to support interpersonal communication with friends that was related to lower levels of loneliness, and e-communication with virtual friends related to increased levels of loneliness.

Due to the correlational nature of this study, it was not clear whether lonely individuals with LD tended to develop more e-communication with people they have never met, thus extending their networking – or whether the communication with virtual friends failed to satisfy their strong need for interpersonal connections, leading to increased loneliness and requiring varied types of social relations.

✿ Conclusions

Awareness of children's difficulties, their unique abilities, special talents and human rights is starting to be the focus of local interest. This chapter's goals were to present the theoretical shift from causal deficit models in conceptualizing LD to a probabilistic risk and protective model (including individuals' struggle against the consequences of their disabilities) and their ability to be empowered. Epidemiological studies showed disagreements on prevalence rates but also clarified the role of genetics and neurology.

This chapter also focused attention on the need to examine interactions between the individuals' abilities and disabilities and contextual environments such as families and educational systems. Studies across disciplines about the balance between disabilities and capacities, and between contextual risks and empowering/supportive environments are to be further developed. These individuals' thoughts, beliefs and emotions, their self-perceptions and the perceptions of significant people in their lives may reflect not only their past experiences with empowering or frustrating challenges, but also their future goals and expectations.

❧ References

1. IDEA 04, IDEA Regulations. *Identification of specific learning disabilities.* Washington, DC: US Department of Education Office of Special Education Programs, 2006.
2. Smith DD. *Introduction to special education: making a difference.* Boston: Allyn & Bacon, 2007.
3. Burns MK, Jacob S, Wagner AR. Ethical and legal issues associated with using response-to-intervention to assess learning disabilities. *Journal of School Psychology* 2008; 46: 263–279.
4. Fawcett AJ, Nicolson RI. Dyslexia, learning and pedagogical neuroscience. *Developmental Medicine & Child Neurology* 2007; 49: 306–311.
5. McDermott PA, Goldberg MM, Watkins MW, *et al.* A nationwide epidemiologic modeling study of LD: risk, protection, and unintended impact. *Journal of Learning Disabilities* 2006; 39: 230–252.
6. Interagency Committee on Learning Disabilities. *Learning disabilities: a report to the US Congress.* Washington, DC, 1987.
7. American Psychiatric Association. *Diagnostic and statistical manual of mental disorders – Fourth edition (DSM-IV).* Washington, DC: American Psychiatric Association, 1994.
8. Gumpel TP, Sharoni V. Current best practices in learning disabilities in Israel. *Learning Disabilities Research & Practice* 2007; 22: 202–209.
9. Fletcher JM, Lyon RG, Fuchs LS, *et al.* Classification, definition and identification of learning disabilities. In Fletcher JM, Lyon RG, Fuchs LS, *et al.*, eds. *Learning disabilities: from identification to intervention.* New York: Guilford Press, 2007.
10. Kerka S. Adults with learning disabilities. ERIC Digest No. 189. Columbus, OH: ERIC Clearinghouse on Adult, Career, and Vocational Education, 2000.
11. Gillberg C, Soderstrom H. Learning disability. *The Lancet* 2003; 362: 811–821.
12. National Joint Committee on Learning Disabilities. Learning disabilities and young children: identification and intervention; a report from the National Joint Committee on Learning Disabilities. *Learning Disability Quarterly* 2007; 30: 63–73.
13. IES. *Demographic and school characteristics of students receiving special education in the elementary grades.* National Center for Education Statistics. Washington, DC: US Department of Education, 2007.
14. Altarac M. Prevalence of learning disability among United States children with asthma and diabetes. *Annals of Epidemiology* 2007; 17: 746–747.
15. Margalit M, Al-Yagon M. The loneliness experience of children with learning disabilities. In: Wong BYL, Donahue M, eds. *The social dimensions of learning disabilities.* New Jersey: Lawrence Erlbaum, 2002.
16. Deshler DD. Adolescents with learning disabilities: unique challenges and reasons for hope. *Learning Disability Quarterly* 2005; 28: 122–125.
17. Blair C, Scott KG. Proportion of learning disabilities placements associated with low socioeconomic status: evidence of a gradient? *Journal of Special Education* 2002; 36: 14–22.
18. Ong-Dean C. High roads and low roads: learning disabilities in California, 1976–1998. *Sociological Perspectives* 2006; 49: 91–113.
19. Margalit M, Otolengi R, Or-Noi A, *et al.* Students with learning disabilities: report of the committee for evaluation of the needs and support for students with learning disabilities. Report submitted to the Minister of Education and Culture and to the Minister of Science, State of Israel, 1997.
20. Isles AR, Humby T. Modes of imprinted gene action in learning disability. *Journal of Intellectual Disability Research* 2006; 50: 318–325.
21. Lyon GR, Fletcher JM, Shaywitz, BA, *et al.* Rethinking learning disabilities. In: Finn CE, Jr., Rotherham RAJ, Hokanson CR, Jr., eds. *Rethinking special education for a new century.* Washington, DC: Thomas B. Fordham Foundation and Progressive Policy Institute, 2001.
22. Williams J, O'Donovan MC. The genetics of developmental dyslexia. *European Journal of Human Genetics* 2006; 14: 681–689.
23. Shalev RS, Manor O, Kerem B, *et al.* Developmental dyscalculia is a familial learning disability. *Journal of Learning Disabilities* 2001; 3: 59–65.
24. Fisher SE, Francks C. Genes, cognition and dyslexia: learning to read the genome. *Trends in Cognitive Sciences* 2006; 10: 250–257.
25. Plomin R, Kovas Y. Generalist genes and learning disabilities. *Psychological Bulletin* 2005; 131: 592–617.
26. Taipale M, Kaminen N, Napola-Hemmi J, *et al.* A candidate gene for developmental dyslexia encodes a nuclear tetratricopeptide repeat domain protein dynamically regulated in brain. *Proceedings of the National Academy of Sciences* 2003; 100: 11553–11558.
27. Galaburda AM, LoTurco J, Ramus F, *et al.* From genes to behavior in developmental dyslexia. *Nature Neuroscience* 2006; 9: 1213–1217.
28. Blumsack J, Lewandowski L, Waterman B. Neurodevelopmental precursors of learning disabilities: a preliminary report from a parent survey. *Journal of Learning Disabilities* 1997; 30: 228–237.

29. Bosse ML, Tainturier MJ, Valdois S. Developmental dyslexia: the visual attention span deficit hypothesis. *Cognition* 2007; 104: 198–230.

30. Breznitz Z. Introduction to this special issue: understanding dyslexia. *Journal of Neurolinguistics* 2005; 18: 89–92.

31. Ram-Tsur R, Faust M, Zivotofsky AZ. Sequential processing deficits of reading disabled persons are independent of inter-stimulus interval. *Vision Research* 2006; 46: 3949–3960.

32. Shalev RS, Manor O, Gross-Tsur V. Developmental dyscalculia: a prospective six-year follow-up. *Developmental Medicine & Child Neurology* 2005; 47: 121–125.

33. Schiff R, Raveh M. Deficient morphological processing in adults with developmental dyslexia: another barrier to efficient word recognition? *International Journal of Research and Practice* 2006; 13: 110–129.

34. Vellutino FR, Fletcher JM, Snowling MJ, *et al.* Specific reading disability (dyslexia): what have we learned in the past four decades? *Journal of Child Psychology and Psychiatry* 2004; 45: 2–40.

35. Margalit M, Tur-Kaspa H. Learning disabilities: neurodevelopment multidimensional model. *Psychology* 1998; 7: 64–76.

36. World Health Organization. *The international classification of diseases – Tenth edition: Classification of mental and behavioral disorders.* Geneva: World Health Organization, 1993.

37. Demonet JF, Taylor MJ, Chaix Y. Developmental dyslexia. *The Lancet* 2004; 363: 1451–1460.

38. Oren R, Breznitz Z. Reading processes in L1 and L2 among dyslexic as compared to regular bilingual readers: behavioral and electrophysiological evidence. *Journal of Neurolinguistics* 2005; 18: 127–151.

39. Friedmann N, Gvion A. Letter form as a constraint for errors in neglect dyslexia and letter position dyslexia. *Behavioral Neurology* 2005; 16: 145–158.

40. Katzir T, Kim Y, Wolf M, *et al.* Reading fluency: the whole is more than the parts. *Annals of Dyslexia* 2006; 56: 51–82.

41. Gross-Tsur v, Shalev R, Manor O, *et al.* Developmental right hemisphere syndrome: clinical spectrum of the nonverbal learning disabilities. *Journal of Learning Disabilities* 1995; 28: 80–86.

42. Rourke BP. Neuropsychology of learning disabilities: past and future. *Learning Disability Quarterly* 2005; 28: 111–114.

43. Snowling, MJ. Specific learning difficulties. *Psychiatry* 2005; 4: 110–113.

44. Lander LK, Bevan A, Butterworth B. Developmental dyscalculia and basic numerical capacities: a study of 8- to 9-year-old students. *Cognition* 2004; 93: 99–125.

45. Fuchs LS, Fuchs D. Mathematical problem-solving profiles of students with mathematics disabilities with and without comorbid reading disabilities. *Journal of Learning Disabilities* 2002; 35: 563–573.

46. Swanson L, Jerman O. Math disabilities: a preliminary meta-analysis of the published literature on cognitive processes. *Advances in Learning and Behavioral Disabilities* 2006; 19: 285–314.

47. Rubinsten O, Henik A. Automatic activation of internal magnitudes: a study of developmental dyscalculia. *Neuropsychology* 2005; 19: 641–648.

48. Bryant DP, Bryant BR, Hammill DD. Characteristic behaviors of students with LD who have teacher-identified math weaknesses. *Journal of Learning Disabilities* 2000; 33: 168–179.

49. Seligman MEP, Csikszentmihalyi M. Positive psychology. *American Psychologist* 2000; 55: 5–14.

50. Margalit M. Second-generation research on resilience: social-emotional aspects of children with learning disabilities. *Learning Disabilities Research & Practice* 2004; 19: 45–48.

51. Beasley M, Thompson T, Davidson J. Resilience in response to life stress: the effects of coping style and cognitive hardiness. *Personality and Individual Differences* 2003; 34: 77–95.

52. Lackaye T, Margalit M, Ziv O, *et al.* Comparisons of self-efficacy, mood, effort, and hope between students with learning disabilities and their non-LD-matched peers. *Learning Disabilities Research & Practice* 2006; 21: 111–121.

53. Snyder CR. Hope theory: rainbows in the mind. *Psychological Inquiry* 2002; 13: 249–275.

54. Shorey HS, Snyder CR, Rand KL, *et al.* Somewhere over the rainbow: hope theory weathers its first decade. *Psychological Inquiry* 2002; 13: 322–331.

55. Morrison GM, Cosden MA. Risk, resilience, and adjustment of individuals with learning disabilities. *Learning Disability Quarterly* 1997; 20: 43–60.

56. Wong BYL. General and specific issues for researchers' consideration in applying the risk and resilience framework to the social domain of learning disabilities. *Learning Disabilities Research & Practice* 2003; 18: 68–76.

57. Finzi-Dottana R, Dekela R, Lavic T, *et al.* Posttraumatic stress disorder reactions among children with learning disabilities exposed to terror attacks. *Comprehensive Psychiatry* 2006; 47: 144–151.

58. Lackaye T, Margalit M. Comparisons of achievement, effort and self-perceptions among students with learning disabilities and their peers from different achievement groups. *Journal of Learning Disabilities* 2006; 39: 432–446.

59. Margalit M. *Loneliness among children with special needs: theory, research, coping and intervention.* New York: Springer-Verlag, 1994.

60. Yu G, Zhang Y, Yan R. Loneliness, peer acceptance and family functioning of Chinese children with learning disabilities: characteristics and relationships. *Psychology in the Schools* 2005; 42: 325–331.

61. Valas H. Students with learning disabilities and low-achieving students: peer acceptance, loneliness, self-esteem, and depression. *Social Psychology of Education* 1999; 3: 173–192.

62. Perrin AJ, Lee H. The undertheorized environment: sociological theory and the ontology of behavioral genetics. *Sociological Perspectives* 2007; 50: 303–322.

63. Al-Yagon M, Mikulincer M. Patterns of close relationships and socioemotional and academic adjustment among school-age children with learning disabilities. *Learning Disabilities Research & Practice* 2004; 19: 12–19.

64. Al-Yagon M. Socioemotional and behavioral adjustment among school-age children with learning disabilities: the moderating role of maternal personal resources. *Journal of Special Education* 2007; 40: 205–218.

65. Margalit M, Heiman T. Family climate and anxiety of families with learning disabled boys. *Journal of the American Academy of Child & Adolescent Psychiatry* 1986; 25: 841–856.

66. Fuller GB, Rankin RE. Differences in the levels of parental stress among mothers of learning disabled, emotionally impaired and regular school children. *Perceptual and Motor Skills* 1994; 78: 583–592.

67. Margalit M, Raskind HM. Mothers' voices on the Internet: perceptions of LD and ADHD. Paper presented at the International Academy of Research on LD. Slovenia, July 2007.

68. Ben-Simhon Y. Testing accommodations for high school students with LD. Report presentation. Jerusalem: Department of Examination, Ministry of Education, 2007 (Hebrew).

69. Swanson L. Searching for the best model for instructing students with learning disabilities. *Focus on Exceptional Children* 2001; 34: 1–14.

70. Kotzer E, Margalit M. Perception of competence: risk and protective predictors following an e-self-advocacy intervention for adolescents with learning disabilities. *European Journal of Special Needs Education* 2007; 22: 443–457.

71. Schreiner MB. Effective self-advocacy: what students and special educators need to know. *Intervention in School and Clinic* 2007; 42: 300–304.

72. Blackhurst AE. Perspectives on applications of technology in the field of learning disabilities. *Learning Disability Quarterly* 2005; 28: 175–178.

73. Harmston KA, Strong CJ, Evans DD. Writing to South Africa: international pen-pal correspondence for students with language-learning disabilities. *Teaching Exceptional Children* 2001; 3: 46–51.

74. Boase J. Horrigan JB, Wellman B, *et al.* The strength of Internet ties: the Internet and e-mail aid users in maintaining their social networks and provide pathways to help when people face big decisions. 2006. Available from: http://www.pewinternet.org/.

75. Raskind MH, Margalit M, Higgins EL. "My LD": children's voices on the Internet. *Learning Disability Quarterly* 2006; 29: 253–268.

76. Sharabi A. Internet and adolescents with LD. Unpublished research. Tel Aviv University, 2007.

Chapter 4

MENTAL DISORDERS AMONG THE ELDERLY POPULATION IN ISRAEL

Perla Werner

In Israel, as in other countries, the proportion of elderly persons in the population is growing. According to estimates of the Central Bureau of Statistics, the proportion of the population aged 65 and over will rise from 10% in 2005 to 12.3% in 2025 (1). This increase will be accompanied by a sharp rise in the number of those aged 65 and older with mental disorders. This expected increase has been labeled as an emergent crisis (2) requiring proper attention.

Although no specific data are available about the costs of mental illness in later life, it is clear that this is becoming a serious public health concern due to the effects on the individual, family and society. Societal effects include an increasing load on the healthcare and social services systems, accompanied by increasing economic costs. Other effects include disability, poorer health outcomes and mortality risk. Finally, psychological effects include stigma, isolation, decreased quality of life and psychological dysfunction such as diminished self-esteem.

Israel's mental health system is not yet prepared to face these prospects. Despite the fact that the percentage of elderly persons who are hospitalized is 16%, only 10% of all hospital units are defined as psychogeriatric units (3). Moreover, only four of 114 community-based mental health clinics in Israel are totally dedicated to the psychogeriatric population (4). Approximately another 25 of the community-based mental health clinics have specialized memory clinics, but most of them work on a partial schedule (5).

Israel is also lagging behind in the training of professional caregivers. While it is estimated that one professional is needed for every 800 to 1,000 persons aged 65 and over (6), in Israel there are only about 110 registered psychogeriatricians, reflecting a ratio of one professional for every 6,000 persons aged 65 and over (3). Moreover, although Israel is in the process of reforming its mental health system (7), limited attention is being given to the elderly population, with its special characteristics and needs.

This chapter presents an overview of the epidemiologic research being conducted on the most prevalent mental health disorders among the Israeli elderly population – including depression, anxiety, dementia and late schizophrenia. Recommendations for future research and action are also presented.

§ Depression

According to the *Diagnostic and Statistical Manual of Mental Disorders – Fourth Edition Revised* (DSM-IV-R) (8), the criteria for major depression include five of the following symptoms present for a period of two weeks – depressed mood, loss of pleasure in most activities, weight loss or gain, insomnia or hypersomnia, psychomotor agitation, fatigue, feelings of worthlessness, guilt, impaired concentration, and suicidal ideation. Symptoms of minor depression include depressed mood during most days for a period of two years and at least two of the following symptoms: poor appetite or overeating, insomnia or hypersomnia, low energy or fatigue, low self-esteem, poor concentration and feelings of hopelessness.

Depression is the most common late-life mood disorder, and although it is similar in both older and younger populations among the elderly it is often hidden in somatic symptoms. Also, depression is characterized by its comorbidity with other medical illnesses (9–10).

Overall, studies in other countries reported that the prevalence of major depression in persons aged 65 and over ranges between .9% and 9.4% in the community-dwelling elderly; between 14% and 42% among the institutionalized elderly; and between 1% and 16% among the elderly living in private households or in institutions (11). As noted, those prevalence studies show great variations, due mainly to the use of varied diagnostic criteria and research methods.

Although there is limited local epidemiological research purported to assess the prevalence of late-life depression, some studies have examined the prevalence rates in specific populations and their risk factors for depression. Results of these studies are summarized below together with an overview of the depression assessment instruments validated in Hebrew.

Depression and depressive symptoms in selected populations

In a study assessing the rate and correlates of depressive symptoms in a sample of 1200 community-dwelling oldest-old (aged 75–94) Jewish residents, Ruskin *et al.* (12) found an estimated 43% rate of depressive symptoms. A lower prevalence of depressive symptoms, 16.8%, was found in a prospective study examining the association between falls and depression among 283 persons aged 60 and over in the city of Beersheba (13). Finally, Geulayov *et al.* (14), in a review article on depression in primary care, summarized prevalence rates cited by several studies that included patients aged 18 to 75. However, no specific rates for the population samples aged 60 and over were given in those studies.

Most research on the topic of depression in the elderly has focused on unique populations, such as immigrants, the Arab-Israeli sector, Holocaust survivors and kibbutz members.

With the high rate of immigration to Israel, particularly in recent decades, research attention focused on the elderly immigrant population has grown accordingly. In a clinical study using an abbreviated version of the Composite International Diagnostic Interview (CIDI-S) (15), Zilber *et al.* examined the prevalence rates of depression among a group of 116 elderly subjects from the former Soviet Union (FSU), 86 of them aged 65 or younger and 30 aged over 65 (16). Their findings showed a higher prevalence rate of major depression in the older as compared to the younger group, 4.8% and 2.0%, respectively. In contrast, rates of dysthymia were closer, 3.7% and 2.9% for the younger and older participants, respectively. The authors also reported that before immigration the incidence of depression was lower in the elderly group, while the reverse was observed in the younger group. These findings suggest that immigration leads to an increase in the incidence of depressive disorders, especially among elderly persons.

Arab Israelis are a significant minority group. High rates of depressive symptoms, based on DSM-IV criteria, were found in a population-based study of elderly Arabs from Wadi Ara who were diagnosed with dementia of both Alzheimer's (AD) type (n=168) and vascular type (n=49) (17). Prevalence rates of depressive symptoms were higher among the latter than among those with AD, 85% and 57% respectively.

Although not directly examining depression, Shemesh *et al.* reported high scores of emotional distress among 824 Arabs aged 60 and above residing in the community (18). Prevalence rates, obtained after establishing suitable cutting points, were especially high for Muslim Arabs (43.4%), followed by Christian Arabs (37%) and Druze (17%). The same study showed a prevalence rate of 21.4% among the 4,231 Jews surveyed.

Holocaust survivors represent another unique population in Israeli society. Several studies have examined depression rates among them, but their results were inconsistent. In a study assessing relationships among hopelessness, depression and suicidality among 464 elderly community dwellers attending five senior-citizen centers near the city of Haifa, Ron reported that Holocaust survivors – who comprised 45% of the study sample – expressed lower levels of depression on the Beck Depression Inventory (19) as compared to those without such an experience (mean scores 1.7 and 2.1 respectively) (19). Those findings were a reversal of the results obtained in a previous study by the same author (20) conducted among a mixed sample of 227 elderly persons residing in the community and 91 in nursing homes, also using the Beck Depression Inventory. In this study, elderly Holocaust survivors reported higher levels of depression scores than elderly people residing in the community (2.7 and 1.3 respectively). Similarly, a study conducted in a long-stay psychiatric setting using the Structured Clinical Interview (SCID) found that 22 of 44 patients who were Holocaust survivors had a diagnosis of affective disorder, compared to five of 30 patients in the comparison group (21). The discrepancy between the studies might stem from methodological differences as well as from different coping mechanisms used by the Holocaust survivors.

Finally, Landau and Litwin (22) compared psychological and somatic symptoms associated with depression – measured by the Zung Self-rating Depression Scale – in a community-based sample of 91 Holocaust survivors and 103 elderly persons aged 75 and above who did not experience the Holocaust. Although they found no statistically significant differences in depression rates between the two groups, those who had experienced the Holocaust reported slightly higher rates of depressive symptoms.

Lastly, elderly persons residing in kibbutzim have also been the focus of research in this area. Blumstein *et al.* (23) compared the depression levels of elderly persons residing in kibbutzim with a suitable national sample. Using the Center for Epidemiological Studies Depression Scale (CES-D), lower depression scores were found among elderly female kibbutz members as compared to elderly women living in other communities.

In sum, the study of depression in special populations of elderly persons in Israel has attracted much research. However, most studies have concentrated on depression symptoms and not on depressive disorders.

Factors associated with depression in the elderly population

Several studies have examined factors associated with depression and depressive symptoms in the elderly population. Among the main factors reported were female gender; widowhood

(19); vascular dementia and Alzheimer's disease (17, 24); anxiety (25); poor self-rated health; poor cognitive status; impaired Activities of Daily Living (ADL); and frequent visits to a physician (13). In a recent review on suicide in the elderly, mood disorders (and especially bipolar disorder) were reported to be one of the main mental disorders associated with suicide in the elderly population in studies in Israel and abroad (26). In Israel, a retrospective, matched, case-controlled evaluation over a 10-year period of elderly bipolar patients showed a greater index of suicide among persons with mood disorder than among those without (27).

Assessment instruments

The following are the most common instruments used for the assessment of depression in the elderly population; they are available in Hebrew and have been validated locally.

The Hamilton Depression Scale (HDS or HAMD) (28) measures the severity of depressive symptoms in individuals, often in people who have already been diagnosed as having a depressive disorder. It is sometimes known as the Hamilton Rating Scale for Depression (HRSD) or the Hamilton Depression Rating Scale (HDRS). Depending on the version used, there are either 17 or 21 items for which an interviewer provides ratings. These include overall depression; guilt; suicide; insomnia; problems related to work; psychomotor retardation; agitation; anxiety; gastrointestinal and other physical symptoms; loss of libido; hypochondriasis; loss of insight; and loss of weight.

The HDS has been widely used in local studies. It was validated by Kertzman et al. (29) in a study of elderly patients, including 50 with primary degenerative dementia and 50 with vascular dementia. Study findings showed the Hebrew version of the HDS to have good criterion validity in the evaluation of depression in patients with dementia.

The Geriatric Depression Scale (GDS) (30), which originally included 30 items but whose shorter form with 15 items (GDS-s) was developed later and shown to have adequate validity in many languages (31), was specially developed for the assessment of depression in geriatric populations.

The GDS-s has been widely used in local studies (13, 32). Its Hebrew version was validated by Zalsman et al. in a study including 27 inpatients (M age=73.3 years) with a diagnosis of major depression, according to the DSM-IV criteria and 21 healthy volunteers (M age=70.3 years) (33). The Hebrew version of the GDS-s has proven to be a valid and reliable instrument for the detection of depression among the geriatric population. It showed high correlation scores with the HAMD (Pearson's correlation=.79, $p <$ .005), as well as high sensitivity for differentiating even mild depression. High *Kappa* values were reported for inter-rater and test-retest reliability (*Kappa*=1.0 and .88, respectively).

The Beck Depression Inventory (BDI) is the most commonly used measure to assess depression (34). It consists of 21 items describing various depressive manifestations, such as sadness, loss of pleasure and pessimism. Total scores range between 0 and 63, with higher scores indicating more severe depression. Although no specific study has examined the validity and reliability of the Hebrew version, the BDI has been used in several studies in the local elderly population and has shown good to excellent internal reliability-consistency, Cronbach's *alpha* ranging from .82 to .88 (19, 20).

The Zung Self-Rating Depression Scale consists of 22 statements that describe the way people sometimes feel (35). An index score is calculated by dividing the total score by 40 and multiplying it by 100. A score of ≥ 70 or greater is considered to indicate depression (36). This screening instrument was translated into Hebrew and showed good internal reliability-consistency in a study with elderly persons, Cronbach's *alpha* = .87 (22).

The Short Zung Interview-Assisted Depression Rating Scale is a modified version including 10 questions on the frequency of symptoms which are rated on a Likert-type scale ranging from 1 = never to 4 = always. Translated into Hebrew and subsequently validated (25), it has shown excellent sensitivity, 71.1%, and specificity, 88.3%, as well as positive and negative predictive value (90.1%) in studies assessing depression in the Israeli elderly (37).

The Center for Epidemiologic Studies – Depression Scale (CES-D) is a 20-item scale designed to measure depressive symptoms experienced in the past week (38). Responses range from 0 to 3 – and the total score, ranging from 0 to 60 – is calculated by adding the scores of all items (after reversing four of them). A score of 16 or greater has been suggested as the cut-off point indicative of probable clinical depression. The CES-D has been translated into Hebrew and has shown excellent internal reliability, Cronbach's *alpha* = .88, in several epidemiological studies (23, 39, 40).

❧ Anxiety disorders

These disorders are characterized by anxious over-concern and include several types, among them generalized anxiety disorder (GAD), panic disorders and obsessive-compulsive disorder (OCD). They are frequently associated with somatic complaints (41) as well as with the following array of symptoms: overwhelming feelings of panic and fear; uncontrollable obsessive thoughts; painful, intrusive memories; recurring nightmares; nausea; sweating; and muscle tension (42) (see chapter 12).

Anxiety disorders may be the most common mental disorders in elderly persons; they can affect twice as many older adults than does depression (43). However, little research has been conducted worldwide and in Israel to assess the prevalence, correlates and treatment of anxiety disorders among the elderly (44).

There are few local studies assessing anxiety in the elderly population. They were aimed at examining the association between anxiety, depression and cognitive decline. Trying to elucidate this relationship, Sinoff *et al.* (45) developed one of the few screening tests for the assessment of anxiety in the elderly – the Short Anxiety Screening Test (SAST). The SAST was developed based on *DSM-IV* criteria (8) and includes, among others, modifications of commonly recurring questions found in other instruments and items exploring somatic symptoms. The instrument includes 10 questions scored from 1 to 4; a total score is calculated by the sum of the scores. A score of 24 or higher is considered as the cut-off point for the diagnosis of anxiety. The SAST was validated in a study including 150 geriatric inpatients and outpatients, and was found to be a valid screening test for detecting anxiety among the elderly (45). The internal consistency of the SAST was Cronbach's *alpha* = .70, and its inter-rater reliability, .80. Additionally, it showed a sensitivity of 75%, a specificity of 79%, and a positive predictive value of 71%. SAST was later used in studies to assess the associations between depression, anxiety, and cognitive impairment (25, 37).

❧ Dementia and Alzheimer's disease

Dementia is the progressive decline in cognitive functioning due to damage or disease of the brain beyond what might be expected from normal aging. The functions particularly affected are memory, attention, language and problem-solving. Alzheimer's disease (AD) is the most common cause for dementia, followed by vascular dementia (46).

The most important age-related disorder, dementia has attracted considerable amount of research worldwide and in Israel. The results of the local studies examining dementia in general and AD in particular are summarized below, together with an overview of the dementia assessment instruments validated in Hebrew and studies assessing the consequences of dementia.

Studies on the prevalence of dementia

The first comprehensive epidemiological study to assess the prevalence of dementia among Jewish-Israeli elderly was conducted in 2002 by Wertman *et al.* on a random sample of 1624 community dwellers aged 65 and over and residing in Jerusalem (47). Following an initial screening for suspected dementia and a further in-depth clinical examination using a clinical protocol developed by the Neuro-Psychogeriatrics Department of Jerusalem's Herzog Hospital in accordance to the diagnostic criteria of *DSM-III-R* and *DSM-IV*, a fifth of the participants (19.2%) were diagnosed with different stages of dementia. When these rates were applied to data on the total elderly community-dwelling population living in Israel by the end of 2002, the numbers reached some 98,000 individuals.

The rate found was higher than those reported by Kahana *et al.* in their study conducted with a population of 1,501 elderly persons over the age of 75 in the coastal city of Ashkelon (48). The total prevalence of dementia in this study was 11%, with rates increasing from 5.9% among those aged 76 up to 26.9% among those aged 90 and over. The difference between the two studies can be explained by the different assessment methods used. In Jerusalem, it was based on a physician examination, while in Ashkelon, on trained medical field workers (nurses or social workers).

As might be expected, higher prevalence rates were found among residents of long-term care geriatric institutions. In a cross-sectional survey of a representative sample of 11 wards in 34 long-term care institutions providing care for the elderly in Jerusalem, 49.9% of the sample was diagnosed with dementia (49).

While these studies referred to all dementias, others have examined specific types of dementia in specific cultural groups. Bowirrat *et al.* reported unusually high prevalence rates (20.5%) of Alzheimer's disease in an epidemiological study of 821 Arab Israelis aged 60 and over residing in Wadi Ara (50). A prevalence rate of 6.0% of vascular dementia was found in the same population (51). These findings are explained by the unique characteristics of this group, such as rural living conditions, environmental hardships, cigarette smoking, and by their unique human genome data (52).

Assessment instruments

A number of instruments are available for the screening of dementia (for a thorough recent review of this topic, see ref. 53). They vary in length, mode of administration and psychometric characteristics (for a review, see ref. 54; specific data are provided below). However, only few of those instruments in their Hebrew version have been appropriately tested and validated.

The Mini-Mental State Examination (MMSE) (55) appears to be the most widely used test for the screening and diagnosis of dementia. It is an 11-item instrument assessing cognitive functioning, with scores ranging from 0 (total cognitive deterioration) to 30 (normal cognitive functioning). The Hebrew version of the Mini Mental State Examination was administered to 36 and 19 elderly persons with and without dementia, respectively. Test-retest reliability scores were calculated as exact agreement rates and ranged from good to excellent for all the items. Strong convergent validity, as measured by the correlation between the MMSE and the CAMCOG (see below, r=.94) was found. Good predictive value was observed, as over three-quarters of the participants were correctly classified as demented or non-demented (56, 57).

The Telephone Interview for Cognitive Status-Modified (TICS-m) is a short instrument, modeled on the Mini-Mental State Examination with the aim of assessing cognitive status over the telephone. The mental functions assessed include orientation, attention, memory, repetition, comprehension and conceptual knowledge (58). Its validated Hebrew version (59) has shown high internal reliability-consistency, Cronbach's *alpha*=.98, as well as excellent convergent validity and sensitivity.

The CAMCOG is a relatively brief neuropsychological battery which forms part of the Cambridge Examination for Mental Disorders of the Elderly (CAMDEX) (60) and assesses a wide range of cognitive functions. The CAMCOG ranges from 0 to 107, with scores lower than 79/80 indicating cognitive impairment. The CAMCOG is the second most popular cognitive test used by Israeli physicians. It was validated by Heinik *et al.* (61) and has shown excellent inter-rater agreement scores, as well as strong convergent validity and predictive characteristics.

Other well-known instruments in use locally – but for which no reliability and validity data have been published – include the Alzheimer's Disease Assessment Scale (cognitive sub-scale) (62), the Modified Mini-Mental State Examination (3MS) (48, 50), the Clock Drawing Test (63) and the Brookdale Cognitive Screening Test (49, 52).

The recent emphasis on the need for early diagnosis of AD highlights the pressing need to develop precise instruments that can be easily and objectively administered and will minimize learning effects. Thus, Israeli researchers have recently been concentrating on the development and validation of computerized tests for the assessment of dementia among the elderly (64). Aharonson *et al.* reported the validity of a computerized method for the diagnosis of mild cognitive impairment by assessing the recall of a pattern and digit symbol substitution (65). Finally, the Mindstreams Mild Impairment Battery is an interactive cognitive test that assesses a wide variety of cognitive domains, including memory; executive function; visual spatial skills; verbal fluency; attention; information processing; and motor skills (66). Results of a Receiving Operating Curve analysis measuring the ability of this instrument to discriminate mild cognitive impairment from cognitively healthy elderly persons showed that the parameters estimated discriminated significantly with an AUC ranging from .70 to .86.

Impact of dementia

The main impact of dementia have also been examined by local researchers. First, the direct and indirect monetary costs associated with caring for persons with AD were examined in community-dwelling and institutionalized patients (67, 68). Seventy-one AD patients who lived in the community, 50 institutionalized AD patients and 50 healthy elderly subjects were interviewed. The interviews covered information about the number of caregivers' hours invested in caring for the patient and amount of expenditures, such as in-house paid help and payments for day care. The annual social cost of caring for a person with AD in Israel was approximately US $17,000, whether the patient lived at home or in a nursing home. The cost components differed in the two groups. For community-dwelling patients, 60% of the cost represented an imputed value of unpaid indirect care compared with 12% for institutionalized patients. Also, in both residences, the private cost was significantly higher than the public cost, i.e., more than 75% of the services provided to patients were paid out-of-pocket. Cost of institutionalization was the major component of the social cost. Additionally, the costs of the disease increased with functional and cognitive deterioration and were especially high for the management of the associated behavioral and psychological symptoms.

In addition, the stigmatic views of the lay public and professionals towards persons with Alzheimer's disease were examined (69. 70). These studies showed that despite anecdotal beliefs regarding the stigma associated with Alzheimer's disease, professionals as well as the lay public reported more positive (such as concern – reported by 60% of the lay public, and desire to help – reported by 72%) than negative emotional reactions (such as irritation – reported by 4% of the lay public, and anger – reported by 10%).

However, one of the hardest consequences of the disease – the burden on the caregivers of the persons with dementia (71, 72) – has attracted limited research attention in Israel. Lowenstein, in a study examining the effects of demographic, ethnic, personal and familial resources on the well-being of children caring for parents with Alzheimer's disease, found that ethnicity and intergenerational relationships were the main predictors of the caregivers' mental health (73). The need remains to expand this line of research locally.

ᕥ Schizophrenia in late life

Although schizophrenia is typical of young adults, it is clear today that it can also appear in or extend into late life. Increased research attention has recently been devoted to schizophrenia in elderly persons, with a special focus on similarities and differences between age groups (74). Diagnostic criteria for schizophrenia in late life are similar to those of early life, and symptoms include delusions; hallucinations; disorganized speech; affective flattening; alogia; and avolition. Although no epidemiological data about the prevalence of late-life schizophrenia are available, a recent Israeli review estimated rates ranging from .1% to 4% (75).

The results of Israeli studies in the area of late-life schizophrenia confirm those of studies worldwide that patients with late-life and very-late-life schizophrenia present stable cognitive and everyday functioning, as compared with younger patients (76); a relatively low base rate of suicide (77); and lower levels of self-stigma than younger populations (78).

In terms of screening instruments, Israeli researchers rely on the Positive and Negative Syndrome Scale (PANSS) (79). This is an interviewer-administered scale scored on the basis of a clinical interview lasting 30 to 45 minutes. It consists of three subscales: positive syndrome scale, negative syndrome scale and general psychopathology scale. The reliability and validity of the PANSS in Hebrew have been established among both adult and elderly schizophrenia patients (80).

ᕥ From epidemiology to mental health action

In view of the anticipated demographic changes worldwide, the number of elderly persons with mental disorders will continue to increase, posing a considerable burden to individuals, professionals and society at large. Importantly, Israel is in the process of undergoing a thorough reform in the delivery of psychiatric care aimed at addressing this problem (7).

Given the relative high prevalence rates of elderly persons with mental disorders, there is an urgent need to expand the research base, particularly in the following areas:

(a) Epidemiological studies assessing the incidence and prevalence of mental disorders among the elderly population are needed, with special attention paid to unique groups, such as Arab Israelis and new immigrants;

(b) Unique correlates of mental illness in the elderly should be identified, such as comorbidity, populations at risk (e.g., elderly persons living alone);

(c) Data obtained through these studies should be geared to provide information and guidelines with regard to the clear definition of policy and priorities that are specifically centered on the needs and unique characteristics of elderly persons with mental disorders;

(d) Knowledge and attitudes regarding discrimination towards elderly persons with mental disorders should be assessed, particularly in relation to the following questions: Are these persons a target for double stigma? Do discriminatory behaviors prevent help seeking in this population? Do professionals' attitudes affect the care that elderly persons with mental disorders receive?

(e) Studies on issues of clinical importance and related to the practice with elderly persons with mental disorders are needed. For example, professionals' knowledge and training regarding the care of elderly persons with mental disorders should be examined and the effectiveness of multi-professional care evaluated;

(f) Evaluation should be conducted of educational programs aimed at providing knowledge about mental disorders among the elderly, specifically those geared to different population groups, such as the lay public, elderly persons with mental disorders and their family members, professionals; and

(g) Assessment of the efficacy of intervention programs for elderly persons with mental disorders should be expanded.

In sum, the field of mental disorders in Israel's elderly population is still in its developing stages. Services geared to the unique needs of this population should be developed. These include mental health services for the elderly in non-hospital-based outpatient settings, nursing homes and community centers for the elderly. Training programs for professionals in the area of psychogeriatrics should be developed. Special attention must be paid to an interdisciplinary mental health care approach for the elderly with mental disorders that include the disciplines of medicine, psychiatry, psychology, psychiatric nursing and clinical social work.

Although old age is not itself a risk factor for mental disorders, increasing numbers of elderly persons will be developing a significant mental health disorder. Israeli society should be prepared to deal with these developments adequately.

This work was partially funded by grant 483/05 from the Israel Science Foundation.

❧ References

1. Central Bureau of Statistics. *Statistical abstract 2006.* Jerusalem: Central Bureau of Statistics, 2006 (Hebrew).

2. Jeste DV, Alexopoulos GS, Bartels SJ, *et al.* Consensus statement on the upcoming crisis in geriatric mental health. *Archives of General Psychiatry* 1999; 56: 848–853.

3. Baruch Y. Psychogeriatrics in Israel. *Gerontology* 2005; 32: 13–20 (Hebrew).

4.   Ministry of Health. Psychiatric care for the elderly [online]. [cited October 1, 2007]. Available from URL: http://www.health.gov.il/download/mental/annual2004/pp84- 89eldery.pdf (accessed October 1, 2007) (Hebrew).

5.   Werner P, Heinik J, Aharon J. Process and organizational characteristics of memory clinics in Israel: a national survey. *Archives of Gerontology and Geriatrics* 2001; 33: 191–201.

6.   Halpain MC, Harris MJ, McClure FS. Training in geriatric mental health: needs and strategies. *Psychiatric Services* 1999; 50: 1205–1208.

7.   Levav I, Lachman M. On the way to psychiatric reform in Israel: notes for an ideological and scientific debate. *Israel Journal of Psychiatry and Related Sciences* 2005; 42: 198–214.

8.   American Psychiatric Association. *Diagnostic and statistical manual of mental disorders – Fourth edition.* Major depressive disorder DSM-IV diagnostic criteria [online]. [cited October 2, 2007]. Available from URL: http://www.iscribe.com/pdf/majorDepDisorderDSM-iv.pdf.

9.   Soref E. The aging of the population and late-life depression – implications for the medical sciences and presentation of one therapeutic modality. *Harefuah* 2007; 146: 38–41 (Hebrew).

10.   Twedell D. Depression in the elderly. *Journal of Continuing Education in Nursing* 2007; 38: 14–15.

11.   Djerner JK. Prevalence and predictors of depression in populations of elderly: a review. *Acta Psychiatrica Scandinavica* 2006; 113: 372–387.

12.   Ruskin PE, Blumstein Z, Walter-Ginzburg A, *et al.* Depressive symptoms among community-dwelling oldest-old residents in Israel. *American Journal of Geriatric Psychiatry* 1996; 4: 208–217.

13.   Biderman A, Cwikel J, Fried V, *et al.* Depression and falls among community dwelling elderly people: a search for common risk factors. *Journal of Epidemiology and Community Health* 2002; 56: 631–636.

14.   Geulayov G, Lipsitz J, Sabar R, *et al.* Depression in primary care in Israel. *Israel Medical Association Journal* 2007; 9: 571–578.

15.   Kovess V, Devigan C, Gysens S, *et al.* Measure of somatization disorders in a French population. *International Journal of Methods in Psychiatric Research* 1993; 3: 121–127.

16.   Zilber N, Lerner Y, Eidelman R, *et al.* Depression and anxiety disorders among Jews from the former Soviet Union five years after their immigration to Israel. *International Journal of Geriatric Psychiatry* 2001; 16: 993–999.

17.   Bowirrat A, Oscar-Berman M, Logroscino G. Association of depression with Alzheimer's disease and vascular dementia in an elderly Arab population of Wadi-Ara, Israel. *International Journal of Geriatric Psychiatry* 2006; 21: 246–251.

18.   Shemesh AA, Kohn R, Blumstein T, *et al.* A community study on emotional distress among Arab and Jewish Israelis over the age of 60. *International Journal of Geriatric Psychiatry* 2006; 21: 64–76.

19.   Ron P. Depression and suicide among community elderly. *Journal of Gerontological Social Work* 2002; 38: 53–70.

20.   Ron P. Depression, hopelessness and suicidal tendency among elderly persons: comparing community-dwelling and institutionalized elderly. *Gerontology* 2001; 25: 83–103.

21.   Terno P, Barak Y, Hadjez J, *et al.* Holocaust survivors hospitalized for life: the Israeli experience. *Comprehensive Psychiatry* 1998; 39: 364–367.

22.   Landau R, Litwin H. The effects of extreme early stress in very old age. *Journal of Traumatic Stress* 2000; 13: 473–487.

23.   Blumstein T, Benyamini Y, Fuchs Z, *et al.* The effects of a communal lifestyle on depressive symptoms in late life. *Journal of Aging Health* 2004; 16: 151–174.

24.   Zalsman G, Aizenberg D, Sigler M, *et al.* Increased risk for dementia in elderly psychiatric in patients with late-onset major depression. *Journal of Nervous and Mental Disease* 2000; 188: 242–243.

25.   Sinoff G, Ore L, Zlotogorsky D, Tamir A. Does the presence of anxiety affect the validity of a screening test for depression in the elderly? *International Journal of Geriatric Psychiatry* 2002; 17: 309–314.

26.   Aizenberg D, Barak Y. Suicides in the elderly. *Gerontology* 2005; 32: 41–47 (Hebrew).

27.   Aizenberg D, Olmer A, Barak Y. Suicide attempts amongst elderly bipolar patients. *Journal of Affective Disorders* 2006; 91: 91–94.

28.   Hamilton M. A rating scale for depression. *Journal of Neurology, Neurosurgery and Psychiatry* 1960; 23: 56–62.

29.   Kertzman SG, Treves IA, Treves TA, *et al.* Hamilton depression scale in dementia. *International Journal of Psychiatric Clinical Practice* 2002; 6: 91–94.

30.   Yesavage JA, Brink TL, Rose TL, *et al.* Development and validation of a geriatric depression screening scale: a preliminary report. *Journal of Psychiatric Research* 1983; 17: 37–49.

31.   Sheik J, Yesavage JA. Geriatric depression scale (GDS): recent evidence and development of a shorter version. In: Brink TL, ed. *Clinical gerontology: a guide to assessment and intervention.* New York: The Haworth Press, 1986.

32.   Cwikel J, Ritchie K. Screening for depression among the elderly in Israel: an assessment of the Short Geriatric Depression Scale (S-GDS). *Israel Journal of Medical Sciences* 1989; 25: 13–137.

33.   Zalsman G, Aizenberg D, Sigler M, *et al.* Geriatric depression scale-short form – validity and reliability of the Hebrew version. *Clinical Gerontology* 1998; 18: 3–9.

34.   Beck AT, Ward CH, Mendelson M, *et al.* An inventory for measuring depression. *Archives of General Psychiatry* 1961; 4: 561–571.

35.   Zung WW. A Self-rating depression scale. *Archives of General Psychiatry* 1965; 12: 63–70.

36.   Tucker MA, Ogle SJ, Davison JG, *et al.* Validation of a brief screening test for depression in the elderly. *Age and Ageing* 1987; 16: 139–144.

37.   Sinoff G, Werner P. Anxiety disorder and accompanying subjective memory loss in the elderly as a predictor of future cognitive decline. *International Journal of Geriatric Psychiatry* 2003; 18: 951–959.

38.   Radloff LS. The CES-D scale: a self-report depression scale for research in the general population. *Applied Psychological Measures* 1997; 1: 385–401.

39. Ben-Ezra M, Shmotkin D. Predictors of mortality in the old-old in Israel: the cross sectional and longitudinal aging study. *Journal of the American Geriatric Society* 2006; 54: 906–911.

40. Zunzunegui MV, Minicuci N, Blumstein T, *et al.* and the CLESA Group. Gender differences in depressive symptoms among older adults: a cross-national comparison. *Social Psychiatry and Psychiatric Epidemiology* 2007; 42: 198–207.

41. Martin LM, Fleming KC, Evans JM. Recognition and management of anxiety and depression in elderly patients. *Mayo Clinic Proceedings* 1995; 70: 999–1,006.

42. Copeland JR, Dewey ME, Wood N, *et al.* Range of mental illness among the elderly in the community. Prevalence in Liverpool using the GMS-AGECAT package. *British Journal of Psychiatry* 1987; 150: 815–823.

43. Hopko DR, Bourland SL, Stanley MA, *et al.* Generalized anxiety disorders in older adults: examining the relation between clinician severity ratings and patient self-report measures. *Depression and Anxiety* 2000; 12: 217–225.

44. Wetherell JL, Le Roux H, Gatz M. DSM-IV criteria for generalized anxiety disorder in older adults: distinguishing the worried from the well. *Psychology in Aging* 2003; 18: 622–627.

45. Sinoff G, Ore L, Zlotogorsky D, *et al.* Short anxiety screening test – a brief instrument for detecting anxiety in the elderly. *International Journal of Geriatric Psychiatry* 1999; 14: 1062–1071.

46. Gühne U, Matschinger H, Angermeyer MC, *et al.* Incident dementia cases and mortality. *Dementia and Geriatric Cognitive Disorders* 2006; 22: 185–193.

47. Wertman E, Brodsky J, King Y, *et al.* An estimate of the prevalence of dementia among community-dwelling elderly in Israel. *Dementia and Geriatric Cognitive Disorders* 2007; 24: 294–299.

48. Kahana E, Galper Y, Zilber N, *et al.* Epidemiology of dementia in Ashkelon: the influence of education. *Journal of Neurology* 2003; 250: 424–428.

49. Feldman H, Clarfield AM, Brodsky J, *et al.* An estimate of the prevalence of dementia among residents of long-term geriatric institutions in the Jerusalem area. *International Psychogeriatrics* 2006; 18: 643–652.

50. Bowirrat A, Treves TA, Friedland RP, *et al.* Prevalence of Alzheimer's type dementia in an elderly Arab population. *European Journal of Neurology* 2001; 8: 119–123.

51. Bowirrat A, Friedland RP, Korczyn AD. Vascular dementia among elderly Arabs in Wadi Ara. *Journal of Neurological Sciences* 2002; 203–204: 73–76.

52. Farrer LA, Friedland RP, Bowirrat A, *et al.* Genetic and environmental epidemiology of Alzheimer's disease in Arabs residing in Israel. *Journal of Molecular Neurosciences* 2003; 20: 207–212.

53. Cullen B, O'Neill B, Evans JJ, *et al.* A review of screening tests for cognitive impairment. *Journal of Neurology, Neurosurgery and Psychiatry* 2007; 78: 790–799.

54. Werner P. A review of instruments for assessing cognitive functioning in the elderly population. *Gerontology* 2001; 28: 103–118 (Hebrew).

55. Folstein MF, Folstein SE, McHugh PR. Mini-Mental State: a practical method for grading the state of patients for the clinician. *Journal of Psychiatric Research* 1975; 12: 189–198.

56. Werner P, Heinik J, Lin R, *et al.* "Yes" ifs, ands and buts: examining performance and correlates of the repetition task in the Mini-mental State Examination. *International Journal of Geriatric Psychiatry* 1999; 14: 719–725.

57. Werner P, Heinik J, Mendel A. Examining the reliability and validity of the Hebrew version of the Mini-mental State Examination. *Aging Clinical and Experimental Research* 1999; 11: 329–334.

58. Brandt J, Spencer M, Folstein M. The telephone instrument for cognitive status. *Neuropsychiatry, Neuropsychology and Behavioral Neurology* 1988; 1: 11–17.

59. Beeri MS, Werner P, Davidson M, *et al.* Validation of the modified Telephone Interview Status (TICS-m). *International Journal of Geriatric Psychiatry* 2003; 18: 381–386.

60. Roth M, Huppert FA, Tym E, *et al.* CAMDEX – *The Cambridge examination for mental disorders of the elderly.* Cambridge: Cambridge University Press, 1988.

61. Heinik J, Werner P, Mendel A, *et al.* The Cambridge Cognitive Examination (CAMCOG): validation of the Hebrew version in elderly demented patients. *International Journal of Geriatric Psychiatry* 1999; 14: 1006–1013.

62. Blesa R, Davidson M, Kurz A, *et al.* Galantamine provides sustained benefits in patients with advanced moderate Alzheimer's disease for at least 12 months. *Dementia Geriatric Cognitive Disorders* 2003; 15: 79–87.

63. Heinik J, Solomesh I, Raikher B, *et al.* Clock Drawing Test-Modified and integrated approach (CDT-MIA): description and preliminary examination if its validity and reliability in dementia patients referred to a specialized psychogeriatric setting. *Journal of Geriatric Psychiatry and Neurology* 2004; 17: 73–80.

64. Korczyn AD, Aharonson V. Computerized methods in the assessment and prediction of dementia. *Current Alzheimer Research* 2007; 4: 364–369.

65. Aharonson V, Halperin I, Korczyn AD. Computerized diagnosis of mild cognitive impairment. *Alzheimer's Dementia* 2007; 3: 23–27.

66. Dwolatzky T, Whitehead V, Doniger GM, *et al.* Validity of a novel computerized cognitive battery for mild cognitive impairment. *BMC Geriatrics* 2003; 3: 1–12.

67. Beeri MS, Werner P, Adar Z, *et al.* Economic cost of Alzheimer disease in Israel. *Alzheimer Disease and Associated Disorders* 2002; 16: 73–80.

68. Beeri MS, Werner P, Davidson M, *et al.* The cost of behavioral and psychological symptoms of dementia (BPSD) in community dwelling Alzheimer's disease patients. *International Journal of Geriatric Psychiatry* 2002; 17: 403–408.

69. Werner P. Social distance towards a person with Alzheimer's disease. *International Journal of Geriatric Psychiatry* 2005; 20: 182–188.

70. Werner P, Davidson M. Emotional reactions to individuals suffering from Alzheimer's disease: examining their patterns and correlates. *International Journal of Geriatric Psychiatry* 2004; 19: 391–397.

71. Korczyn AD, Davidson M. Quality of life in Alzheimer's disease. *European Journal of Neurology* 1999; 6: 487–489.

72. Ory M, Yee JL, Tennstedt SL, *et al.* The extent and impact of dementia care: unique challenges experienced by family caregivers. In: Schulz R, ed. *Handbook of dementia caregiving: evidence-based interventions for family caregivers.* New York: Springer, 2000.

73. Lowenstein A. Caring for parents with Alzheimer's disease: comparing perceptions of physical and mental health in the Jewish and Arab sectors in Israel. *Journal of Cross-Cultural Gerontology* 1999; 14: 65–76.

74. Folsom DP, Lebowitz BD, Lindamer LA, *et al.* Schizophrenia in late life: emerging issues. *Dialogues in Clinical Neurosciences* 2006; 8: 45–52.

75. Barak Y, Knovler CH. Late onset schizophrenia. *Gerontology* 2005; 32: 33–40 (Hebrew).

76. Mazeh D, Zemishlany Z, Aizenberg D, *et al.* Patients with very-late onset schizophrenia-like psychosis: a follow-up study. *American Journal of Geriatric Psychiatry* 2005; 13: 417–419.

77. Barak Y, Knobler CH, Aizenberg D. Suicide attempts amongst elderly schizophrenia patients: a 10-year case-control study. *Schizophrenia Research* 2004; 71: 77–81.

78. Werner P, Aviv A, Barak Y. Self-stigma, self-esteem and age in persons with schizophrenia. *International Psychogeriatrics* 2007; 23: 1–15.

79. Kay SR, Fishbein A, Opler LA. The Positive and Negative Syndrome Scale (PANSS) for schizophrenia. *Schizophrenia Bulletin* 1987; 13: 261–276.

80. Barak Y, Shamir E, Weizman R. Would a switch from typical antipsychotics to risperidone be beneficial for elderly schizophrenic patients? A naturalistic, long-term, retrospective, comparative study. *Journal of Clinical Psychopharmacology* 2002; 22: 115–120.

Chapter 5

THE EPIDEMIOLOGY OF MENTAL HEALTH DISORDERS AMONG ARABS IN ISRAEL

Alean Al-Krenawi

Mental illness in the Arab world bears stigma and is often considered taboo. In fact, a common Arabic term to describe mental illness is *majnun*, which derives from the term *jinn*, defined as a supernatural spirit that unlike the concept of "possession" associated with the Middle Ages, can be either good or evil. It has the power to assume human and animal forms. In other words, although a person may be perceived as being "possessed," this may be by a good or an evil spirit (1).

Nonetheless, the consequences of the stigma often associated with mental illness may be harsh, affecting the marriage ability of relatives and leading to social exclusion and marginalization of individuals with mental illness and of their families. In high-context societies, governed by collectivist rather than Western individualistic principles, the price of social exclusion is particularly high. Thus, mental illness is often concealed – and treatment, if sought, may be limited to the realm of traditional healing. Regarding the recognition and treatment of mental illness, Arab populations living in Western societies are caught between traditional beliefs and Western approaches. In Israel, the situation of the Palestinian Arab minority is especially compounded as a result of their complex and tenuous relationship with the state.

This chapter surveys the historical and current trends of mental illness in the Arab world, in general, and among the Palestinian Arab minority in Israel, in particular. The chapter commences with a review of global psychiatric manifestations and methods in the Arab world, followed by a short historical description of the situation of the Arab sector in Israel. Subsequently, the chapter focuses on Palestinian Arabs in Israel and mental health, including a review of epidemiological studies. Specific highlighted topics include substance abuse, the psychological impact of polygamy and blood vengeance.

✥ Psychiatric manifestations and methods in the Arab world

In the Arab world, somatization – defined as the expression of psychological distress through physical symptoms – is a widespread phenomenon. Somatization shields people coping with emotional or mental problems from the mental illness-related stigma that pervades Arab culture. Indeed, those who do not "pull their weight" need reasonable justification and, since mental distress is culturally unacceptable, many of those suffering from mental distress resort to physical complaints. El-Islam (2) addressed the somatization of mental distress, noting that the most common manifestations include chest and lower-back pain; the latter is often associated with masculinity. A cross-cultural comparison of depression in Egyptian and Western populations found that among Egyptians, somatization and physical symptomatology were prevalent, while mental distress was rare.

In turn, somatization presents one of the foremost "first-filter" challenges facing mental health professionals – that is, to assist patients in recognizing and accepting their mental health problems and seeking appropriate care. To deal with psychological difficulties, people suffering from depression turn to general practitioners – or in some cases to traditional healers. In the Arab world, healers are considered powerful cognitive and social constructions and thus are often favored over general health providers (3, 4). Traditional healers in many Arab societies thus constitute an additional obstacle to receiving appropriate mental health treatment.

Arab families are more involved than their Western counterparts in all aspects of family members' health and illness and demand adherence to the Islamic code of conduct. Those who deviate from this code are referred to mental evaluation by the family's elders, who rid the family of the shame of a rebellious member (2). For example, the emphasis in Egyptian society is on family function, and all members of the family must contribute to the general good.

However, collective social structure as described above may have meaningful mental health advantages. For example, studies show that in developing countries, schizophrenia has a better outcome then in industrialized countries (5). A main factor that may account for this difference is the extended family structure prevalent in developing societies. Research indicates that persons within an extended family structure who have schizophrenia are more likely to accept medical treatment, have social contacts with family members and be accepted by other families despite their occasional odd behaviors. Also, there may be more opportunities for labor for ill people in agricultural settings.

Schizophrenia appears in all cultures and countries but somewhat varies with regard to its manifestations and the nature of symptoms. When comparing differences among Egypt, the US and the UK, researchers found that in Egypt, incongruity of affect was the primary diagnostic symptom for schizophrenia, while in the US, formal thought disorder and delusions were paramount. Reports on disease manifestations in the UK resembled those in Egypt to a greater extent; this similarity may be explained by the predominately British training of Egyptian psychiatrists. In Egypt, delusions tend to focus on religious issues as well as on social and sexual restrictions. A similar trend appears regarding hallucinations – the content in Egypt is primarily religion-based, while in the UK the content tends to be instructional (6).

With regard to treatment settings, Arab countries and the West differ as well. While in Western cultures, day programs are common treatment options for persons with schizophrenia, in Arab countries, the extended family may yield more favorable results (7, 8).

Those differences extend to other domains as well. Many Western tools for psychiatric and psychological evaluations are inappropriate for use with Arab populations. For example, suicide is condemned by Islam, thus questions about suicidal thoughts/intentions may be considered offensive. Analogous problems of cultural adequacy have been reported with regards to screening and diagnostic instruments for children. For example, Thabet *et al.* (9) used the Strengths and

Difficulties Questionnaire (sDQ) developed in UK (10) to examine the mental health profile of Palestinian Arab children living in the Gaza Strip. The authors found that the published factor structure was not entirely appropriate for their samples. Although general factors of conduct, emotional behavior, hyperactivity, and peer-relationship problems were applicable, certain items had different meanings for the Palestinian children than for Western children and their parents, including being unhappy, scared or distracted; stealing; or being picked on or bullied. Emotional problems such as aches, nervousness, clinging and worries were rated differently in preschool subsamples than in samples of previous Western studies. Another difference involves treatment. In many Arab cultures, it is believed that every symptom must be treated with pre-scribed medications and that each medication works exclusively on one symptom. Psychological therapy, such as cognitive behavioral therapy or psychoanalysis, might be rejected altogether if offered independently of pharmacological therapy (26).

✷ Palestinian Arabs in Israel

Since the establishment of the State of Israel in 1948, Palestinian Arabs have experienced op-pression, trauma, social exclusion and related socioeconomic and political problems. Indeed, the Arab term for the events of 1948 is *Al-Nakbah* (Arabic for catastrophe), representing the loss of homeland, the disintegration of society, the frustration of national aspirations and the beginning of a process of cultural disintegration (11). The psychosocial and economic conse-quences of the period were severe: homes, livelihoods and political power were lost, families were displaced and separated and communities were destroyed. *Al-Nakbah* is considered the moment when a part of the Palestinian people became homeless, a predicament associated with a deep sense of insecurity. Accordingly, a house key became a symbol of the former home and the hoped-for return to that home and to normality (11).

Between 1948 and 1966, Palestinian Arabs in Israel lived under military administration. Israeli and world scholars report the continuing traumatic impact of social exclusion (12). Pal-estinian Arabs in Israel find themselves in a difficult and complicated reality. They primarily perceive themselves as Palestinians. Many have first- and second-degree relatives in the oc-cupied territories and most identify nationally and emotionally with the Palestinian people in these territories (13).

By the end of 2007, the Palestinian Arab minority reached slightly over 1.44 million of the total Israeli population of 7.24 million. The Muslim Arabs included slightly over 1.17 million people; the difference was comprised of Christian Arabs, Druze and other small groups (www. cbs.gov.il, accessed July 2008). The vast majority reside in all-Arab towns and villages located in three main areas: the Galilee in the north, the "Triangle" in the center and the border that separates Israel from the West Bank.

Differences exist with regard to the quality of life of Palestinian Arabs and Jews in Israel (14). Over 100 Palestinian Arab villages in Israel lack official government recognition. More than 54,000 Palestinian Arabs, in the south, live in villages under threat of destruction, their development is halted and do not appear on any map (15). Over 66% of Palestinian Arab chil-dren live under the poverty line, compared with 24% of Jewish children (16). A study by aDVA (Center for Information on Equality and Social Justice in Israel) noted that on average, the in-come of Palestinian Arabs in Israel is lower than that of Jewish Israelis. In fact, relative to the average income, proportionally, this income has been declining since 1995 (17).

In May 2001, a conference held at the residence of Israel's president revealed that 42% of Palestinian Arab families in Israel are poor compared to 14% of Jewish families. Despite the achievements of Israel's education system in general, there are great disparities between Palestinian Arabs and Jews with respect to infrastructure, funding allocations, number of pupils per class and academic achievement. Educational funding allocations, as well as other municipal and social services, disproportionately harm Palestinian Arabs in Israel. For instance, of the 50 localities that received the lowest state allocation for education, 41 were Arab-Israeli town or cities (18).

Although the general condition of Palestinian Arabs in Israel is poorer than that of the Jewish population, over the years this sector has enjoyed a better health system and improvements in quality of life. Life expectancy in the Palestinian Arab society has been increasing since 1975, and infant mortality had been decreasing (19) (tables 1 and 2).

Table 1. Life expectancy of Jews and Palestinian Arabs in Israel. Years 1975–2006

Gender	1975		1990		2006	
	Jewish Israelis	Palestinian Arabs in Israel	Jewish Israelis	Palestinian Arabs in Israel	Jewish Israelis	Palestinian Arabs in Israel
Women	74.5	71.5	78.8	75.8	82.7	78.1

Table 2. Infant mortality per every 1000 live births in Jews and Palestinian Arabs in Israel. Years 1980–2006

1980		1990		2006	
Jewish Israelis	Palestinian Arabs in Israel	Jewish Israelis	Palestinian Arabs in Israel	Jewish Israelis	Palestinian Arabs in Israel
12.1	24.4	7.8	14.6	3.1	8.3

Noteworthy, the 10 cities with the lowest infant mortality rates are all Jewish cities, with the exception of the mixed Jewish-Arab city of Akko. In contrast, the 10 Israeli cities with the highest infant mortality rate are home to Palestinian Arabs with a Muslim majority.

A comparison with the neighboring Arab countries shows that infant mortality rates are lower and life expectancy higher among Palestinian Arabs in Israel (table 3) (19).

Table 3. Current life expectancy in years and infant mortality per every 1000 live-births among Palestinian Arabs in Israel and in neighboring Arab countries

Measures	Jordan	Egypt	Lebanon	Syria	Israel
Life expectancy – men	69	66	68	70	74.6
Life expectancy – women	73	70	73	75	78.1
Infant mortality	22	28	27	14	8.3

ᛸ Palestinian Arabs in Israel: mental health

The factors reviewed in the previous section contribute significantly to the social and mental wellbeing of Palestinian Arabs in Israel. In particular, the following psychosocial variables are highlighted: perception of the mental health services as an instrument of social control, mental health problems associated with Arab cultural practices such as polygamy, and economic problems and experiences of social exclusion resulting from the residual political conflict.

Current mental health literature shows that Palestinian Arab service users tend to underutilize health services, in general, and mental health services, in particular (20–22). This health-seeking behavior has been attributed to cultural sensitivity and religious belief, two factors that have substantial influences on Palestinian Arabs' attitudes toward formal mental health services. However, few studies (8, 23–28) examined the mediating factors of individuals' decisions to seek treatment for mental health reasons. A number of barriers that may induce the individual to avoid seeking formal services were observed in these studies. One such barrier is the historical relationship between psychiatry and religion. This relationship has been dubious at best and outright antagonistic at worse. Although there are certain exceptions (higher education and acculturation levels), it is safe to assume that most Palestinian Arabs view mental health in a negative light and, consequently, the utilization of mental health services is relatively rare, particularly for women. The traditional Arab view does not make much distinction among psychiatrists, psychologists or other professionals in the mental health field. All mental health professionals are viewed suspiciously, since such professionals tend to discard religious values and fail to see such values as a "true" source of solace and healing. Within such a context, it is difficult to establish trust (27). Another significant factor found to influence help-seeking behavior is, as noted above, the stigma attached to mental health problems (23, 24, 27). As a result of potential stigma, mental illness is often denied and constitutes a long-term predicament in the Arab individuals' lives, excluding them from professional treatment and intervention.

Authors (e.g., 25) claimed that Arabs tend to deny the existence of mental health problems because they believe the problem will shame their families and harm individual wellbeing within their community. Perhaps, most importantly, there is a political dynamic at play, influencing the intervention process. Palestinian Arabs in Israel have had limited historical exposure to the helping professions. In the case of Palestinian Arabs in Israel, the more extended introduction of helping professional practices coincides with the establishment of the State of Israel – an event viewed by many as yet another example of colonial regimes extending back to the Crusades, the Ottoman Empire, the British Empire and the Egyptian occupation (26).

The past colonial processes have upset social structures, community relations and – indeed – all areas of Arab life. The most recent example of what many perceive along this continuum – the establishment of the State of Israel – may be viewed negatively. Therefore, the mental health systems – funded and usually implemented by state institutions – may be perceived as coercive and unhelpful, despite the implementers' good intentions. To compound the problem, mental health services are frequently unavailable in Palestinian Arab communities, often necessitating travel outside the community (28), further reinforcing feelings of estrangement.

In addition, some studies concluded that the use of non-native practitioners in mental health settings may decrease the individuals' willingness to seek help. In their study in Saudi Arabia, Al-Subaie and Alhamad (25) attributed underutilization to the fact that mental health service practitioners were non-Saudis and did not speak Arabic, a situation that may also mimic the situation in Israel when Arabic-speaking mental health practitioners or cultural mediators are not always available. This induced Arabs with mental distress to more conveniently seek treatment from traditional practitioners who share their identity and speak their language (8, 24).

❧ Epidemiological studies

Studies on the differential causes, triggers, manifestations and treatment of mental health disorders among Palestinian Arabs and Jews in Israel is developing slowly. The following section reviews the existing data (see also chapters: 1, 2, 9–11 and 16).

Depression and anxiety

In 2004, the Ministry of Health conducted a wide-scale national health survey (also reviewed in other chapters) of approximately 5,000 subjects that examined mental health issues such as mood and anxiety disorders end emotional distress. One of the survey's beneficial outputs included the ability to compare prevalence rates of the Jewish and Palestinian Arab populations in Israel (see also chapter 11). Findings indicate that Palestinian Arabs in Israel suffer moderately more from depressive and anxiety disorders than their Jewish counterparts (table 4). Interestingly, while both Palestinian Arab women and men showed higher rates of depression than Jewish women and men, Palestinian Arab men showed higher rates of anxiety disorders than Jewish men, but Palestinian Arab women exhibited lower anxiety rates than Jewish women (29).

Table 4. Arab and Jewish Israelis by any anxiety and any affective disorder or any of the disorders combined (%) (29).

Population groups	n	Any affective disorder* % (95% CI)	Any anxiety disorder** % (95% CI)	Any affective or anxiety disorder** % (95% CI)
Israeli Arabs	659	8.2 (6.2–11.0)	3.3 (2.2–5.0)	11.1 (8.7–14.2)
Men	324	6.2 (3.8–9.4)	3.7 (2.1–6.5)	10.2 (7.0–14.7)
Women	335	10.5 (7.3–14.8)	3.0 (1.5–5.8)	12.0 (8.6–16.7)
Israeli Jews	3332	5.9 (5.1–6.8)	3.2 (2.6–3.9)	9.3 (8.3–10.3)
Men	1662	4.7 (3.8–5.8)	2.8 (2.1–3.8)	8.4 (7.2–9.8)
Women	1670	7.1 (5.9–8.5)	3.6 (2.8–4.6)	10.1 (8.6–11.7)

Overall gender difference: p = .0008. Overall Arab Israelis/Jewish Israelis difference: p = .06
**Overall gender difference: ns. Overall Arab Israelis/Jewish Israelis difference: ns.*

Attempted suicides

A study mapping suicide attempts among Palestinian Arabs and Jews in Israel that was conducted in the emergency room of a hospital in the Galilee found more than twice as many suicide attempts among Palestinian Arabs in Israel (24.4 per 100,000 persons), compared to Jews (11 per 100,000). In addition, suicide attempts among Palestinian Arab men evenly spanned all age groups, whereas among Jewish-Israeli men attempts rose dramatically after the age of 40. Suicide attempts for Jewish-Israeli women rose gradually with age, whereas the rate for Palestinian Arab women peaked in the 20 to 29 age group. The researchers hypothesized that infliction of self-harm among Palestinian Arabs in Israel is more a way to externalize emotions than an actual attempt to end one's life. Along with the delineated differences, it was found that both Jews and Palestinian Arabs use the same methods and locations and have similar numbers of past episodes (30).

Suicide

Among those aged 15 years and older between 1996 and 2000, the suicide rate for Jewish Israelis was 3.2 times higher than for Palestinian Arabs in Israel. This finding may be the result of great adherence in the Arab community in Israel to the Islamic strict prohibition of taking one's life, such an act would interfere with the work of Allah. This could be concluded from several places in the Koran.

Suicide is most common among the population group of young people aged 15 to 24. Nearly 45% of all the suicides committed by Palestinian Arabs in Israel are adolescents, in contrast to the general Israeli population, in which adolescent/young adult suicide stands at 17%. The lowest recorded suicide rates are among Palestinian Arab women, .9 per 100,000, compared to Palestinian Arab men, 4.7, and Jewish women, 3.7 (31) (see chapter 16).

Emotional distress/demoralization

The primary informational source regarding emotional distress (ED) is the General Health Questionnaire (GHQ). The GHQ indicated significantly higher ED levels among Palestinian Arabs in Israel than among their Jewish counterparts (29).

Shemesh *et al.* (31), examining ED scores among Palestinian Arab and Jewish elderly in Israel (aged 60 and over), found that scores were highest among Muslim Arabs, followed by Christian Arabs, Jews and Druze. The authors speculated that the higher ED scores among elderly Palestinian Arabs in Israel were associated with their minority status affiliation, as well as with rapid social transformations. They also entertained the notion that a cultural response style may be a possible explanation. Interestingly, these factors – possibly operating with regard to emotional distress – did not influence the risk of suspected psychopathology since no differential risk was noted after adjustments for confounders.

Post-traumatic stress reactions

A study about the impact of terrorism on Jews and Palestinian Arabs in Israel found that exposure to terrorism was significantly related to post-traumatic stress disorder (PTSD) and depressive symptoms, and that Palestinian Arabs reported significantly higher levels of both, PTSD (M difference = 3.10) and depressive symptoms (M difference = 1.49) than Jews (33).

In another study conducted by researchers from Tel Aviv University, a sample of 148 Palestinian Arab students (aged 19 to 27) completed questionnaires about their past traumatic life experiences and self indication of stress symptoms and stress response. Findings showed that those students were exposed to relatively low levels of terrorism-related traumatic events but to high levels of nationality-related stressful events. In addition, 25% of the students suffered from acute stress disorder, and their levels of psychiatric symptoms exceeded norms for the general population (34). Another study, which considered politically contextualized violence in the Palestinian Authority since the onset of the *Al-Aqsa Intifada* in September 2000, showed an outbreak of PTSD and depression, as well as problems in family functioning and social exclusion. Family functioning was found to be significantly compromised, and individuals experienced psychological trauma, depression, social exclusion and economic deprivation. The authors concluded that while mental health therapy was pursued in the cases studied, the political arena is the ultimate source for the resolution of these issues (35, 36).

Substance abuse

A number of studies (see chapters 8, 9 and 10) examined substance abuse from varying perspectives. In a study examining the relation between binge drinking and socioeconomic status (SES) among Jewish and Palestinian Arab adults in Israel (aged 18 to 40), the prevalence of binge drinking was highest among Arab men (21.4%), followed by Jewish men (15.2%), Arab women (7.3%) and Jewish women (4.0%) (37). SES was assessed using education, household income and occupation. A positive correlation was found between household income and occupation to binge drinking for Palestinian Arab men and women, while the opposite correlation was found for Jews. Researchers submitted that religion and religiosity are the main reason for these results, explaining that Jewish culture encourages controlled alcohol consumption on defined occasions, while in Islamic culture, alcohol drinking is completely prohibited. Therefore, alcohol is not as common or easy for Palestinian Muslim Arabs in Israel to purchase. Also, researchers believed that Palestinian Arabs in Israel with higher SES tend to drink more because they are more exposed to cultural norms outside of their community and might drink in excess due to the absence of social drinking norms (37).

A study of substance abuse and violence among Jewish and Palestinian Arab sixth- to tenth-grade pupils in Israel found that daily smoking, illicit drug abuse, history of drunkenness and binge drinking were the best predictors of violent behavior, across age, gender and ethnicity. It was also found that girls, especially Palestinian Arab, were more likely to participate in violent behavior due to substance use compared with boys, even though they were less likely to use such drugs in general (38).

In a study mapping the reasons for not drinking alcohol that was conducted among four different religious groups of adolescents in Israel – Jews, Muslims, Druze and Christians – it was found that for Muslims and Druze, religion comprised the main reason for not consuming alcohol (about 19% of participants gave "religious intolerances of alcohol use" when citing one reason for not drinking alcohol). This finding was consistent across ages in both groups. An interesting finding was the second reason given by the respondents (approximately 19%) that drinking alcohol harms health (39). A different study conducted among Palestinian Arab adolescents in Israel regarding similar topics found that although religion plays a role in limiting alcohol consumption, it has little effect on substance abuse. Not surprisingly, the highest rates of illicit substance abuse was found among adolescents whose degree of religiosity was very low, but high rates of substance abuse were also found among adolescents whose degree of religiosity was very high. The authors explained these results by pointing to the stronger influence of peers and the social environment compared to the influence of religion or parents on illicit drug use and abuse (40).

A number of studies conducted in different Palestinian Arab communities in Israel found that drug and alcohol consumption was associated with various psychosocial factors such as being male, having a tolerant attitude toward drug use, perceiving drugs as not dangerous, being secular, having low family cohesion and showing either low or high family adaptability (40, 41).

In a study examining the prevalence rates of substance abuse among Bedouin adults and adolescents in Israel, it was found that 14% consumed alcohol and 11.1% used illicit drugs (41). Alcohol consumption was found to be lower among the Bedouin than the Jewish-Israeli population – once again, probably due to the Islamic prohibitions on alcohol use. Substance abuse among adults stood at a rate similar to that of the general Israeli population. Specific drugs – such as narcotics and hallucinogens – were found to be used among Bedouin Arab adults at a rate twice higher than that of the general population. Among adolescents, the numbers were much higher than among adults; 21.9% of adolescents consumed alcohol and 20.4% used illicit drugs during the past year. Substance abuse rates among Bedouin Arab adolescents were recorded as more than double that of the same age group in the general Israeli population. In addition, the findings showed that Bedouin adolescents used specific drugs at rates three to eight times higher than their Jewish counterparts. General substance abuse was found to be higher among adolescents who attended school compared to those who dropped out, and the use of specific drugs such as narcotics and hallucinogens, was found to be 2.5 times higher than the rate of usage among the same age group who dropped out of school (table 5). These findings contrast with findings regarding other Israeli populations that showed higher substance abuse rates among those who dropped out of school. Researchers believe that higher parental monitoring and involvement in the child's life as well as the child involvement in productive activities that relate to agricultural and family responsibilities explain the lower rates of drug use among adolescents who dropped out of school (41).

Table 5. Past year prevalence rates (%) of use of substances among Bedouin adolescents by school status (41)

Type of drug	Students n = 295	School drop outs n = 145	Total N = 440
Any alcohol	23.3	20.5	21.9
Wine	17.4	13.7	15.5
Beer	18.3	15.7	17.0
Liquor	19.0	13.7	16.3
Any drugs	27.7	13.1	20.4
Prescribed medications	19.6	10.7	15.2
Sleeping pills/sedatives	15.5	9.4	12.5
speed	16.4	5.8	11.1
Cannabis	18.0	12.7	15.4
Hashish	16.4	10.7	13.5
Marijuana	16.4	9.2	12.8
Other drugs	25.4	9.9	17.6
Methadone	17.8	7.0	12.4
Heroin/opium	16.9	5.6	11.3
Cocaine	15.8	5.6	10.7
Crack	15.9	3.7	9.8
LSD	16.4	7.0	11.7
Ecstasy	15.9	5.5	10.7
PCP/Poppers	14.0	3.3	8.7

Furthermore, Bedouin Arabs living in recognized settlements showed higher substance abuse rates than those residing in unrecognized traditional agrarian villages; a fact that may be attributed to the stress, family and social disintegration, as well as unemployment involved in the transition from a rural to an urban lifestyle (41).

In a study conducted among the general Palestinian Arab school population in Israel (ages 12 to 18), alcohol and drug consumption rates were significantly lower among Palestinian Arabs who were not Bedouins than among Bedouin Arab adolescents. This study also found that children of well-educated parents used alcohol at higher rates than those whose parents had a high school education or less. The authors explained this as being the result of the poor returns that many Palestinian Arabs in Israel obtain for an academic education and the economic hardship that parents have to contend with despite their academic education (40).

✿ Psychological impact of polygamy and blood vengeance in the Arab world

Arab society in Israel has a few internal cultural characteristics that may impact on the mental health of its members, in addition to the external factors alluded earlier.

Arab culture has a long history and brings with it many ancient customs and traditions. Many of these do clash with some of the values of the State of Israel, which supports modernity and a connection to the Western world. In this context, two traditional Arabic customs – polygamy and blood vengeance – still practiced by some Palestinian Arabs in Israel, particularly of the Muslim faith, are major risk factors to the mental health of the individuals living in the shadow of these traditions.

Polygamy

Al-Krenawi and Slonim-Nevo (42) examined the impact of polygamous marriage on the psychological, social and educational functioning of Bedouin Arab children, mothers and husbands in the south of Israel. Palestinian Arab society in Israel is comprised of various ethnic and religious subgroups, among them Bedouin Arabs. This group differs on account of mutual traditions, history and family affiliation. Bedouin refers to all the nomadic tribes of the Middle East and North Africa. Bedouins not only boast a specific lifestyle but also adhere to a social organization and values that differentiate the Bedouin from city dwellers and agrarians.

Findings demonstrated that children from polygamous families show more mental health problems and social difficulties than their peers from monogamous families; they also exhibit lower academic achievement and more problematic relationships with their fathers. Similarly, women in polygamous families present with more mental health problems than wives in monogamous families. In addition, men with more than one wife exhibit more mental health problems than their peers in monogamous relationships. A later study identified a number of different ways and techniques that enable family members to come to grips with polygamy, thus improving family functioning. Among these are acceptance of polygamy as God's wish or destiny, equal allocation of resources among both families by the husband, separation between the two households, avoidance of "minor" conflicts and disagreements, maintaining respect for the other wife and allowing open communication among all siblings and among children and the other mother.

Blood vengeance

Blood vengeance is deeply rooted in Arab culture (as illustrated by the saying "blood can be erased only by blood") and still exists in the Arab world today. Examples include several killings in the Negev and central regions of Israel, Jordan, the Gaza Strip and the West Bank (43). In the Arab world, revenge is considered a person's right and duty. Vengeance is a means of restoring symmetry to a social exchange that has become unbalanced through an act of murder (44). Blood vengeance is not regarded as an individual matter that a person undertakes on his own or for emotional or other personal reasons. Rather, it is viewed as a collective guarantee provided by the group to all its members (45).

A study about vengeance was conducted at the Juarish elementary school in the city of

Ramle. This particular school was selected because of the ongoing stress that the children faced over the decade prior to the study and the fact that most of the children belong to one of the feuding *hamulas* (Arabic for extended families). The study participants demonstrated higher levels of distress and symptomatic behavior as compared to the Israeli norms. Girls reported higher anxiety levels than the boys, who were more willing to continue the feud of blood vengeance. The symptoms among the Juarish adolescents were similar to those observed among children and adolescents exposed to warfare, thereby indicating the massive adverse psychological affects of exposure to the ongoing blood feud on children and adolescents (46).

֍ From epidemiology to mental health action

Examining the historical and current trends of mental illness in the Arab world, in general and among the Palestinian Arab minority in Israel in particular, yields a number of important conclusions. On a general level, the subject of mental illness among Arabs – both those living in Arab societies and those residing in Western nations – is stigma-laden and taboo. Thus, Arabs tend not to seek the assistance of Western-based psychological and psychiatric approaches to mental illness and may either conceal the situation or turn to traditional healers for help.

The situation in Israel is particularly complex and tenuous as a result of the unique status of Arabs in Israel as noted earlier. The Palestinian Arab population in Israel has since the inception of the state been undergoing a process of rapid transformation. The Palestinian Arab population in Israel enjoys various benefits of Western society including lower infant mortality rates, higher education levels and longer life spans. However, on the other hand, its situation is significantly worse then that of the Jewish population with regard to every realm (socioeconomic, education, health and welfare).

This complex predicament coupled with the characteristics of general Arab culture as described in this chapter have numerous ramifications on the mental wellbeing of Palestinian Arabs in Israel and on the way mental illness is manifested and treated.

How Palestinian Arabs in Israel understand and relate to mental health, including their help-seeking practices, brings to light the need for culturally appropriate interventions. The majority of treatment options available to Palestinian Arabs in Israel are not suitable to meeting the unique requirements of this population. First, while the Israeli establishment offers an array of Western treatment practices for mental distress and mental illness, Palestinian Arabs in Israel are faced with accessibility issues due, in part, to geographical limitations but also – and more importantly – to both externally and internally imposed cultural limitations. Among such cultural limitations are the fear of social stigma that accompanies those suffering from mental health disorders in the Arab world, the negative perception of mental health issues and mental health professionals stemming from the Islamic religion and the biased perception that the mental health system and helping professionals are part of a grand scheme to perpetuate the State of Israel's control over its Arab citizens. Second, the programs and treatment options that exist today are not suited to the special needs of the Palestinian Arab population in Israel. Risk factors such as polygamy and blood vengeance are not taken into account. In addition, issues such as substance abuse or anxiety and emotional distress that are prevalent in the community are not sufficiently addressed.

The complex situation of the Palestinian Arab minority in Israel calls for modifications, adaptations and the revamping of programs by institutions that provide mental health support in these communities. First, in light of the dire poverty plaguing this society, persistent levels of inadequate education and the growing prevalence of certain mental disorders, larger resources should be allocated to guarantee that mental health programs and institutions become available to the Arab-Israeli community. Also adequate resources should be allocated towards education campaigns for reducing widespread ignorance about mental disease and the stigma placed on those contending with mental illness and their families.

Reducing stigma and taboo will undoubtedly increase treatment-seeking rates. Second, treatment options should be tailored to suit the Arab community. New intervention models should be implemented that take in to consideration the special characteristics of this population such as the influences of polygamy and blood vengeance or the greater need for discretion (so that the patients may avoid the stigma associated with mental illness). In fact, the entire therapeutic approach needs to be reevaluated. One fundamental question that needs to be asked involves the ethnic, cultural and professional characteristics of the treating professional. Currently, most of the helping professionals working with the Arab population are Jewish Israelis, some of whom are not trained with regard to the life realities of the patient. Furthermore, many Palestinian Arabs in Israel have limited day-to-day contact with Jews and are thus uncomfortable with a Jewish therapist. Admittedly, having a Palestinian Arab therapist does not automatically guarantee greater understanding of or consideration for the Arab patient. Therefore, one of the most urgent issues to be contended with in the field of mental health services for the Palestinian Arab community in Israel involves the training of helping professionals in accordance with the community's comprehensive needs. Such culturally tailored modification in the current status will greatly improve the possibilities of truly helping to mitigate the suffering of those in need.

✸ References

1. Okasha, A. History of mental health in the Arab world. In: Okasha A, Maj M, eds. *Images in psychiatry: an Arab perspective.* Cairo: Scientific Book House, 2001.
2. El-Islam MF. Social psychiatry and the impact of religion. In: Okasha A, Maj M, eds. *Images in psychiatry: an Arab perspective.* Cairo: Scientific Book House, 2001.
3. Okasha A. Mental health services in the Arab world. *Arab Studies Quarterly* 2003; 25: 39–52.
4. Al-Krenawi A, Graham JR, Dean YZ, *et al.* Cross-national study of attitudes toward seeking professional help: Jordan, United Arab Emirates (UAE) and Arabs in Israel. *International Journal of Social Psychiatry* 2004; 50: 102–114.
5. Hopper K, Harrison G, Janca A, *et al.*, eds. *Recovery from schizophrenia: an international perspective.* New York: Oxford University Press, 2007.
6. Okasha, A. Mental health in Egypt. *Israel Journal of Psychiatry and Related Sciences* 2005; 42: 116–125.
7. Khalil AH. Schizophrenia across Arab culture. In: Okasha A, Maj M, eds. *Images in psychiatry: an Arab perspective.* Cairo: Scientific Book House, 2001.
8. Al-Krenawi, A. Mental health practice in Arab countries. *Current Opinion in Psychiatry* 2005; 18: 560–565.
9. Thabet AA, Stretch D, Vostanis P. Child mental health problems in Arab children: application of the strengths and difficulties questionnaire. *International Journal of Social Psychiatry* 2000; 46: 266–280.
10. Goodman R. The Strengths and Difficulties Questionnaire: a research note. *Journal of Child Psychology and Psychiatry* 1997; 38:581–586.
11. Sa'di AH. Catastrophe, memory and identity: *Al-Nakbah* as a component of Palestinian identity. *Israel Studies* 2002; 7: 175–198.
12. Ghanem A. State and minority in Israel: the case of ethnic state and the predicament of its minority. *Ethnic and Racial Studies* 1998; 21: 428–447.
13. Ruhana N. *Palestinian citizens in an ethnic Jewish state: identities in conflict.* New Haven: Yale, 1997.
14. Government of Israel. State Comptroller's Report, No. 52B, 2002. [cited August 1, 2003]. Available from URL: http://www.mevaker.gov.il.
15. Government of Israel. Central Bureau of Statistics. *Statistical abstract of Israel 2006*, No. 58. Jerusalem: Central Bureau of Statistics, 2007.
16. National Insurance Institute of Israel. *Annual survey: poverty and inequality.* Appendix. 2007. Available from URL: http://www.btl.gov.il.

17. Swirski S, Konor-Attias E. *Israel: a social report 2001* [online]. [cited August 1, 2003]. Available from URL: http://www.adva.org/englishd.html.

18. Government of Israel. State Comptroller's Report, 1997 No. 48, p. 319 [online]. [cited August 1, 2003]. Available from URL: http://www.mevaker.gov.il.

19. Government of Israel. Central Bureau of Statistics, *Statistical abstract of Israel*, 2006 Tables No. 3.22, 3.25, 3.30 [cited August 1, 2003]. Available from URL: http://www.cbs.gov.il.

20. Al-Krenawi A, Graham RJ. Gender and biomedical/traditional mental health utilization among the Bedouin Arabs of the Negev. *Culture, Medicine and Psychiatry* 1999; 23: 219–243.

21. Savaya R. The under-use of psychological services by Israeli Arabs: an examination of the roles of negative attitudes and the use of alternative sources of help. *International Social Work* 1995; 41: 195–209.

22. Al-Krenawi A, Graham JR, Ophir M, et al. Ethnic and gender differences in mental health utilization: the case of Muslim Jordanian and Moroccan Jewish Israeli out-patient psychiatric patients. *International Journal of Social Psychiatry* 2001; 47: 42–54.

23. Al-Krenawi A, Graham JR. Culturally-sensitive social work practice with Arab clients in mental health settings. *Health Social Work* 2000; 25: 9–22.

24. Al-Krenawi A. Explanation of mental health symptoms by the Bedouin Arabs of the Negev. *International Journal of Social Psychiatry* 1999; 45: 56–64.

25. Al-Subaie A, Alhamad A. Psychiatry in Saudi Arabia. In: Al-Issa I, ed. *Al-Junun: mental illness in the Islamic world.* Madison, CT: International Universities, 2000.

26. Barakat H. *The Arab world: society, culture, and state.* Los Angeles: University of California, 1993.

27. Savaya R. The under-use of psychological services by Israeli Arabs: an examination of the roles of negative attitudes and the use of alternative sources of help. *International Social Work* 1995; 41: 195–209.

28. Savaya R. Political attitudes, economic distress, and the utilization of welfare services by Arab women in Israel. *Journal of Applied Social Sciences* 1997; 21: 111–121.

29. Levav I, Al-Krenawi A, Ifrah A, et al. Common mental disorders among Arab-Israelis: findings from the Israel National Health Survey. *Israel Journal of Psychiatry and Related Sciences* 2007; 44: 104–113.

30. Ashkar K, Giloni C, Grinshpoon A, et al. Suicidal attempts admitted to a general hospital in the Western Galilee: an inter-ethnic comparison study. *Israel Journal of Psychiatry and Related Sciences* 2006; 43: 137–145.

31. Ministry of Health, Department of Information. *Suicide in Israel.* Jerusalem: Ministry of Health, 2006.

32. Shemesh AA, Kohn R, Blumstein T, et al. A community study on emotional distress among Arab and Jewish Israelis over the age of 60. *International Journal of Geriatric Psychiatry* 2005; 21: 64–76.

33. Hobfoll SE, Canetti ND, Johnson RJ. Exposure to terrorism, stress related mental health symptoms, and defensive coping among Jews and Arabs in Israel. *Journal of Consulting and Clinical Psychology* 2006; 74: 207–218.

34. Msallam N, Ginzburg K, Lev-Shalem L, et al. The psychological effects of *Intifada Al Aqsa*: acute stress disorder and distress in Palestinian-Israeli students. *Israel Journal of Psychiatry and Related Sciences* 2005; 42: 96–105.

35. Al-Krenawi A, Graham JR, Sehwail M. Mental health and violence/trauma in Palestine: implications for helping professional practice. *Journal of Comparative Family Studies* 2004; 35: 185–209.

36. Al-Krenawi A, Lev-Wiesel R, Sehwail MA. Psychological symptomatology among Palestinian adolescents living with political violence. *Child and Adolescent Mental Health Journal* 2007; 12: 27–31.

37. Neumark YD, Rahav G, Jaffe DH. Socioeconomic status and binge drinking in Israel. *Drug and Alcohol Dependence* 2003; 69: 15–21.

38. Molcho M, Harel Y, Dina LO. Substance use and youth violence. A study among sixth to tenth grade Israeli school children. *International Journal on Adolescents* 2004; 16: 239–251.

39. Moorea M, Weiss S. Reasons for non-drinking among Israeli adolescents of four religions. *Drug and Alcohol Dependence* 1995; 38: 45–50.

40. Azaiza F, Bar-Hamburger R, Moran M. Psychoactive substance use among Arab adolescents at Israel. *Journal of Social Work Practice in Addictions* 2008; 8: 21–43.

41. Diamond GM, Farhat A, Al-Amor M, et al. Drug and alcohol use among the Bedouin of the Negev: prevalence and psychosocial correlates. *Addictive Behaviors* 2008; 33: 143–151.

42. Al-Krenawi A, Slonim-Nevo V. Mental health aspects of Arab-Israeli adolescents from polygamous versus monogamous families. *Journal of Social Psychology* 2002; 142: 446–460.

43. Al-Munjed. *Arabic dictionary.* Beirut: Daar El-Mashreq Publishers, 1975 (Arabic).

44. Rieder J. The social organization of vengeance. In: Donald B, ed. *Toward a general theory of social control: fundamentals.* Toronto: Academic Press, 1984.

45. Jabbur JS. *The Bedouins and the desert: aspects of nomadic life in the Arab east.* New York: State University of New York Press, 1995.

46. Al-Krenawi A, Slonim-Nevo V, Maymon Y, et al. Psychological responses to blood vengeance among Arab adolescents. *Child Abuse and Neglect* 2001; 25: 457–472.

Chapter 6

THE EPIDEMIOLOGY OF MENTAL HEALTH
PROBLEMS AMONG IMMIGRANTS IN ISRAEL

Julia Mirsky

Five decades of research into the association between migration and mental health has yielded two contrasting hypotheses. The classical acculturation-stress hypothesis (also known as migration-morbidity hypothesis) maintains that migration, particularly from one country to another, causes distress because it disrupts family and other support networks; exposes the migrant to an unfamiliar environment and, at times, to prejudice and discrimination; and may lead to low socioeconomic status. Consequently, the migration-morbidity hypothesis predicts, at least at the beginning of the process, a greater risk for mental health problems among immigrants compared to nonimmigrants (1). Numerous findings support this hypothesis (2–4). In contrast, the selection hypothesis – or the healthy-immigrant hypothesis – states that healthier (and younger and better-educated) individuals are more likely to emigrate from their homeland (5). These immigrants are strongly motivated to cope with the hardships of transition, including the experience of unemployment, underemployment and poverty. Their expectation that these difficulties will be finally overcome may act as a protective factor (6). This hypothesis predicts equal or lower risk for mental health problems among immigrant compared to nonimmigrants. As earlier, also this hypothesis is supported by numerous research findings (5, 7, 8).

A strict research model for testing these hypotheses calls for a comparison of the mental health of immigrants to that of a cohort of nonimmigrants in their country of origin. Understandably, those comparative data are often unavailable. In addition, the migration-morbidity hypothesis calls for a longitudinal research design that is not only complex and costly but often unfeasible due to the high mobility of immigrants in the initial stages of their resettlement. Because of these constraints, the majority of studies compare the mental health of immigrants to that of nonimmigrants in their host country. Obviously, these two populations may differ not only in the migration experience, but in many other variables (for example, in coping assets such as networking or sense of mastery in their native society). This may partly account for the inconsistency in research findings.

❧ Immigration to Israel

A number of attributes of the Israeli context make it possible for local studies to add substantial insight to the research on migration and mental health. First, immigration policies grant every Jew the right to immigrate to the land settled by his/her ancestors and to become a citizen immediately. This policy creates a population of immigrants with various subgroups that may not be accessible for research in countries that enforce selective immigration policies.

Second, upon entering the country, immigrants are registered in the Population Registry of the Ministry of Interior. To secure the benefits they are entitled to receive early in their absorption process – a period that varies according to the various privileges available such as housing, education and Hebrew-language-study benefits, immigrants must keep their registration updated. The Population Registry and the relatively small size (about 7.5 million people) and close-knit nature of the Israeli society make it easier than in other counties to trace immigrants in follow-up studies.

Third, since 1989 over one million immigrants from the former Soviet Union (FSU) arrived in Israel (9). Their large numbers offer unique opportunities for epidemiological and other types of studies.

Fourth, a national psychiatric case register (PCR), which maintains records of all admissions and discharges to inpatient and day hospital services, provides important information on psychiatric disorders in the general population (10). In addition to this unique database on persons with psychiatric disorders, the Israel National Health Survey (INHS) was carried out in 2002–2003. The INHS constitutes the first countrywide study designed to estimate the true prevalence rates of common mental disorders and psychological distress in the adult population.

INHS, reviewed in other chapters with regard to mental and behavioral disorders in different populations, also included an immigrant subsample. Importantly, this study was carried out in conjunction with the World Mental Health (WMH) Survey (11), which included 27 countries – thus it offers an invaluable opportunity for cross-national comparisons.

This chapter primarily reviews Israeli epidemiological studies, emphasizing the local contribution to the subject of immigrants' mental health. Initially, it will address findings on the prevalence rates of psychological distress and psychiatric morbidity. Subsequently, it will address a number of risk factors that have been identified among immigrants.

❧ Early studies on Western and Oriental immigrants

Most of the early studies included immigrants from Europe or Western countries, Africa (generally, North Africa) and Asia. The studies were of a clinical type or based on psychiatric hospitalizations. They did not rely on representative samples or advanced screening and diagnostic procedures (12). Given their research limitations, their findings were inconsistent.

The studies reported higher rates of mental illness among immigrants compared to the native born (13, 14). Yet, in one study, the highest rate of schizophrenia was found among native-born Israelis as compared to both Western and Oriental immigrants (15). Higher rates of mental illness were typically found among Oriental than among Western immigrants (13, 14). Only one study reported reversed results (16). Oriental immigrants were found more likely to show schizophrenia (14, 17) and alcohol-related problems (18), while Western immigrants were more likely to suffer from mood disorders – specifically depression (17), bipolar disorders (19) and suicide (20).

Despite their methodological limitations, those early studies brought attention to the possible differences in mental health status between the more affluent immigrants from Europe and other Western countries and the more socioeconomically and educationally disadvantaged Oriental immigrants. A later study that compared second-generation immigrants in these two large groups using more advanced research methods and instruments shed light on a classical epidemiological issue – the social causation versus the social selection explanations in the etiology of certain psychiatric disorders. The results of this study (also reviewed in chapters 11 and 14) indicated that social selection factors may be more important for schizophrenia, while social causation factors may be more important for depression in women and antisocial personality and substance use disorders in men (21).

❧ Recent studies on immigrants from the former Soviet Union

Starting from the mid 1980s, the majority of studies focused on immigrants from the FSU. Over one million immigrants arrived in Israel from the FSU since 1989; they now comprise over 14% of the general population (9). These circumstances created unique research opportunities as well as drawbacks. Due to the large numbers, it was possible to study adequate samples as well as subgroups that are typically underrepresented among immigrants (for example, unaccompanied minor immigrants) (22). The nature of emigration from the FSU presents exceptional opportunities for the study of one ethnic group of immigrants in different host environments, as large numbers of FSU residents have settled in different countries such as the US and Germany. At the same time, the focus on one ethnic group imposes limits to generalizations, since culture-specific factors may affect its psychological reactions. In the case of FSU immigrants, there is evidence for cultural specificity, such as more stigmatic views of psychiatric disorders and avoidance of seeking help from mental health professionals – presumably determined by their previous life under a totalitarian regime (23–25). The following review is presented here while keeping these advantages and limitations in mind.

Psychological distress

The first psychiatric epidemiological study of immigrants in Israel that relied on rigorous sampling procedures and applied advanced screening and diagnostic instruments was conducted between the years 1983 and 1985. The nationally representative sample in this study included 273 immigrants from the former Soviet Union who arrived in the country between 1972 and 1984. Respondents were assessed with the demoralization subscale of the Psychiatric Epidemiologic Research Interview (PERI-D) (26). This study, like many others that followed, focused primarily on psychological distress and not on discrete psychiatric disorders. It found a significantly higher level of psychological distress (anxiety, depression and somatization symptoms) in the immigrant sample as compared to a matched subsample of non-immigrant respondents, immigrants' PERI-D mean scores ranged from 1.1 to 1.2 while Israeli respondents scores (N = 2455) ranged from .8 to 1.0 (26). This study was replicated in 1990 with a nationally representative sample of 600 immigrants who arrived between 1989 and 1990. Higher scores of psychological distress were also found in this sample compared to an Israeli sample, immigrant men's PERI-D M score = 1.0, SD = .1 compared to Israeli men's (n = 1139) M score = .8, SD = .1. Immigrant women's M score = 1.3, SD = .1 compared to Israeli women's (n = 1216) M score = 1.0, SD = .6 (27). In 1995, a follow-up study was conducted on this sample, and similarly elevated scores of psychological distress were found; immigrant men's PERI-D *M* score = 1.1, *SD* .6; women's *M* score = 1.4, *SD* .7 (28).

Finally, the INHS, which included a subsample of 844 FSU immigrants who arrived in the country since 1989, identified significantly higher level of psychological distress in this population group (12-GHQ men's *M* score = 20.1, *SE* = .03; women's *M* score = 22.5, *SE* = .05), compared with the Israeli-born Jewish population (12-GHQ men's *M* score = 16.9, *SE* = .06; women's *M* score = 18.5, *SE* .05) (29).

Several other studies have focused on FSU immigrants in Israel using standard screening instruments and based on large community samples. Although none of them included representative samples, their findings corroborate those of the above-mentioned epidemiological studies. They all indicate higher psychological distress in immigrant samples than among their Jewish-Israeli counterparts. For example, statistically significant higher psychological distress was found in a sample of 560 immigrant university students than among their Israeli-born peers (Brief Symptom Inventory (BSI) *M* scores among immigrant: males = .8, *SD* = .5; females = 1.0, *SD* = .5; Israeli-born males = .7, *SD* = .6; females = .8, *SD* = .5) (30). In a sample of 376 elderly immigrants and 392 nonimmigrants, negatively significant differences were found regarding hopelessness, helplessness and depression among immigrants compared to nonimmigrants (31). Also, in a telephone survey of a random sample of 760 immigrant and nonimmigrants adult females, 52% of immigrants reported depressive symptoms in contrast to 38% among nonimmigrants (32). A number of other studies also identified elevated levels of psychological distress among immigrants (33–39). Additional support for these findings comes from studies of other manifestations of psychological ill-feelings among immigrants, such as lower quality of life (40), high level of alcohol-related symptoms (41,42), and suicide ideation (39).

Psychiatric disorders

As noted above, prior to the recent INHS findings, data on psychiatric disorders among immigrants were based on the national psychiatric hospitalization case register. FSU immigrants were reported to show slightly higher rates of hospitalization compared to the general Jewish-Israeli population: for example, .35 per 1,000 residents compared to .24 per 1,000 for the year 1990 (43).

Initially, a relatively high hospitalization rate of immigrants was found among first hospitalizations. Most first hospitalizations took place closer to arrival, which may be an indication of the effect of social-cultural stresses, or of the existence of premigration psychopathology. The rate of immigrants among first hospitalizations decreased steadily over the years, while their rate among repeated hospitalizations increased thus identifying a group with chronic mental disorders (Y. Lerner, personal communication).

Findings from the INHS indicate higher prevalence rates of psychiatric morbidity in the community among FSU immigrants compared to native-born Jewish Israelis. This study was based on a nationally representative sample that included 884 first-generation immigrants from the FSU. The study applied the WMH survey version of the Composite International Diagnostic Interview (CIDI) (11) and assessed anxiety, mood and substance abuse disorders. Prevalence estimates were determined by whether respondents' past or current symptoms met the 12 month – and/or lifetime – diagnostic criteria for disorders listed in the *Diagnostic and Statistical Manual of Mental Disorders – Fourth Edition* (DSM-IV).

Statistically significant higher 12-month prevalence rates of common psychiatric disorders were found among the immigrants in contrast to the native-born population. Immigrants were almost one-and-a-half times more likely than the Israeli born to suffer from any disorder (men: immigrants, 9.5% vs. Israeli born, 8.7% OR = 1.4, 95% CI 1.1–1.3; and women: immigrants, 12.5% vs. Israeli born, 9.5% OR = 1.4, 95% CI 1.3–1.5). Immigrant men were one-and-a-half times more likely than Israeli-born men to suffer from mood disorders (immigrants, 5.6% vs. Israeli born, 4.4% OR = 1.6, 95% CI 1.4–1.7). Similarly for immigrant women, although the odds ratio was slightly lower than among men (immigrants, 8.6% vs. Israeli born, 7.2% OR = 1.2, 95% CI 1.1–1.3). Immigrant women were one-and-a-half times more likely than Israeli-born women to suffer from anxiety disorders (4.8% vs. 3.0% OR = 1.5, 95% CI 1.3–1.7), while among men, the prevalence rate of anxiety disorders was higher for the Israeli born; immigrants .9% vs. Israeli born 2.9% (OR = .4, 95% CI .3–.5) (29).

A recent, but still unpublished study (44), based on the psychiatric case register found higher incidence rates of schizophrenia among immigrants from all countries than among native-born Jewish Israelis. The more disadvantaged Oriental immigrants had higher incidence rates than the more advantaged Western immigrants. Also, higher rates of schizophrenia were found in the first as compared to the second generation of immigrants. These findings showed an association between migration and schizophrenia and the role of social causation in this link.

In light of the association between immigration and psychiatric morbidity, it is surprising that a later age of first hospitalization was found among immigrants from all countries compared to native-born Israelis (25, 44). This delayed effect of immigration on the age of first admission was not found among second-generation immigrants (25). The most likely explanation is that immigrants may be reluctant to seek mental health help and may be underdiagnosed because culturally sensitive mental health services are not always available. This cultural barrier hindering help-seeking is not relevant for second-generation immigrants who are both more socially integrated and identified with the prevailing mental health beliefs systems.

ᔐ Risk factors for psychological distress

The mental health of immigrants may be affected by numerous objective variables like life events (28) and subjective experiences such as identification with the host society (45) as well as by demographic characteristics and pre- and post-migration factors. This section addresses the most widely researched risk factors for immigrant mental health in Israel: gender, age, premigration traumatization, postmigration social networks and the length of residence in the country.

Gender

As in most epidemiological studies, immigrant women – like the native born – in Israel also report higher psychological distress than men (27, 36, 38). Different stressors and protective factors appear to affect the mental health of immigrant men and women. For example, women's psychological distress was found to be more affected by psychosocial factors such as family problems, while men's wellbeing was more affected by employment problems (34, 37). Like in many foreign studies, it remains unclear whether the fact that women report higher psychological distress reflects their higher vulnerability or their higher readiness to admit psychological distress and to seek help.

Age

A positive association was found between age and psychiatric disorders in a study of a representative sample of 140 FSU immigrants assessed with the World Health Organization's Composite International Diagnostic Interview (CIDI-S, a short version of the CIDI). The 12- month prevalence rate of any psychiatric disorder among immigrants under the age of 65 was 7.0%, while for immigrants over the age of 65 this rate was double, 14.8% (46). Age-specific negative effects of migration were also found in this study. Before immigration, yearly incidence rates of affective disorders were lower for older than for younger adults: ages 18–39, .2%; ages 40–65, .1%; ages 65 and older, .0% – a finding consistent with the literature. After immigration, however, higher yearly incidence rates of affective disorders were found among older as compared to younger adults: ages 18–39, .5%; ages 40–65, 1%; and ages 65 and older, 1.3% (46). An increase in psychological distress scores was found among immigrants over the age of 65 five years after migration (PERI-Demoralization M scores males, baseline = 1.1, SD = .6; after five years = 1.3, SD = .6; females baseline = 1.3, SD = .6; after five years = 1.6, SD = .7). In the younger age group, psychological distress remained at its baseline level (28). Other studies support these findings (47). The elderly immigrants were also found to be more distressed than the non-immigrant elderly (31). Poor physical health or chronic illnesses were found to be correlated with psychological distress. Therefore, it is possible that it is not age *per se* that is the risk factor in migration, but rather the health status of elderly immigrants (28, 46).

Contrary to the popular belief that the transitions of migration are easier on children and adolescents, research findings indicate that immigrant adolescents suffer higher psychological distress than do their native-born peers. For example, higher statistically significant Brief Symptom Inventory (BSI) M scores were found in a sample of 560 immigrant adolescents as compared to a general sample of 840 Jewish adolescents (male adolescent immigrants = .8, SD = .4; female adolescents = 1.0, SD = .5; male non-immigrant adolescents = .7, SD = .5; female adolescents = .8, SD = .5) (30). Other studies support these findings (48, 49). Noteworthy, elevated psychological distress was found not only in first-generation immigrant adolescents but also in the second generation. Adolescents also express their distress as impairment of functioning and in antisocial behavior. Indeed, the rates of school dropout are much higher among immigrant adolescents than among their native-born peers. For example, in the 2006–2007 school years, the dropout rate among immigrant pupils in seventh grade was 3%, while among non-immigrant pupils it was 1.0%. Dropout rates in eighth grade were 5% and 2%, and in tenth grade – 8% and 3% respectively (50). Immigrant adolescents are also overrepresented among juvenile delinquents. For example, in 2005 immigrants constituted 10.6% of all children and adolescents in Israel, but 18% of the male and 29% of the female minors were suspected in criminal cases (50). Studies from other countries suggest these are universal phenomena (51, 52).

⸆ Previous traumatization: the Chernobyl nuclear reactor accident

For many FSU immigrants, the 1986 nuclear reactor accident in Chernobyl, Ukraine, that caused many health problems is considered a major pre-immigration trauma. Immigrants who came from its proximity reported higher rates of psychological symptoms (post-traumatic stress disorder, depression, somatization, anxiety, obsessive-compulsive symptoms) than immigrants from distant areas. For example, the SCL-90 (a measure of psychological distress) scores of three groups of immigrants were compared: those coming from highly exposed areas (n = 137), from less-exposed areas (n = 240), and a matched comparison sample of immigrants from outside the contaminated areas (n = 331). Statistically significant associations were found between exposure and level of distress M scores. For depression: high exposure group = 15.3, SD = 9.8; less exposed group = 14.9, SD = 9.8; and comparison group = 11.4, SD = 9.5. For anxiety: high exposure = 5.4, SD = 4.6; less exposure = 4.7, SD = 4.1; and comparison = 3.8, SD = 3.6 (53). Interestingly, in another study, no effect of exposure to Chernobyl's nuclear radiation was found when "exposure" was defined based on the actual radiation level in the respondents' place of residence. However, when the criterion was defined as "100 km. around Chernobyl," although not all areas within this radius were actually contaminated, exposure had a significant effect on psychological distress. It appeared that subjectively defined "proximity to Chernobyl" was operating as a risk factor for psychological distress (27).

With the passage of time and as their adjustment to Israel improved, levels of psychological distress among Chernobyl survivors decreased. In a follow-up study on the abovementioned sample conducted five years later, there was already no effect of radiation exposure resulting from the Chernobyl accident (28). In another follow-up study of 520 respondents, after seven and 10 years following the accident, a significant decline was observed in the depression and PTSD scores (54). An interaction effect was found between age and time of interview – a more moderate decrease in depression scores among the group over 55 years of age (55). However, in a sociological study that utilized semi-structured interviews 15 years following the accident, Chernobyl survivors reported being significantly more distressed than other immigrants of the same gender and age (56). This finding suggests that Chernobyl survivors' distress may have not disappeared entirely but, rather, that it had declined below a diagnosable threshold. Studies on Chernobyl survivors in other countries provide support to the notion that psychological consequences of this disaster persist, especially in complex life transitions like migration (57–58).

Social and familial support

Social support in the host environment, typically defined as a subjective feeling of having someone to whom the immigrant can turn for help, has been recognized as a protective factor. Lack of social support, particularly from the family, was found in many studies to be associated with various manifestations of psychological distress in immigrants (23, 26–28, 30, 34, 35, 37, 59–61). In contrast, intact family support is conducive to a better long-term adjustment of individual family members (30, 49, 62, 63).

Since perceived social support is a subjective experience, it may be determined by personality traits and cognitive appraisal style. However, there is also objective evidence that having no family in the new country is a risk factor in migration (27, 43, 60). For example, in a study based on a random sample of 241 married and 241 unmarried immigrant mothers, the levels of social support were significantly lower among the single mothers. Accordingly, mean distress scores were significantly higher among single = 1.5, SD = .8 compared to married mothers = 1.2, SD = .7, p < .001). Multivariate analysis on distress showed that the beneficial effect of social support was significantly greater for married mothers than for single mothers (61).

The importance of social support is illustrated in a study on unaccompanied adolescents who immigrated to Israel within the framework of a structured educational program. Lower psychological distress M scores measured by the BSI was found in a sample of 235 unaccompanied immigrant adolescents = .6, SD = .5 than in a sample of 310 immigrant adolescents who immigrated with their parents and were living with them = .8, SD = .5, p < .001. Perceived group support and positive relationships with adult staff (surrogate parents) were the major predictors of psychological wellbeing (22) and seem to have compensated for the absence of parental care. These results were replicated in another study on this immigrant group (64).

Length of residence

Psychological adjustment in migration is a lengthy and dynamic process, and its manifestations may change over time. The classical 'U'-shaped curve model that predicts an initial psychologically benign phase, followed by deterioration and a final recovery (65), has been disputed for decades in the immigration literature. Loose definitions of time since migration and the paucity of longitudinal designs may account for the failure to reach a clear understanding of the dynamics of psychological reactions in migration over time. In Israel, mass migration from the FSU that took place over a span of 15 years allows for a fine definition and assessment of the time factor in cohorts, as well as in longitudinal designs. The latter are more feasible in Israel as indicated above.

Most findings of Israeli studies point to the persistence of psychological distress among immigrants during the first years after migration. A comparison of three cohorts of Soviet immigrants who arrived between 1972 to 1984 and have been in the country one to three, four to six and over seven years showed a persistence of psychological distress even after seven years (PERI-D M scores, N = 273: 1–3 yrs. = 1.1, SD = .6; 4–6 yrs. = 1.2, SD = .6; and 7 yrs. and above = 1.2, SD = .7). A similar pattern was observed in a sample of 415 Soviet immigrants to the US (26).

Local longitudinal studies provide similar findings. In a one-year follow-up survey on recently arrived immigrants no decrease in psychological distress was observed over the baseline (36). In a two-year follow-up conducted in the US, 45% continued to suffer from the depressive symptoms that they had initially; 26%, became depressed; and in 30% of the sample group, the depression lifted (59). In a follow-up Israeli study covering four years following migration no significant improvement in psychological well-being was found (48). Also, in a follow-up study on a nationally representative sample five years after immigration, although there was significant improvement in the objective measures of adjustment (such as employment, housing and mastery of the new language), psychological distress was as high as in the first year after migration (28).

These findings seem to indicate that migration may be a very prolonged process that puts individuals at risk for psychological distress for many years. Interestingly, in a sample of patients undergoing colonoscopy in an Israeli hospital, it was found that respondents who immigrated more than 40 years prior to the study scored better than native born on most physical and psychological well-being indicators (33). Possibly, reaching the recovery part of the U-curve of adjustment in migration may take a number of decades.

A number of studies hypothesized that psychological adaptation in migration is a curvilinear process and may include specific risk periods, somewhat like the U-shape hypothesis. In one research study that included repeated assessment of psychological distress among immigrants over 60 months after immigration, a two-phase temporal pattern was identified – an escalation phase characterized by an increase in distress until the seventh month after arrival, followed by a reduction phase that led to a decline returning to initial levels of distress (39).

Another four-year longitudinal study of a group of 61 adolescents, whose psychological distress was assessed with the BSI at three points of time, identified a similar temporal pattern. The initial experience of adolescent immigrants in the first year after arrival was typified by mild distress (depression = .5, SD = .5; anxiety = .4, SD = .6). Two years thereafter, minimal deterioration occurred in their psychological well-being (depression = .6, SD = .6; anxiety = .5, SD = .6). The recovery phase took place in the fourth year following migration (depression = .4, SD = .4; anxiety = .4, SD = .6) (48). A similar pattern of initially mild distress with deterioration in the second year and later improvement was found in a sample of unaccompanied adolescents (63) and in a sample of late adolescents of FSU immigrants living in Israel (66).

⸹ Cross-national studies on FSU immigrants

Although an exclusive focus on FSU immigrants limits how much one could generalize about the Israeli studies' findings, the special circumstances of this wave of migration discussed earlier enable cross-national study designs. One of the limitations of single-ethnic studies is the fact that cultural background may affect the immigrants' psychological reactions and thus render them culturally specific rather than universal. The elevated psychological distress and psychiatric morbidity among Israeli immigrants from the FSU may be attributed to high baseline levels in their country of origin. No systematic and reliable data on the population's psychological condition in the former Soviet Union are available. Nevertheless, in view of the social disintegration that followed the preceding totalitarian regime, it may be possible to assume that the psychological wellbeing of FSU residents was lower than that of residents of Western countries. Indeed, Russians appear to report being unhappy more often than people of other nations. It was suggested that they do so not only because of their external circumstances, but also because of a negative cognitive bias that affects the way they perceive their lives (67). In an epidemiological study conducted in the Ukraine, prevalence rates of alcoholism among men and depression among women were higher than in comparable European surveys (68). This indication of high baseline rates should be interpreted with caution, as it is not clear whether those general rates also had applied to the Jewish minority in the FSU.

Premigration mental health

There is some evidence that the distress of FSU immigrants in Israel is higher than that of their non-immigrant counterparts in the FSU. For example, higher rates of suicidal ideation were found among FSU immigrants in Israel than in comparison samples in the FSU. Using a door-to-door procedure, 788 Russian-born Jewish immigrants in Israel were compared with a sample of Jewish respondents in the former Soviet Union (N = 411). The one-month prevalence rate of suicide ideation in the immigrant sample, 15.1%, was significantly higher than that in the Russian controls, 6.6%. A total of 5.5% of immigrants, but only .5% of controls, had made a suicide attempt at some time in their lives (69). Another study of over 200 adolescents indicated that six-month rates of suicide ideation and attempts among immigrant adolescents (ideation, 10.9%; attempts, 10.4%) were higher than among their counterparts in the former Soviet Union (ideation, 3.5%; attempts, 4.4%). The rates among the immigrants were closer to those found among Israeli-born adolescents (ideation, 8.7%; attempts, 8.7%) (70).

In a recent study, psychological distress among adolescent immigrants from the FSU (first and second generation) was compared to that of their peers, Jewish and non-Jewish, in the FSU.

The level of general psychological distress and of specific symptoms was higher in the Israeli groups than in the FSU groups. The *M* BSI scores for non-Jewish Russian adolescents (n = 212) were .8, *SD* = .1; for Jewish adolescents in the FSU (n = 184) = .9, *SD* = .1; for first-generation immigrants from the FSU in Israel (n = 63) = 1.2, *SD* = .1; and for second-generation immigrants (n = 64) = 1.0, *SD* = .1 (71).

The above studies show that the common ethnic origin of immigrants in Israel and their Russian counterparts does not result in similar levels of psychological distress. Therefore, the findings raise the possibility that psychological distress of FSU immigrants is not ethnically-related but rather linked to the experience of immigration.

Post-migration environmental factors

Once the gates of FSU opened for emigration, millions of FSU citizens dispersed all over the world including Israel, Germany and the US. FSU emigrants also arrived in Israel and in the US in the 1970s. These circumstances have created ample opportunities for cross-national research on FSU immigrants. The results of these studies shed lights on interactions between different variables affecting the psychological adjustment of immigrants.

The first cross-national study – a derivative of the nationwide epidemiological study in the 1980s – compared psychological distress among Soviet immigrants in Israel with their counterparts in the US. A lower level of psychological distress was found among immigrants in Israel than in the US as follows: PERI-D *M* scores in the US = 1.6, *SD* = .8; in Israel = 1.2, *SD* = .7 (26). These findings were corroborated in a later study that compared depression scores of women immigrants from the FSU in Israel and in the US. Immigrants in the US were more depressed than their counterparts in Israel (72). In the 10 years that passed between the two studies, the immigrant cohort changed considerably and so did the circumstances in the Soviet Union, which in the meantime ceased to exist. What apparently persisted were the differences between the two host environments, Israel and US. It is difficult to determine which environmental variables operated as risk or as protective factors. For example, one may expect that the size and resources of the US would make it better able to accept new immigrant groups and that the security situation in Israel may act as an additional stressor. Possibly, the interaction with other environmental variables counterbalances risks and opportunities.

An interesting point of view on the interaction between environmental factors and immigrants' psychological adjustment is illuminated in a comparative study of FSU immigrants in Israel and Germany. There are similarities between the circumstances involved in immigration in both countries. In the 1990s, they received almost similar numbers of FSU immigrants (1.63 million of ethnic Germans in Germany and 1.2 million Jews in Israel). FSU immigrants are considered in both countries as "repatriates" who receive considerable financial support. However, in Germany, these immigrants constitute a small minority that dispersed over a very large society and are expected to mingle. In contrast, in Israel they constitute a sizeable proportion of the population, often settle in close proximity to each other and maintain cultural enclaves. A comparative study of FSU immigrants in Israel and Germany found no difference in their psychological distress but identified two distinct social adaptation styles. Immigrants in Israel were less likely to engage themselves in their new society; their mastery of the new language was more limited and their willingness to socialize with nonimmigrants was lower than that of their counterparts in Germany. Paradoxically, FSU immigrants in Germany, who apparently were making greater efforts to enter the new society, were more likely to feel discrimination than did their counterparts in Israel (73). This study suggested that the effect of environmental factors on psychological wellbeing may be mediated by the coping style of immigrants who adjust their coping strategies to different circumstances.

Another comparative study that monitored psychological distress measured by the BSI among adult and adolescent immigrants in Israel and Germany over four years identified a different set of environmental effects. Initially, a similar level of psychological distress characterized immigrants in both countries (in Israel, M scores: adults = .5, SD = .4; adolescents = .6, SD = .3; in Germany, M scores: adults = .4, SD = .3; adolescents = .5, SD = .3 with either no change or no deterioration in wellbeing in the second year after migration (in Israel: adults = .5, SD = .5; adolescents = .5, SD = .3; in Germany: adults = .5, SD = .4; adolescents = .5, SD = .4). However, in the fourth year, significant differences were observed in the distress trajectories between immigrants in the two countries and between the two age groups. While the distress M scores of adult immigrants in Germany improved = .4, SD = .4, the wellbeing of their counterparts in Israel decreased = .6, SD = .4). Among adolescents, the tendency was reversed. While among adolescent FSU immigrants in Israel a recovery in the M scores occurred in the fourth year = .4, SD = .3, the psychological wellbeing of their counterparts in Germany did not improve = .5, SD = .4 (48). The relative psychological wellness enjoyed by adult FSU immigrants in Israel can be explained by their relatively large numbers. This enabled them to resist social pressures to sever their ties with their past culture and profit from higher levels of social support. The very same circumstances, however, may create more intense conflicts for adolescents who may be torn between the two cultures.

❧ Immigrants from Ethiopia

This group attracts much research attention because of the wide gap between their cultural background and the predominant Western culture of Israel, compounded by the trauma that many experienced on their way to Israel. This immigrant community is spread throughout the country, and comprises about 100,000 people (9). Different reasons, including language barriers, have precluded comprehensive epidemiological studies. Only small-scale studies were conducted, and findings have often been inconsistent.

One community study showed a high incidence of psychological symptoms among these immigrants and their persistence after five years of residence in Israel. However, the severity of symptoms decreased with time. A correlation was found between the rate of their symptoms and suffering on the way to Israel. A high incidence of symptoms was also related to increased age, low levels of education and living at far from an Ethiopian community (74, 75). Another community study found lower psychological distress among Ethiopian as compared to FSU immigrants. Ethiopian immigrants were characterized by a higher level of paranoid ideation symptoms, while FSU immigrants exhibited a significant higher degree of hostility and anxiety (76).

Because of the cultural background of Ethiopian immigrants, it is likely that Western-based screening and diagnostic instruments can not accurately estimate psychological distress in this population. Specific cultural somatization – the use of the body as a metaphor for personal distress – was identified among Ethiopian immigrants in medical practice (77). A community study with Ethiopian and non-Ethiopian service providers for these immigrants showed a pattern of somatization of emotional problems through symptoms, usually centered on the head, chest and stomach. Ethiopian immigrants had difficulty in differentiating between physical and emotional complaints. They believed that emotional distress derives principally from external factors, including supernatural powers (78).

A study that analyzed the National Insurance Institute's national registry comprising 1,004 children diagnosed with pervasive developmental disorder (PDD) found that the rate of this disorder was much lower among Ethiopian-born children as compared to native Israelis, immigrant children from other countries and Israeli-born children of Ethiopian descent. Curiously, birth and childhood in a rural, non-Western environment would appear to be a protective factor for PDD (79).

Clinical studies also revealed the cultural specificity of Ethiopian immigrants. For example, adolescents of Ethiopian origin hospitalized in mental health centers had significantly higher rates of dissociative disorders than other Israeli adolescents as well as significantly lower rates of the major functional psychoses, nonspecific depressive symptoms and anxiety symptoms (80). Clinical studies also identified two culture-bound psychiatric syndromes: One is possession by "Zar" spirits (expressed among other things in involuntary movements, mutism and incomprehensible language) (81). The other culture-bound syndrome is "brain fag" referred to by Ethiopian immigrants as "overworking of the head" due to the strain of studying (82).

In light of these culture-specific idioms of distress, misunderstandings often take place between Ethiopian immigrant patients and Western-trained clinicians. For example, the "Zar" has been misinterpreted as representing symptoms of neurological or psychiatric disorders and led to inappropriate psychiatric admissions and misdiagnosis of such cases as major psychiatric disorders (77). To promote communication between the two, a Culturally Sensitive Psychiatric Screening Instrument for Detecting Emotional Problems among Ethiopian immigrants was developed based on the WHO Self-Reporting Questionnaire (SRQ), a psychiatric screening instrument to assess populations in developing countries (83)

The timely detection of psychological distress among Ethiopian immigrants is especially important in view of the relatively high suicide rates that have been repeatedly reported in this population (84). Suicide rates found among Ethiopian immigrants were higher than those of the general Israeli population and much higher than in other Jewish immigrant populations, 1.9–4.6 vs. .6–.8 per 10,000 (85). The profile of a high suicide risk among Ethiopian immigrants was that of a married man up to 40 years old, usually involved in a marital conflict, who appears depressed but does not communicate suicidal intent and who frequently visits his general physician (85). Adolescent Ethiopian immigrants were also found at risk for suicidal behavior (86). In addition to directing aggression towards themselves, Ethiopian immigrants' distress may be manifested in aggression directed towards family members. Immigrants from Ethiopia are highly overrepresented among intimate famicide offenders. In the years 1990 to 1995, while their proportion in the population was .9%, their proportion among intimate femicide offenders was 9.1% (87).

✿ From epidemiology to mental health action

Israeli studies have identified the existence of an association between migration and mental problems. Higher psychological distress and psychiatric morbidity have been consistently found among immigrants compared to those born in Israel. These findings support the migration-morbidity hypothesis that predicts a greater risk for mental health problems among immigrants compared to nonimmigrants. Israel, being one of the few countries in the world that does not implement selective migration policy for Jews, provides valuable evidence on the mental risks of migration. These risks may perhaps be minimized when selective immigration policy is implemented and only the better-adjusted individuals are allowed in, which is contrary to current ideology of "ingathering of the exiles". At the same time, the Israeli case illustrates that in an environment where the social status of immigrants improves and they are allowed to advance in their social integration, the risk for mental health problems diminishes and is not transmitted to subsequent generations.

As far as specific risk factors are concerned, Israeli studies support some general findings such as women reporting higher psychological distress than men and considerable psychological distress among adolescent immigrants. However, there are a number of unique contributions: first, the fact that many FSU immigrants have been residing in the Ukraine and Belarus at the time of the Chernobyl accident made it possible to shed some light on the interaction between previous traumatization and migration. Findings consistently indicate that the Chernobyl reactor trauma made individuals more vulnerable to the stresses of migration. There is evidence that with time, the level of psychological distress among survivors of the Chernobyl disaster drops in some cases below a diagnosable threshold, but it does not disappear completely.

The crucial role of social support – a stress-buffering factor in migration – has been illustrated in many Israeli studies. It may even compensate for the absence of family in the case of unaccompanied adolescent immigrants. Also, the supportive nature of the host society serves to explain relatively low levels of psychological distress among immigrants in contrast to findings from other countries.

Perhaps the most important contribution of Israeli studies is the exploration of immigrants' mental health over the course of time since migration. It appears that some methodological merits of Israeli longitudinal studies (such as more precise definition of length of residence in the host country and repeated assessment points) and the focus on adolescents help to shed some light on the dynamic nature of adjustment in migration. The findings suggest that the adaptation may be a prolonged process that puts immigrants at risk for psychological distress for many years. Most studies reveal the persistence of psychological distress among immigrants, at least during the first five years following arrival and of appropriate programs of intervention.

Many studies illustrate a curvilinear process with an initially benign stage, a subsequent deterioration in wellbeing (around the second and third years following migration) when immigrants are particularly at risk for mental health problems and a possible recovery phase starting from the fourth and fifth year following arrival.

Another interesting insight comes from cross-national studies of FSU immigrants in Israel and in Germany. These studies highlight the effects of environmental and social risk factors (lack of social support networks or pressure to adjust to the majority group) on the psychological wellbeing of immigrants. However, they also suggest that these effects may be mediated by the coping style of immigrants who can adapt to different circumstances.

The most important limitation of recent Israeli studies refers to the fact that the majority of them focus on one ethnic group, the immigrants from the FSU. Although efforts have been made in some studies to control for ethnicity and although it is quite likely that many of the phenomena uncovered may be universally applicable, replication of these studies with other immigrant populations is necessary.

Research on the small group of Ethiopian immigrants in Israel illustrates some phenomena typical to immigrant from developing countries in Western societies. The cultural gaps between the two cultures may create specific risks not only to the mental health but also to the lives of such immigrants. Timely detection of psychological distress of those immigrants necessitates the implementation of culturally-appropriate diagnostic instruments.

❧ References

1. Bratter JL, Eschbach K. Race/ethnic differences in nonspecific psychological distress: evidence from the National Health Interview Survey. *Social Science Quarterly* 2005; 86: 620–644.
2. Pernice R, Brook J. Refugees' and immigrants' mental health: association of demographic and post-immigration factors. *Journal of Social Psychology* 1996; 136: 511–519.
3. Bengi-Arslan L, Verhulst FC, Crijnen AAM. Prevalence and determinants of minor psychiatric in Turkish immigrants living in the Netherlands. *Social Psychiatry and Psychiatric Epidemiology* 2002; 37: 118–124.
4. Dalgard O, Thapa S, Hauff E, *et al.* Health and disability: immigration, lack of control and psychological distress: findings from the Oslo Health Study. *Scandinavian Journal of Psychology* 2006; 47: 551–558.
5. Flores G, Brotanek J. The healthy immigrant effect. *Archives of Pediatrics and Adolescence Medicine* 2005; 159: 295–297.
6. Beiser M. The health of immigrants and refugees in Canada. *Canadian Journal of Public Health* 2005; 96: 30–44.
7. Alderete E, Vega A, Kolody B, *et al.* Lifetime prevalence of and risk factors for psychiatric disorders among Mexican migrant farm workers in California. *American Journal of Public Health* 2000; 90: 608–614.
8. Gee EM, Kobayashi KM, Prus SG. Examining the healthy immigrant effect in mid- to-later life: findings from the Canadian community health survey. *Canadian Journal of Aging* 2004; Suppl S55–S63.
9. Central Bureau of Statistics. *Statistical abstracts of Israel.* Jerusalem: Central Bureau of Statistics, 2006.
10. Lichtenberg P, Kaplan Z, Grinshpoon A. The goals and limitations of Israel's psychiatric case register. *Psychiatric Services* 1999; 50:1043–1048.
11. Kessler RC, Ustun TB. The World Mental Health (WMH) Survey Initiative Version of the World Health Organization (WHO) Composite International Diagnostic Interview (CIDI). *International Journal of Methods in Psychiatric Research* 2004; 13: 93–121.
12. Lerner Y. Psychiatric epidemiology in Israel. *Israel Journal of Psychiatry and Related Sciences* 1992; 29: 218–228.
13. Halevi HS. Frequency of mental illness among Jews in Israel. *International Journal of Social Psychiatry* 1963; 9: 268–282.
14. Eaton, WW, Levav I. Schizophrenia, social class and ethnic disadvantage. A study of first hospitalization among Israeli-born Jews. *Israel Journal of Psychiatry and Related Sciences* 1982; 19: 289–302.
15. Maoz B, Levy S, Brand N, *et al.* An epidemiological survey of mental disorders in a community of newcomers to Israel. *Journal of the College of General Practitioners* 1966; 2: 267–284.
16. Rahav M, Goodman A, Popper M, *et al.* Distribution of treated mental illness in the neighborhoods of Jerusalem. *American Journal of Psychiatry* 1986; 143: 1249–1254.
17. Miller L. Culture and psychopathology of Jews in Israel. *Psychiatric Journal of the University of Ottawa* 1979; 4: 302–306.
18. Snyder C, Palgi P, Eldar P, *et al.* Alcoholism among Jews in Israel: a pilot study I. Research rationale and a look at the ethnic factors. *Journal of the Study of Alcohol* 1982; 43: 623–654.
19. Gershon E, Liebowitz J. Sociocultural and demographic correlates of affective disorders in Jerusalem. *Journal of Psychiatric Research* 1975; 12: 37–50.
20. Miller L. Some data on suicide and attempted suicide of the Jewish population in Israel. *Mental Health Society* 1976; 178–181.
21. Dohrenwend B, Levav I, Shrout P, *et al.* Socioeconomic status and psychiatric disorders: the causation-selection issue. *Science* 1992; 255: 946–952.
22. Mirsky J. Post-migratory milieu and the psychological wellbeing of adolescent immigrants. *European Journal of Social Work* 2007; 10: 353–367.
23. Levav I, Kohn R, Flaherty JA, et al. Mental health attitudes and practices of Soviet immigrants. *Israel Journal of Psychiatry and Related Sciences* 1990; 27: 131–144.
24. Sharlin S. Soviet immigrants to Israel: users and non-users of social work services. *International Social Work* 1998; 41: 455–463.
25. Rabinowitz J, Fennig, S. Differences in age of first hospitalization for schizophrenia among immigrants and nonimmigrants in a National Case Registry. *Schizophrenia Bulletin* 2002; 28: 491–499
26. Flaherty J, Kohn R, Levav I, *et al.* Demoralization in Soviet-Jewish immigrants to the United States and Israel. *Comprehensive Psychiatry* 1088; 29: 588–597.
27. Zilber N, Lerner Y, Psychological distress among recent immigrants from the former Soviet Union to Israel. I. Mediating factors. *Psychological Medicine* 1996; 26: 493–501.
28. Lerner Y, Kertes J, Zilber N. Immigrants from the former Soviet Union, five years post-immigration to Israel: adaptation and risk factors for psychological distress. *Psychological Medicine* 2005; 35: 1805–1814.
29. Mirsky J, Kohn R, Levav I, *et al.* Psychological distress and psychiatric morbidity among immigrants from the former Soviet Union in Israel: findings from the Israel National Health Study. *Journal of Clinical Psychiatry* 2008; 69: 1715–1720.
30. Mirsky J. Psychological distress among immigrant adolescents: culture specific factors in the case of immigrant students from the former Soviet Union. *International Journal of Psychology* 1997; 32: 221–230.

31. Ron P. Depression, hopelessness and suicidal ideation among the elderly: a comparison between veterans and new immigrants. *Illness, Crisis & Loss* 2007; 15: 25–38.

32. Gross R, Brammli-Greenberg S, Remennick L. Self-rated health status and healthcare utilization among immigrant and non-immigrant Israeli Jewish women. *Women's Health* 2001; 31: 53–69.

33. Anson O, Pilpel D, Rolnik v. Physical and psychological well-being among immigrant referrals to colonoscopy. *Social Science and Medicine* 1996; 43: 1309–1316.

34. Baider L, Ever-Hadani P, Kaplan DeNour A. Crosssing new bridges: the process of adaptation and psychological distress of Russian immigrants in Israel. *Psychiatry* 1996; 59: 175–183.

35. Ritsner M, Ponizovsky A, Ginath Y. Changing patterns of distress during the adjustment of recent immigrants: a one-year follow-up study. *Acta Psychiatrica Scandinavica* 1997; 95: 494–499.

36. Ritsner M, Ponizovsky A, Kurs R, et al. Somatization in an immigrant population in Israel: a community survey of prevalence, risk factors, and help-seeking behavior. *American Journal of Psychiatry* 2000; 157: 385–392.

37. Ritsner M, Ponizovsky A, Nechamkin Y, et al. Gender differences in psychological risk factors for psychological distress among immigrants. *Comprehensive Psychiatry* 2001; 42: 151–160.

38. Ritsner M, Ponizovsky A. Psychological symptoms among immigrant population: a prevalence study. *Comprehensive Psychiatry* 1998; 39: 21–27.

39. Ritsner M, Ponizovsky A. Psychological distress through immigration: the two-phase temporal pattern? *International Journal of Social Psychiatry* 1999; 45: 125–139.

40. Amir M, Ayalon L, Varshavsky S., et al. Motherland or home country: a comparative study of quality of life among Jews from the former Soviet Union who immigrated to Israel, Jews in Russia, and Israeli non immigrants. *Journal of Cross-Cultural Psychology* 1999; 30: 712–721.

41. Hasin D, Rahav G, Meydan J, et al. The drinking of earlier and more recent Russian immigrants to Israel: comparison to other Israelis. *Journal of Substance Abuse* 1999; 10: 341–353.

42. Hasin D, Aharonovich E, Liu X, et al. Alcohol dependence symptoms and alcohol dehydrogenase 2 Polymorphism: Israeli Ashkenazis, Sephardics, and recent Russian immigrants. *Alcoholism: clinical & experimental research* 2002; 26: 1315–1321.

43. Lerner Y, Popper M. Trends in psychiatric hospitalization in the years 1986–1990 and projection till 1995. *Harefuah* 1993; 125: 75–79 (Hebrew).

44. Kohn R, Levav, I. Schizophrenic disorders among first and second-generation immigrants. (Unpublished manuscript).

45. Epstein A. The impact of Jewish identity on the psychological adjustment of Soviet Jewish Immigrants in Israel. *Israel Journal of Psychiatry and Related Sciences* 1996; 33: 21–31.

46. Zilber N, Lerner Y, Eidelman R, et al. Depression and anxiety disorders among Jews from the former Soviet Union five years after their immigration to Israel. *International Journal of Geriatric Psychiatry* 2001; 16: 993–999.

47. Ritsner M, Ponizovsky A. Age differences in the stress process of recent immigrants. *Comprehensive Psychiatry* 2003; 44: 135–141.

48. Mirsky J, Slonim-Nevo V, Rubinstein L. Psychological wellness and distress among recent immigrants: a four-year longitudinal study in Israel and Germany. *International Migration* 2007; 45: 151–173.

49. Slonim-Nevo V, Sharaga Y. Psychological and social adjustment of Russian born and Israel born Jewish adolescents. *Child and Adolescent Social Work* 2000; 17: 455–475.

50. Kimhi M, Ben-Arie A, Cohen S. *Immigrant children in Israel 2007.* Jerusalem: Ministry of Immigrant Absorption and National Council for Children Welfare, 2007.

51. Liebkind K, Jasinskaja-Lahti I. Acculturation and psychological well-being among immigrant adolescents in Finland: a comparative study of adolescents from different cultural backgrounds. *Journal of Adolescent-Research* 2000; 15: 446–469.

52. Birman D, Trickett E, Vinokurov A. Acculturation and adaptation of Soviet Jewish refugee adolescents: predictors of adjustment across life domains. *American Journal of Community Psychology* 2002; 30: 585–607.

53. Cwikel J, Abdelgani A, Rozovski U, et al. Long-term stress reactions in new immigrants to Israel exposed to the Chernobyl accident. *Anxiety, Stress & Coping* 2000; 13: 413–439.

54. Cwikel J, Abdelgani A, Goldsmith J, et al. Two-year follow-up of stress related disorders among immigrants to Israel from the Chernobyl area. *Environmental Health Perspectives* 1997; 105 (Suppl 6): 1545–1550.

55. Cwikel J, Abdelgani A, Rozovski U. Coping with the stress of migration among new immigrants to Israel from Commonwealth of Independent States (CIS) who were exposed to Chernobyl: the effect of age. *International Journal of Aging and Human Development* 1998; 46: 305–318.

56. Remennick L, Immigrants from Chernobyl-affected areas in Israel: the link between health and social adjustment. *Social Science and Medicine* 2002; 54: 309–317.

57. Perez Foster R, Goldstein M. Chernobyl disaster sequelae in recent immigrants to the United States from the former Soviet Union (FSU). *Journal of Immigrants and Minorities Health* 2007; 2: 115–124.

58. Rahu K, Rahu M, Tekkel M, et al. Suicide risk among Chernobyl cleanup workers in Estonia still increased: an updated cohort study. *Annals of Epidemiology* 2007; 16: 917–919.

59. Aroyan K, Norris A. Depression trajectories in relatively recent immigrants. *Comprehensive Psychiatry* 2003; 44: 420–427.

60. Ponizovsky A, Safro S, Ginath Y, et al. Suicide ideation among recent immigrants: an epidemiological study. *Israel Journal of Psychiatry and Related Sciences* 1997; 34:139–148.

61. Soskolne V. Single parenthood, occupational drift and psychological distress among immigrant women from the former Soviet Union in Israel. *Women's Health* 2001; 33: 67–84.

62. Mirsky J, Baron-Draiman Y, Kedem P. Social support and psychological distress among young immigrants from the former Soviet Union in Israel. *International Social Work* 2002; 45: 83–97.

63. Slonim-Nevo V, Mirsky J, Rubinstein L. The impact of family relations on the psychological adjustment of recent immigrants to Israel and Germany. *The Journal of Child and Family* (in press).

64. Tartakovsky E. A longitudinal study of acculturative stress and homesickness: high-school adolescents immigrating from Russia and Ukraine to Israel without parents. *Social Psychiatry and Psychiatric Epidemiology* 2007; 42: 485–494.

65. Oberg K. Culture shock: adjustment to a new cultural environment. *Practical Anthropology* 1960; 7: 177–182.

66. Walsh S, Shulman, S. Splits in the self following immigration: an adaptive defense or a pathological reaction. *Psychoanalytic Psychology* 2007; 24: 355–372.

67. Veenhoven R. Are the Russians as unhappy as they say they are? *Journal of Happiness Studies* 2001; 2: 111–136.

68. Bromet E, Gluzman S, Paniotto V, *et al.* Epidemiology of psychiatric and alcohol disorders in Ukraine: findings from the Ukraine World Mental Health Survey. *Social Psychiatry and Psychiatric Epidemiology* 2005; 40: 681–690.

69. Ponizovsky A, Ritsner M. Suicide ideation among recent immigrants to Israel from the former Soviet Union: an epidemiological survey of prevalence and risk factors. *Suicide and Life Threatening Behavior* 1999; 29: 376–392.

70. Ponizovsky A, Ritsner M, Modai I. Suicidal ideation and suicide attempts among immigrant adolescents from the former Soviet Union to Israel. *Journal of the American Academy of Child & Adolescent Psychiatry* 1999; 38: 1433–1441.

71. Slonim-Nevo V, Sharaga Y, Mirsky J, *et al.* Ethnicity versus migration: two hypotheses about the psychosocial adjustment of immigrant adolescents. *International Journal of Social Psychiatry* 2006; 52: 41–53.

72. Miller MA, Gross R. Health and depression in women from the former Soviet Union living in the United States and Israel. *Journal of Immigrant Health* 2004; 6: 187–196.

73. Slonim-Nevo V, Mirsky J, Nauck B, *et al.* Social participation and psychological distress among immigrants from the former Soviet Union: a comparative study in Israel and Germany. *International Social Work* 2007; 50: 56–64.

74. Arieli A, Aycheh S. Psychopathology among Jewish Ethiopian immigrants to Israel. *Journal of Nervous and Mental Disease* 1992; 180: 465–466.

75. Arieli A, Aycheh S. Psychopathological aspects of the Ethiopian immigration to Israel. *Israel Journal of Medical Sciences* 1993; 29: 411–418.

76. Ginath Y, Vendiamino B. Safro S, *et al.* Cross-cultural study of psychological distress among Ethiopian and Russian immigrants to Israel. *European Psychiatry* 1996; 11 (Suppl 4) 265s.

77. Andermann L. Ethiopian Jews meet Israeli family physicians: a study of cultural somatization. *Transcultural Psychiatry* 1996; 33: 333–345.

78. Youngmann R, Menuchin-Itzigsohn S, Barasch M. Manifestations of emotional distress among Ethiopian immigrants in Israel: patient and clinician perspectives. *Transcultural Psychiatry* 1999; 36: 45–63.

79. Kamer A, Zohar AH, Youngmann R, et al. A prevalence estimate of pervasive developmental disorder among immigrants to Israel and Israeli natives – A file review study. *Social Psychiatry and Psychiatric Epidemiology* 2004; 39: 141–145.

80. Ratzoni G, Ben Amo I, Weizman T, et al. Psychiatric diagnoses in hospitalized adolescent and adult Ethiopian immigrants in Israel. *Israel Journal of Medical Sciences* 1993; 29: 419–421.

81. Grisaru N, Budowski D, Witztum E. Possession by the "Zar" among Ethiopian immigrants to Israel: psychopathology or culture-bound syndrome? *Psychopathology* 1997; 30: 223–233.

82. Durst R, Minuchin-Itzigsohn S, Jabotinsky-Rubin K. "Brain-fag" syndrome: manifestation of transculturation in an Ethiopian Jewish immigrant. *Israel Journal of Psychiatry and Related Sciences* 1993; 30: 223–232.

83. Youngmann R, Zilber N, Kaveh N, et al. Development of a culturally sensitive psychiatric screening instrument for detecting emotional problems among Ethiopian immigrants in Israel. *Harefuah* 2002; 141: 10–16 (Hebrew).

84. Shoval G, Schoen G, Vardi N, et al. Suicide in Ethiopian immigrants in Israel: a case for study of the genetic-environmental relation in suicide. *Archives of Suicide Research* 2007; 11: 247–253.

85. Arieli A, Gilat I, Aycheh S. Suicide among Ethiopian Jews: a survey conducted by means of a psychological autopsy. *Journal of Nervous and Mental Disease* 1996; 184: 317–318.

86. Ratzoni G, Blumensohn R, Apter A, et al. Psychopathology and management of hospitalized suicidal Ethiopian adolescents in Israel. *Israel Journal of Medical Sciences* 1991; 27: 293–296.

87. Landau S, Hattis Rolef S. Intimate femicide in Israel; temporal, social and motivational patterns. *European Journal on Criminal Policy and Research* 1998; 6: 75–90.

Chapter 7

The psychiatric epidemiology of the after-effects of the Holocaust among Israeli survivors and their offspring

Itzhak Levav

World War II (WWII) ended in Europe on May 8, 1945 – but the psychopathological impact on the survivors lingered beyond their liberation. Painful fresh memories, further amplified by the traumatic events that followed, gave room to emotional wounds that took years to heal, if at all. The assaults by the Nazis on the Jewish people in Europe and Africa during the war varied in form, intensity and length. They included several domains, among them (1, 2):

(a) physical, such as beatings, physical illnesses, insufficient sleep, extreme food deprivation, exposure to strenuous temperatures and forced labor;
(b) psychological, such as bereavement, witnessing of cruelest events, fear of death, insult to self-worth and dehumanization;
(c) psychosocial, such as the collapse of the social support group, confinement and financial losses; and
(d) cultural-religious, such as anti-Semitic acts of different types, among them perverse discriminatory laws and the need to hide one's Jewish identity.

Those severe experiences were further compounded by other events following liberation, such as pogroms upon the survivors' return to the places of former residence and the ordeals of their clandestine immigration to prestate Israel (1).

As a result, psychiatrists called to care for the survivors had to coin a new term, the KZ (concentration camp) syndrome to encompass the manifold psychopathological wounds and early scars caused by so many and repeated assaults (3).

Subsequently, mental health professionals' attention extended to the second generation of survivors, since they began to suspect that the overwhelming psychopathological aftereffects of the Holocaust might be be transmitted to their children (2).

What was/is the impact of the above traumas on the survivors and their offspring, as it has been captured by epidemiological studies conducted in Israel? Given the criteria of inclusion followed in this book, the very large number of clinical studies conducted in Israel, as documented by bibliographical lists and reviews that are almost outdated by the time of their publication (e.g., 4–6), will be omitted here.

⸎ Psychopathology among the first generation of Holocaust survivors

Eitinger's epidemiological inquiry remained for many years the only one that investigated psychiatric syndromes in selected community settings – but mixed with clinic samples (3). Thus it only partially meets the inclusion criteria followed in this review. Better suited to fully meet the criteria is a recent epidemiological study (7). All other community-based studies have relied on screening measures that ascertained nonspecific psychopathology i.e., emotional distress or demoralization (2). In addition to both groups of studies, where the dependent variable consisted of either psychiatric disorders or emotional distress, there is a third one that explored the vulnerability of Holocaust survivors to renewed traumas, such as war-related events and the diagnosis or treatment of a life-threatening illness. Those three groups of studies will be dealt in that order.

⸎ Psychiatric disorders as dependent variable

At the end of WWII, the literature on post-traumatic stress disorder (PTSD) that multiplied in recent years both in Israel (see chapters 12 and 13) and abroad was not available. As noted above, psychiatrists who examined survivors had to face a new mental condition in civilians for which they had no accepted definition. Also, the etiology of such a condition was not entirely clear. Initially, the presence of comorbid physical disorders, the effect of protracted starvation and the knowledge that survivors suffered from head traumas resulting from beatings led professionals to posit that the condition was primarily physical rather than psychological or, at best, mixed (3). Eitinger was not the only clinician who argued that (8). Given so much ambiguity, psychiatrists simply labeled the survivors' condition KZ syndrome (the acronym for concentration camp in German) alluding, simply, to where it originated (9).

Would such a syndrome match the category of PTSD in the *Diagnostic and Statistical Manual of Mental Disorders – Fourth Edition* (DSM-IV) category of PTSD – or, alternatively, the category bearing the more suggestive denomination " enduring personality change after catastrophic experience," as in the *International Classification of Diseases – Tenth Edition* (ICD-10)? The likely answer to this question is, yes, but only partially. Eitinger identified 11 symptoms as characteristic of the KZ syndrome where the number of symptoms present in any combination was correlated with the degree of certainty that the syndrome was indeed present (9). Of Eitinger's 11 symptoms, a few overlap with the A to D criteria of PTSD, 309.8, of the DSM-IV. Levav noted that some of those items might be regarded as residual symptoms of a pathological grief reaction, thus raising the possibility that the KZ syndrome included both PTSD and bereavement-related symptoms (2). The personal losses that the survivors endured (Eitinger, in the interviews he conducted with survivors in the Israeli component of his study, found that almost all respondents had lost family members) – with few or no possibilities for adequate mourning (3) – would make that notion possible.

Eitinger studied three paired samples of populations in Israel and Norway. In Israel, the samples were selected from psychiatric hospitals (n = 396), psychiatric clinics (n = 92), and kibbutzim (n = 66). In Oslo, the samples were from psychiatric hospitals (n = 96), claim compensation offices (n = 152); and former prisoners (n = 50). All six groups had been subjected to differing degree of persecution, from mild to very severe. Eitinger found differing proportion of the concentration camp syndrome by group. In Israel: among the inpatients, the rate was 26.8%; in the clinic patients, 55.4%; and among the fully functioning kibbutz members, 34.9%. In Norway, the proportion among the inpatients was 36.4%; among claimants, 80.9%; and 6.2%, in fully functioning former war prisoners.

The second fully-based community study, described here at some length, was part of the Israel National Health Survey (INHS) (7). This study included both Holocaust survivors and a suitable comparison group. Given the time elapsed from WWII, it might remain as the only study that examined relevant psychiatric diagnoses, such as depressive and anxiety disorders. In addition, it explored emotional distress (reported in the next section); sleep disturbances; complaints of pain; body mass index (BMI) and selected self-reported chronic medical conditions; smoking; and mental health services utilization.

The methods of the INHS are described in other chapters. Here it suffices to note that the Holocaust group included European Jews who lived in a Nazi-ruled country. The comparison group was comprised of both, European-born Jews who arrived before 1939 and had not lived under a Nazi regime and Israeli-born respondents whose fathers were of similar origin.

The interview schedule relevant to this study included:

(a) sociodemographic variables (such as age, gender, origin, marital and employment status, education, income and degree of religious observance);

(b) the World Mental Health Survey version of the Composite International Diagnostic Interview (CIDI) (14). CIDI enabled diagnosing selected psychiatric disorders according to ICD-10 and DSM-IV. The following ones were assessed: anxiety disorders (panic disorder, generalized anxiety disorder-GAD, agoraphobia without panic disorder and post-traumatic stress disorder-PTSD); and affective disorders (major depressive disorder and dysthymia). Prevalence rates were estimated when respondents' psychopathology met the 12-month and lifetime diagnostic criteria for DSM-IV disorder. For each disorder, a screening sub-questionnaire was administered. All participants answering positively to a specific screening item were asked the questions in the respective diagnostic section of the main questionnaire. Organic exclusion criteria were taken into account in determining DSM-IV diagnoses;

(c) questions about sleep disturbances. To meet criteria, respondents had to report at least one difficulty in falling and/or staying asleep, and/or waking up too early. The disturbance/s had to be present during the preceding 12 months almost nightly, and for a period of two weeks or more; and

(d) exposure to traumatic events, to adjust for the possible effects of stressful events on outcome variables excluding those Holocaust-related.

The group of survivors included 145 individuals; of those, 55 had been in concentration camps; 36, in ghettos or in hiding; and 54, fled their country under a Nazi regime (14 of them before the war begun). In the comparison group there were 143 subjects: 31 born in Europe and 112 born in Israel to European-born fathers. Survivors were significantly older (M age = 74.6, SD = 6.9) than those in the comparison group (M age = 69.0, SD = 8.5; p < .001). There were significant age differences among the three Holocaust subgroups F(7.71), p < .01. Survivors who lived in ghettos or in hiding were significantly younger than those in the other two subgroups (p < .01), and closer in mean age to the subjects in the comparison group. The percentage of survivors with higher education was significantly lower than in the comparison group (23% and 47%, respectively, *p* < .001).

Half of the survivors defined themselves as secular, in contrast to 70% of the comparison group (*p* < .001). There were no significant inter-group differences in gender and marital status. On average, survivors were 17.5 years old (*SD* = 6.8) upon immigration to Israel. Survivors who were in ghettos or in hiding (*M* age = 14.9, *SD* = 6.4) were significantly younger upon immigration than those from concentration camps (*M* age = 20.4, *SD* = 5.5, *p* < .01), but not from survivors who fled their country (*M* age = 16.5, *SD* = 7.3).

Survivors lived apart from one or both parents below the age of 16 with greater frequency than individuals of the comparison group (26% and 16%, respectively; *p* = .055).

Exposure to traumatic events

The frequency of exposure to at least one traumatic event in the past was significantly higher in the survivor than in the comparison group, 94% and 83%, respectively (OR = 3.2, 95% CI 1.4–7.2), but the difference was all related to the Holocaust. Accordingly, this variable remained uncontrolled.

Anxiety disorders

Statistically significant differences for the combined anxiety disorders between survivors and their counterparts were noted for both lifetime (16% and 4%, Odds ratio (OR) = 4.8, 95% Confidence interval (CI) 1.8–12.4) and 12-month prevalence rates (7% and 1%, OR = 12.1, 95% CI 1.5–99.3). These differences remained significant after controlling for age, religious observance and education (OR = 6.8, 95% CI 1.9–24.2; and OR = 22.5, 95% CI 2.5–204.8, respectively). When specific anxiety disorders were examined, PTSD, agoraphobia and generalized anxiety disorder were not statistically significant between the two groups. There were no differences between the three Holocaust subgroups with regard to anxiety disorders.

Depressive disorders

Surprisingly, in view of past losses, no statistically significant differences were found between both survivors and comparison groups for lifetime and 12-month prevalence rates of depressive disorders, both unadjusted and adjusted for confounders.

Sleep disturbances

The percentage of survivors who reported at least one sleep disturbance was twice higher (62%; N = 90) than for individuals of the comparison group (33%; N = 46) (OR = 3.4, 95% CI 2.0–5.6). This difference remained highly significant following control for age, education, religious observance and past year anxiety and mood disorders (OR = 2.5, 95% CI 1.4–4.4).

❧ Emotional distress or psychiatric symptoms as dependent variable

Several epidemiological studies were conducted in different community-based settings using psychiatric screening scales such as an abbreviated Cornell Medical Index (10), the SCL-90 (11) and the 12-General Health Questionnaire (12), as well as a number of different measures of mental health, e.g., the Impact of the Event Scale (13). Those studies span a number of years, 25 to 60 years after the war, and included both middle-aged and elderly respondents. Importantly, most surveys were conducted in contexts totally independent from secondary gains that could have compromised reliability.

An early study limited to women aged 45 to 54 was conducted about 25 years after the end of the war (14). The authors used a battery of items measuring diverse health domains, including mental health, to assess adaptation to menopause: (a) overall menopausal symptoms, "psychic menopausal symptoms," "psychosomatic" and "somatic menopausal symptoms"; (b) overall ratings by physicians, comprising of physical and emotional symptoms and functioning; (c) wellbeing, self-evaluation of overall life situation and coping, and mood and worries scales; and (d) role satisfaction.

Their study included 287 subjects drawn from the Population Register who were born in Central European countries; of those, 77 were survivors. The household-based protocol included a semi-structured psychiatric interview.

According to the respondents' general practitioners, 33% of the survivor randomly included in the survey was in a worse health status than the non-Holocaust comparison group (10%). Lower moods were reported by 61% and 46%, respectively. For the worry scale, a proxy for anxiety, the respective proportions were 56% and 30%. All those differences were statistically significant.

In conclusion, the group of survivors evidenced poor adaptation to the psychological problems of the climacteric period. However, the authors also pointed out that a considerable proportion of the survivors were rated by the physicians as being in excellent or quite good health for women of their age. The successful adaptation of women who had been victims of traumatic events is an issue that has been taken up partially by Israeli researchers, but only many years later.

Levav and Abramson (15) studied adult women and men who had survived concentration camps (n = 360) and a suitable comparison group of European-born individuals who had not been in concentration or extermination camps but could have been in Nazi-occupied countries (n = 1070). Members of both groups, who resided in a stable neighborhood of Jerusalem, were administered an abbreviated version of the Cornell Medical Index (CMI), a screening instrument developed in the war years by US researchers (10). This shortened version, which measures feelings of anxiety, sadness and hopelessness, was tested and found to possess adequate validity and reliability.

The interviews took place during the years 1969 to 1971, about 25 years after the end of WWII. Women and men survivors' mean CMI scores were statistically significantly higher than those of the comparison group, following adjustments for age, educational level and respondent's appraisal that she/he had gone through a hard life. Fifteen years later, a group of investigators studied residents of the same neighborhood (16). They compared survivors both men (n = 130) and women (n = 158) of M ages = 68.0 years, SD = 9.0, and 67.2 years, SD = 8.0, respectively, with a group of European-born Jews that had been not been exposed to the Holocaust (n=486). Of this group, 202 were men and 284 were women, M ages = 69.0 years, SD = 8.7; and 69.0 years, SD = 9.6, respectively. They used the same abbreviated CMI scale as earlier. In addition, they used the 27-item demoralization scale of the Psychiatry Epidemiology Research Interview (PERI), whose psychometric properties had been researched previously in Jerusalem (17). The female group of survivors reported poorer emotional health (CMI M score = 2.0, SD = 2.0; PERI M score = 32.7, SD = 16.1) than the comparison group (CMI M score = 1.5, SD = 1.9; PERI M score = 28.8, SD = 14.8). The level of statistical significance was p < .05, adjusted for age but uncontrolled for education.

This difference in emotional health was not found among men. In turn, men survivors, but not women survivors, reported statistically significant poorer self-appraisal of health (M score = 2.4, SD = .9) than non-Holocaust-exposed men (M score = 2.2, SD = .01). Interestingly, survivors of both gender tended to appraise their overall life situation as better than the comparison group, although the differences did not reach statistical significance.

Carmil and Carel's study (18) included a large number of survivors that had been exposed to all types of Holocaust situations (N = 2159) and a suitable comparison group (N = 1150). Subjects were medically screened in a health organization for reasons totally unrelated to their past experiences. Physical health measures such as cholesterol, blood glucose and systolic blood pressure did not differ between both groups of individuals. Emotional distress was measured with a set of items extracted from the battery of questions routinely presented to the screened individuals tapping anxiety, depression, fears, loss of emotional control due to anger and sleeping problems. In addition, respondents were asked whether currently or in the past had serious psychological problems or were seen regularly by a psychologist or a psychiatrist. The results showed that there were statistically significant differences between both groups of women, but not for men, for all items – except sleep disturbances.

Other Israeli studies focused almost exclusively on elderly subjects that had been children, adolescents or young adults during WWII. The case of the elderly is special since this is a time of life where the individual may look both inwards and back, as noted by the Book of Ecclesiastes in the Bible. Those reminiscences may bring the past with renewed strength. The picture that emerged from community-based studies in which those survivors were compared with European-born Israelis who did not undergo the Holocaust showed impairments in some, but not in all areas of psychological and social functioning.

In the more recent INHS (7), emotional distress was measured using the GHQ-12. The time frame for the items was referenced to the previous 30 days. The internal reliability consistency was measured by Cronbach's *alpha*, .83. The mean score for the survivors = 19.9, SD = 6.1) was statistically higher than that of the comparison group = 16.7, SD = 4.8 (p < .001), adjusting for demographic variables.

Previous to the INHS, Landau and Litwin (20) studied 400 community residents aged 75 years or older who were selected from the Population Register in 1997, including individuals residing in settings for independent older adults. Of them, 194, or 50%, agreed to be interviewed. The index group of survivors immigrated after 1945 (n = 91) and the comparison group, presumably all born in Europe, arrived before that year and did not go through the Holocaust. The two groups were closely similar with regard to sociodemographic characteristics. The dependent variables included measures of physical health, mental health (indicators of affect, depression and life satisfaction) and an inventory of PTSD symptoms (13). The modifying variables of social support (21), locus of control (22) and an adapted social network schedule (23) were included.

The results differed by gender. While men had statistically higher mean scores of PTSD symptoms, women reported higher physical morbidity, less physical capacity and lower self-rated health. Similar personal resources were found in both studied groups.

Shmotkin *et al.* (24) noted that "survivors fared worse than prewar European-born Israelis in certain but not all psychosocial domains." As mentioned above, Collins *et al.* (16) found in their community-based study poorer self-appraised health in men and increased emotional distress in women survivors compared with suitable controls, but no higher mortality within a 10-year period. Only Ben-Zur and Zimmerman (25), who did not cover psychopathology, found impairment with regard to negative affect and ambivalence over emotional expression, and lower results on psychosocial adjustment.

Lastly, a research team studied 43 Holocaust survivors recruited from survivors' organizations and 44 individuals who were in Israel during WWII or in countries not involved in the war (the sampling origin of the latter was not specified) (26). Both groups were administered the PTSD Inventory (13); the SCL-90 (11); and the WHOQOL-Bref, which measures quality of life (27). In addition, candidates for the comparison group were administered a list of stressful life events. To maximize the specificity of the comparison, those respondents were selected for the study if one of the items was positive.

Results showed statistical significant differences for PTSD M score (survivors = 4.8, SD .4; comparison = 3.1, SD = 1.1); and four subscales of the SCL-90 (depression, anxiety, somatization, and anger-hostility). They all were higher among survivors. WHOQOL-Bref was lower for survivors in three (physical, psychological and social) of the four domains explored.

The largest community study conducted in Israel is summarized henceforth at some length (28). This study examined emotional distress and other health dimensions, such as self-reported chronic health conditions, sleep problems and social activities, among both elderly survivors and a suitable comparison group living in the community. This study, part of a comprehensive health and social survey, was conducted in 1997 to 1998. Respondents, who were aged 60 years and above at the time of fieldwork, had been between seven to 28 years of age by the end of WWII. The sample was weighted back to the population based on the proportion of respondents in each stratum using the 1995 census; the estimated population totaled 703,910 individuals; of them, about 280,000 Holocaust survivors.

The interview schedule covered, among other items:(a) sociodemographic information (including place of birth and year of immigration); (b) emotional distress, measured by a modified version of the 12-GHQ (12), which used a dichotomous Yes/No answer; the time frame referred to "recent times." Cronbach's *alpha* internal reliability for the scale was .85 for the survivors and .80 for the comparison group; (c) self-reported diagnosed chronic illnesses and conditions (hypertension; heart attack, myocardial infarction; stroke; diabetes; asthma; herniated disc; cataracts; glaucoma; cancer; hip or pelvic fracture, osteoporosis; Parkinson's disease); (d) sleep problems (difficulty in falling asleep, difficulty in staying asleep and early-morning awakening); (e) visits to the family physician in the preceding six months; (f) social activities (attendance to a social club or to lectures, movies, theatre, concerts or other events such as sports, involvement in volunteer work, and engagement in hobbies); and (g) life satisfaction (with life in general and the way time is spent).

Exposure to the Holocaust was measured using a single item: "Did you live in a country under Nazi occupation?" If positive, the respondent was asked whether he/she had stayed in a ghetto, gone into hiding, sent to a work camp or extermination camp, or been in none of these situations; the more severe situation was coded. To avoid bias arising from secondary-gain effects, questions about the Holocaust were included within sections that addressed a variety of other issues. The interviews were conducted in Hebrew in the respondent's home. Emotional distress was measured by the sum of positive GHQ responses and analyzed as a continuous variable. Sleep disturbances were analyzed either as absent or at least one of them present. Chronic diseases/conditions were analyzed by the presence of none, one, two or three and more. Both dimensions of life satisfaction were combined into one variable.

The survivors in the sample were 896, which upon weighting back to the Jewish population of corresponding ages represented 145,437 persons. The respective figures for the comparison group were 331 and 51,231. Table 1 describes selected sociodemographic characteristics of both groups. Statistically significant inter-group differences were found for marital status (survivors included more divorced/separated and widowed persons than the comparison group) and for years of education (more survivors were in the 0 to 8 years category than the comparison group).

Table 1. Holocaust survivors and comparison group by sociodemographic characteristics and number of chronic health conditions (%), unweighted between weighted samples (28)

Variables	Survivors		Comparison group			
	Unweighted n = 896	Weighted N = 145,437	Unweighted n = 331	Weighted N = 51,231		Sig.
Gender	n	%	%	n	%	%	$x^2 = .03$, df = 1, $p = .85$
Gender	n	%	%	n	%	%	$x^2 = .03$, df = 1, $p = .85$
Women	436	48.7	55.0	155	46.8	54.5	
Men	460	51.3	45.0	176	53.2	45.5	
Age groups							$x^2 = 5.12$, df = 4, $p = .28$
60–64	94	10.5	14.3	39	11.8	16.8	
65–69	142	15.9	19.5	57	17.2	20.7	
70–74	216	24.1	25.8	58	17.5	20.6	
75–79	240	26.8	22.0	88	26.6	20.3	
80+	204	22.8	18.3	89	26.9	21.6	
Marital status							$x^2 = 17.69$, df = 4, $p = .001$
Married	556	62.1	63.2	214	64.6	65.5	
Never married	23	2.6	2.0	16	4.8	4.4	
Divorced / separated	31	3.5	3.0	3	.9	.3	
Widowed	286	31.9	31.7	98	29.6	29.8	
Years of education							$x^2 = 32.52$, df = 5, $p < .0001$
0	13	1.5	1.5	7	2.1	1.6	
1–4	92	10.3	9.7	10	3.0	3.5	
5–8	267	29.8	28.6	68	20.5	20.4	
9–12	328	36.6	37.5	126	38.1	37.4	
13–15	89	9.9	10.2	60	18.1	18.4	
16+	107	11.9	12.4	60	18.1	18.6	
Chronic health conditions							$x^2 = 8.73$, df = 3, $p = .03$
None	173	19.3	19.3	85	25.7	26.5	
1	299	33.4	33.2	111	33.5	34.0	
2	233	26.0	26.0	76	23.0	21.8	
3+	191	21.3	21.5	59	17.8	17.7	

Table 2 gives details on the survivors' exposure to war situations. There were more men who had been in labor camps, $p < .0001$. Survivors that had been in ghettos or extermination camps had fewer years of education.

Table 2. Holocaust survivors and comparison group by sociodemographic characteristics and type of WWII experience, weighted percent (28)

Variables	Survivors					Comparison group
	Ghetto	Hiding	Work camp	Death camp	Other*	
	n = 56	n = 113	n = 184	n = 187	n = 356	n = 331
Gender						
Women	36.1	35.2	71.2	44.3	38.0	45.5
Men	63.9	64.8	28.8	55.7	62.0	54.5
Age groups						
60–64	10.7	23.0	5.0	5.5	21.0	16.8
65–69	21.6	21.6	13.3	18.3	22.0	20.7
70–74	25.2	21.2	30.9	40.3	17.7	20.6
75–79	27.1	21.2	25.6	20.5	20.6	20.3
80+	15.4	13.0	25.3	15.4	18.7	21.6
Marital status						
Married	53.6	69.3	70.4	60.6	61.0	65.5
Never married	3.3	.5	1.2	1.0	3.4	4.4
Divorced / separated	2.6	.7	2.5	4.4	3.2	.3
Widowed	40.5	29.5	25.9	34.0	32.4	29.8
Years of education						
0	–	3.7	1.7	–	1.9	1.6
1–4	12.0	5.8	15.5	10.1	7.7	3.5
5–8	41.7	25.8	33.8	32.1	23.3	20.3
9–12	34.2	38.1	27.9	43.6	38.9	37.4
13–15	6.4	12.1	10.7	9.0	10.8	18.4
16+	5.6	14.5	10.4	5.2	17.4	18.6
Chronic health conditions						
None	16.5	15.8	17.4	19.7	21.4	26.5
1	39.9	40.9	28.3	23.2	35.6	34.0
2	15.8	25.3	29.8	26.1	26.0	21.8
3+	27.8	18.0	24.4	28.0	17.0	17.7

Exposed to the Holocaust but in none of the other specific situations.

Emotional distress

Survivors had a statistically significant higher M emotional distress score = 2.7, SE = .1, than their counterparts = 2.1, SE .1, $p < .003$). This difference remained statistically significant across gender ($p < .004$); marital status ($p < .005$); age groups ($p < .002$); and chronic health conditions ($p < .02$); and barely for years of education ($p < .06$) (table 3).

Table 3. Holocaust survivors and comparison group by mean emotional distress scores 2nd demographic variables (28)

Variables	Survivors (1)			Comparison group (2)			(1) vs. (2)
	M	SE	Sig.	M	SE	Sig.	Sig.
Total	2.7	.1	–	2.1	.1	–	.0028
Gender							.0035
Women	3.0	.1	1.0	2.3	.1	1.0	
Men	2.3	.1	.0001	2.0	.1	.2241	
Age groups							.0018
60–64	1.6	.2	1.0	1.4	.1	1.0	
65–69	1.9	.2	.3545	1.6	.1	.6572	
70–74	2.6	.2	.0013	1.7	.1	.3797	
75–79	3.2	.2	.0001	2.0	.2	.0719	
80+	4.1	.3	.0001	4.1	.3	.0001	
Marital status							.0047
Married	2.2	.1	1.0	1.8	.1	1.0	
Not married	3.5	.2	.0001	2.7	.2	.0030	
Years of education							.0564
0–8	3.6	.15	1.0	2.6	.10	1.0	
9–12	2.3	.13	.0001	2.3	.11	.4866	
13–15	2.1	.14	.0001	2.0	.05	.2063	
16+	1.5	.07	.0001	1.3	.04	.0015	
Chronic health conditions							.0214
None	1.4	.10	1.0	1.4	.08	1.0	
1	2.3	.13	.0001	1.8	.09	.1418	
2	2.7	.14	.0001	2.4	.11	.0091	
3+	4.4	.17	.0001	3.7	.18	.0001	

1.0 = reference group

The mean score was higher for survivors who had been in ghettos (2.8, $SE = .1$, $p < .18$); hiding (3.2, $SE = .2$, $p < .01$); forced labor (3.1, $SE = .2$, $p < .01$) and extermination camps (2.9, $SE = .2$, $p < .04$), compared to survivors who had lived in Nazi-occupied countries but were in none of those situations (2.2, $SE = .1$). Pair-wise comparisons between those in a ghetto, in forced labor and in extermination camps were not statistically significant.

Other health-related dimensions

Except for visits to the family physician in the preceding six months and for some social activities, the following variables did show statistically significant differences between both groups: sleep problems ($p < .0002$); number of chronic medical conditions ($p < .02$); hobbies ($p < .01$); participation in social clubs ($p < .005$); and attendance to lectures and movies ($p < .0005$) and volunteer work ($p < .0001$). In all these situations, the results were less favorable among the survivors. "Satisfaction with life" and "satisfaction with the way time is spent" were significantly reported as more favorable in the comparison group than among survivors, $p < .04$ and $p < .05$ respectively.

Emotional distress

The authors applied a multivariate analysis to control for confounding variables. The model included the following variables: survivor/comparison groups, gender, age groups, educational groups, marital status and number of chronic health conditions. The respective effect of the variables on emotional distress is shown in table 4. The direct effect of the variable Holocaust, that was present in the bivariate analysis, lost its statistical significance ($p < .11$) adjusting for variables affected by the Holocaust, such as the number of chronic medical conditions and years of formal education. Similarly, only the effect of hiding remained highly significant, after all other variables in the model were controlled ($p < .002$).

Table 4. Predictive model for emotional distress scores among Holocaust survivors vs.comparison group, weighted data (28)

Variables	Beta	SE	Sig.
WWII experience			.105
Holocaust	-.2	.2	.105
Comparison*			1.0
Gender			.0081
Women	-.4	.1	.0081
Men*			1.0
Age groups			.0001
60–64*			1.0
65–69	-.1	.2	.7739
70–74	.3	.2	.1488
75–79	.6	.3	.0141
80+	1.7	.3	<.0001
Marital status			.0141
Married*			1.0
Not married	.5	.2	.0141
Years of education			.0001
0–8*	–		1.000
9–12	-.8	.2	.0001
13–15	-1.0	.2	.0001
16+	-1.2	.2	.0001
Chronic health conditions			.0001
None*	–		1.0
1	.6	.2	.0020
2	1.0	.2	.0001
3+	2.2	.3	.0001

*Reference group

Other health-related dimensions

The multivariate analyses that included the same set of controlled variables as above showed significant differences for sleep disturbances ($p < .001$); and for social activities (participation in a social club, $p < .001$; attendance to lectures/movies, $p < .03$; engagement in volunteer work, $p < .001$).

♪ The Holocaust as a risk factor when facing new threats

Shuval (29), who studied immigrants residing in transit camps during the early years of Israel, showed that while the war trauma had not immunized survivors to the strains of life in the transit accommodations, past experience seemed to have hardened them, thus enabling satisfactory coping. She used the term "steeling effect." Rutter (30) made a similar claim in a discussion on resilience, suggesting that past trauma could facilitate coping successfully when the person faces a new stressful event. However, other authors have posited past traumas as a risk factor.

In more recent years, two sets of studies identified the Holocaust as a risk factor when survivors were confronted with a life-threatening situation such as war and the diagnosis/treatment of cancer. However, as noted below, in some of the research studies, the differences between the survivors and their counterparts were of marginal significance when confounding variables were controlled. Also, some of the early studies had some limitations with regard to the samples – both index cases and comparisons – and baseline measures. With time, those limitations were better addressed.

The threat of war-related events

Solomon and Prager (31) studied the psychopathological reaction to the Iraqi Scud missiles during the 1991 Gulf War among both elderly Holocaust survivors (n = 61; M age = 68.3) and elderly individuals that had not been in Europe during WWII (n = 131, M age = 72.9). The subjects answered a questionnaire including sociodemographic items; a scale measuring "sense of safety"; a state-trait anxiety inventory; and psychological distress during war time. In all four dependent variables taken singly, the elderly survivors scored worse than their counterparts. Since the Holocaust survivors were younger, had fewer years of formal education, were closer to the bomb sites, and were more religious than their counterparts, the authors performed a multivariate analysis controlling for these variables. The results still showed significant differences ($p < .05$).

Dekel and Hobfoll (32) conducted a theory-driven study purported to ascertain the vulnerability of Holocaust survivors to renewed war stress. They relied on the Conservation of Resources theory that submits that individuals seek, retain and protect resources. Psychological stress occurs when personal and/or interpersonal resources are lost, threatened or invested without return. Survivors, who have been exposed to losses of resources during the WWII, were at risk of becoming symptomatic when exposed again to major threats such as the terrorist attacks that took place during the *Al-Aqsa Intifada* (insurrection, in Arabic) that begun at the end of September 2000. In 2003, the authors selected 102 Holocaust survivors listed in organizations for survivors. Their interview schedule included several measures such as Holocaust experiences, additional stressful events, loss of psychosocial resources, distress measures e.g., the PTSD inventory (13) and the Brief Symptom Inventory-BSI (33). Nearly one in five survivors was exposed to direct or indirect acts of terror. Because the authors did not include a comparison group, they borrowed mean scores from another local study (34). Survivors had statistically significant distress scores than the norm used for comparison. However, none of the comparisons were adjusted for relevant variables such as education. Despite these limitations, what remains of interest is that survivors who experienced severe losses (such as loss of spouse or children during WWII) had higher scores in both the PTSD inventory and in the summary results of the BSI when they faced additional losses during the *Al-Aqsa Intifada*.

The threat of a malignant disease

Psycho-oncologists based at Hadassah Medical Center in Jerusalem have conducted a number of successive tests from 1984 to 2007 aimed at studying the effect of the Holocaust on survivors who had been diagnosed or were under treatment for cancer.

The first study (35), intended as exploratory, included a small sample of patients with cancer who survived the Holocaust (n = 26) and European-born subjects (n = 24) who were loosely defined as the "no camp" group. There were no differences between both groups with regard to schooling, religiosity, physical ability, awareness of the diagnosis and type of cancer. The comparison group included more women than men; this difference would make some of the tests even more conservative since women often score higher than men in emotional distress. The only structured scale used in this study measured psychological mood during the preceding month. The origin and the psychometric properties of this scale, however, were not reported. Uncontrolled analysis showed statistical significant lower mood scores among the survivors. Given its cross-sectional design, no conclusion was extracted because the survivors could have been in a lower initial status.

The second study utilized a more adequate methodology (36). In this study, survivors (n = 53), in active treatment or in follow-up for cancer, were compared with patients with cancer "who have had no [preceding] severe life threats." The latter patients had more children than the Holocaust group and, importantly for the effect of this variable on some scales, more years of education, $M = 12.8$, $SD = 4.4$, compared to 11.6, $SD = 3.4$, respectively; the differences were not significant. The time elapsed since cancer diagnosis was survivors, $M = 45$ months, and comparison, 50 months. Both groups were similar with regard to cancer status. The measures used were the IES-Impact of Event Scale (avoidance/intrusion subscales) (13), the BSI-Brief Symptom Inventory (33) for distress, and the PAIS-Psychosocial Adjustment to Physical Illness Scale (37) to assess the impact of cancer on functioning.

Avoidance and intrusiveness mean scores were higher among the survivors. Similar results were found for BSI mean scores. As for PAIS, the differences did not reach statistical significance.

A third study attempted to overcome the lack of baseline information, unavailable in the previous inquiries (38). Holocaust survivors who had cancer (n = 57) were compared with non-randomly selected survivors free of cancer (n = 50). In this study, only the BSI scale (33) was applied. Survivors with cancer showed significant higher mean scores in nine of the 10 BSI subscales. The lack of control for education in the multivariate analysis and of information of the degree of traumatization during the Holocaust turned this study into one which is not entirely definitive.

The last study (39) reported by this research group is more complex; it is also relevant for the section on offspring of Holocaust survivors (see below). This study included four groups of mother-daughter pairs, as follows: (a) patients with breast cancer whose mothers were Holocaust survivors (n = 20); (b) similar type of patients with "no traumatized mothers" (n = 19); (c) cancer-free daughters of survivors (n = 22); (d) cancer-free daughters of "non-traumatized mothers (n = 20).

Except for a larger percentage of married mothers in group (c) and a 20% presence of Israeli born among the "non-traumatized mothers," there were no other statistical differences with regard to sociodemographic variables. No additional information was provided with reference to the origin and further characteristics of the samples. Respondents were administered the

BSI (33); the IES (13); MAC-the Mental Adjustment to Cancer Scale (40), a 40-item instrument to measure coping styles with regard to cancer; and the PFS-Perception of Family Support (41). All scales and subscales had adequate reliability coefficient measures.

The results showed that the daughters with cancer whose mothers were Holocaust survivors had statistically significant higher distress sores than their cancer-free counterparts, and higher than daughters whose mothers were "non-traumatized." The analysis of the comparison of mothers who were survivors with daughters with and without cancer did not show statistical differences. Mothers and daughters in group (a) had higher IES scores than those from the "non-traumatized" group (b). MAC was equal in both groups of daughters, groups (a) and (b).

Hantman and Solomon (42), who also tested the vulnerability of Holocaust survivors to cancer, included a novel research dimension in their inquiry. They explored the survivors' reactions to the Holocaust according to three categories of overall coping styles, known as the "victims," the "fighters" and "those who made it" (43).

As above, the first objective of their study was to establish the differential degree of reaction to the stress of cancer in the survivors and their counterparts. The second objective explored the survivors' reactions according to their overall coping style. The study took place 55 years after WWII. Convenient samples of patients, both survivors (n = 150) and non-survivors who had lived in European countries during WWII but not under Nazi occupation (n = 50), were selected from hospital-based oncology services. The comparison group had higher levels of education and religiosity than the survivor group, but both groups did not differ with regard to stage or type of cancer. As in previously described studies, the authors used the 17-item PTSD inventory (44), the SCL-90 (11), the PAIS (37) and a questionnaire purported to explore coping with the aftermath of the Holocaust. Statistically significant results were found for the intrusion and avoidance subscales of the PTSD scale. No differences were found with regard to the mean scores of the SCL-90 and the PAIS.

The frequency of the survivors' coping groups was: "victims", 17.3%; "fighters", 39.3%; and "those who made it", 43.4%. A one-way Manova showed that the mean number of PTSD symptoms increased in that order, 5.1, 7.6 and 10.5, respectively. The SCL-90 results were rather similar – the "victims" had higher scores in three subscales, somatization, depression and anxiety. PAIS did not show marked different results. Of highest interest is the group of "those who made it," which outperformed the comparison group in some measures, a truly resilient group of survivors.

֍ From research to data

The epidemiology of the mental health impact of the Holocaust on the survivors has attracted and continues to attract the attention of Israeli researchers. The reasons are obvious, survivors constitute a visible group in society despite their advanced age and dwindling numbers. Their psychological suffering, mental disability and vulnerabilities but also admirable adaptation and contribution to society are an indivisible part of the professional and nonprofessional ethos in the country.

What has been the main epidemiologic contribution of Israeli researchers to the field? This question will be disaggregated as follows:

What types of research have been done on the aftereffects of the Holocaust, and how were they conducted? What were the research results and how were they interpreted?

As noted earlier, there were three main topics addressed in the epidemiological research conducted locally – the presence of psychiatric disorders among community residents; the presence of emotional distress; and the Holocaust experience as a risk factor for renewed stressful events such as those generated by life-threatening events (war or cancer). Many studies were driven by theory, while other studies derived theoretical notions from their research findings.

What types of research have been conducted and how were they done?

It may be surprising that – despite clinicians' concern for the survivors on account of both their demand for psychiatric help and the need to answer their reparation claims – only a single study explored the association between Holocaust experiences and psychiatric disorders in the community (7). The authors found that anxiety disorders, emotional distress and sleep disturbances were more frequent among survivors living in the community than among their counterparts. Other dimensions of morbidity investigated (not reported above) – mood disorders, pain, selected self-reported cardiovascular problems, obesity and smoking – were not significantly different in the two groups. All health dimensions analyzed were controlled for relevant variables. The psychopathological problems found did not seem to result from learning about symptoms in the clinical context, since the survivors who were interviewed used mental health services no differently from their counterparts, and secondary gains were unlikely.

As noted above, most community studies conducted in Israel (and the same is for abroad) used scales to measure nonspecific psychopathology. Admittedly, those scales had good psychometric properties and are adequate indicators of psychopathology, but they do not generate psychiatric diagnoses. The size of the samples included in the studies varied; some of them were relatively small but others (such as ref. 28) included large number of respondents that provided adequate statistical power. Also, the source of the study samples differed. A serious limitation was created by the inclusion of survivors from lists of their organizations

Obviously, Holocaust survivors constitute a heterogeneous group, yet in some research this issue has been glossed over. For example, Fennig and Levav (45), and to some extent Shemesh *et al.* (28), showed that there was a "dose-effect" of the traumatic experiences. Survivors who had been in more adverse situations like extermination camps had higher distress scores than those in relatively lesser traumatic situations, as in ghettos. Deckel and Hobfoll (32) did address another aspect of the heterogeneity of the psychological trauma of the Holocaust: in their study they took into account the extent of the personal and interpersonal losses to assess the psychological impact of renewed stress related to terror. A few authors considered the differential impact of the trauma when they explored the effect of individuals' ages during the Holocaust – but no careful empirical comparisons were made.

An important research problem addressed in Israeli epidemiological studies is the vulnerability or protection granted by past experiences to the survivor when facing life-threatening stressors. The stressors selected for investigation – war and cancer – carry the necessary weight to explore those untoward reactions. The evidence seems to indicate (31, 36, 38, 42) that the past leaves both psychological and biological traces. Those dormant traces are awakened when the trigger has a life-threatening quality.

However, it is not only vulnerability that has been found among survivors, but also resilience (as has been noted in 14, 29). Yet, the exploration of resilience remains limited in Israel. The exceptions are few and include an early inquiry by Fennig and Levav, that explored the protective effect of current social supports on emotional distress among women attending a primary care clinic (45). Of late, Hantman and Solomon (42) investigated typologies of coping styles to ascertain their differential protective effects when the survivor had cancer.

What were the research results and how to interpret them?

Notwithstanding the limitations of Eitinger's pioneer study (3), he was able to show that KZ syndrome was identifiable among individuals living in Norway (a country that knew no belic conflict after WWII) and Israel (which has faced armed hostilities and terror before and since the establishment of the state in May 1948). Recall here that the largest wave of survivors arrived in Israel in 1948 and 1949 while the War of Independence was raging. Roughly half of the Israeli fighting force in the second stage of that war consisted of Holocaust survivors.

Analogously, the studies on nonspecific psychopathology and especially those exploring post-traumatic symptoms (particularly of the intrusion and avoidance domains) showed higher mean scores among survivors than suitable counterparts after adjustments were made for potential confounders, such as education (usually, survivors had a lower educational level). With the ageing of survivors and the passage of the years since the Holocaust, the results are less clear since the survivors, who are elderly by now, are those who were best able to resist the wear and tear of life. In addition, biases arising from the research design could affect the results, since the institutionalized elderly were not included in the later community studies; conceivably, those interviewed in the community were the healthiest of the group, if institutionalization was more frequent among survivors as they aged.

The bivariate analysis of one community survey on the elderly, which was conducted 55 years after the end of WWII (28), showed that the survivors had higher emotional distress than the comparison group. In turn, the multivariate analysis indicated that the effect of the traumatic experiences on emotional distress seemed to be accounted by other Holocaust-dependent variables, such as fewer years of education and number of self-reported chronic health conditions.

The findings of this study (28) showed that even among resilient survivors emotional distress scores were significantly higher than among European-born respondents who did not live in Nazi-occupied countries. Also, the number of chronic health conditions affecting the survivors was larger than among respondents from the comparison group, assuming that help-seeking and medical care received were equal between the two groups. (This reservation loses strength since the results showed that visits to the primary care physician did not differ between the groups during the preceding six months). As noted earlier, the sampling method excluded survivors residing in institutions for the infirm; conceivably, their inclusion would have generated even higher mean emotional distress scores.

Studies showed that sleep disturbances were more common among survivors. Other authors identified the same finding among survivors (3, 46); conceivably, these sleep problems are lingering manifestations of clinical or subclinical post-traumatic disorders no longer fully present. Lastly, this study showed the late negative effect of the Holocaust on being engaged in pleasurable activities favored generally by European-born Israelis. It would appear that while the group of elderly survivors investigated by Shemesh *et al.* (28) may have adapted successfully to life in many respects, other areas of life rarely investigated in epidemiological studies were also affected.

In conclusion, despite the noted research limitations, the aggregated results are fully convincing, Holocaust survivors included in random samples and interviewed about conditions unrelated to compensation claims presented more psychopathology than relevant comparison groups. Furthermore, survivors seem to constitute an at-risk population group when they face life-threatening events. Luckily, however, the affected survivors with psychopathology are far from being the majority.

§ Psychopathology among the second-generation of Holocaust survivors

As years since WWII elapsed, clinicians begun to report that second-generation survivors presented psychopathology possibly linked to their parents' experiences (4). This was not entirely surprising, the Holocaust-related severe adversities noted above, including hastily contracted marriages after liberation to recreate the lost family, were thought to have impaired the survivors' parental abilities (2). Accordingly, authors raised the hypotheses that child-rearing processes such as separation-individuation (47) and attachment (48) might have been disrupted.

Today, the picture that emerges from a vast literature on the mental health of children of Holocaust survivors is more complex. The community-based epidemiological inquiries summarized below, which are not based on help-seeking, cast a shadow of doubt on the clinical findings. Indeed, reviewers (49) have noted that clinical and community studies fail to concur. Whereas "clinical studies tend to present a specific psychological profile that includes a predisposition to PTSD, various difficulties in separation-individuation and a contradictory mix of resilience and vulnerability when coping with stress," community surveys "do not show that the offspring of the survivors differ from well-selected comparison populations." Admittedly, the clinical studies were not uniform with regard to their findings nor they were all free from methodological shortcomings (50). As noted by reviewers, several clinical studies failed to support the notion that psychopathology in the first generation was generally transmitted to the second. Yet, for many practitioners, the existence or lack thereof of the "second-generation syndrome" has not reached closure, especially since a set of well-designed studies has identified vulnerability factors in the offspring, such as when diagnosed with breast cancer (51) and following exposure to war actions. Some exceptions, however, were also reported (52, 53).

As in the previous section of this chapter, the studies covered here address two central themes – psychiatric symptoms and disorders ascertained during community-based psychiatric epidemiology studies, as well as vulnerability to psychopathology when survivors' children face highly stressful life events.

§ Psychiatric symptoms and disorders

Study 1

Schwartz *et al.* (54) used data collected in a 1980s epidemiological study to examine a possible trans-generational transmission of psychiatric disorders to survivors' children. Their examination was guided by a theoretical framework that enabled the formulation of alternative research predictions.

Initially, the authors discarded the possible genetic transmission of disorders since they considered it unlikely that Jews with severe psychiatric disorders had greater chances of surviving traumatic events during and after the war, and then raise a family. The most likely explanation was a non-genetic transmission. This would result from social learning and modeling expressed in an excess of disorders in survivors – such as anxiety, depression or PTSD ("direct or specific transmission") – or be due to a generic deficit or vulnerability expressed by no particular disorder that contributed to the excess of psychiatric morbidity among the offspring ("indirect or nonspecific transmission").

The study they conducted yielded psychiatric diagnoses. Respondents, both offspring of survivors and the comparison group, were included in a large cohort of native Israelis born between 1949 and 1958 whose parents had immigrated from Europe or North Africa (see chapters 11 and 14). Respondents were asked about parents' Holocaust experience. In the first part of a two-stage study design, all respondents were screened with the PERI (17), together with anamnestic questions purported to elicit past or current psychiatric disorders. All respondents who were found to be "positive" in the first stage and 18% of those found "negative" were interviewed by psychiatrists using a modified lifetime version of the Schedule of Affective Disorders and Schizophrenia, known as SADS-I (55). Both stages had remarkable high response rates, 94% and 91%, respectively.

The authors took as "cases" those respondents whose fathers and mothers were in labor or concentration camps and immigrated to Israel after 1945. Respondents with parents of European origin who had immigrated before 1945 and were not in ghettos, hiding or camps were included in the "comparison group." The selection criterion that was adopted attempted to maximize the contrast between both groups (respondents who had one parent in the Holocaust or were only in a ghetto or in hiding were excluded).

In the first or screening stage, 957 individuals met the criteria for the comparison group and 271 for the category of survivor's offspring. In the second or diagnostic stage, the respective numbers were 476 and 147. Results were weighted to the inverse of the sampling probabilities.

The dependent variables were obtained from both stages. In the first stage the following symptoms scales were derived: demoralization or emotional distress; enervation; false beliefs and perceptions; suicidal ideation; anti-social behaviors; problems with drinking; and schizoid traits. Two additional scales were included – the Impact of Events Scale (13) and a purposely designed 23-item scale of symptoms of PTSD. In the second stage, the diagnoses that were extracted were based on the RDC-Research Diagnostic Criteria, including the identification of the symptom of guilt wherever it was present, such as in major depression disorder. Statistical power in this study was generally adequate. Confounders, such as education, marital status and others, were taken into account based on findings in the literature on survivors and their children.

The analysis for the year prevalence revealed no differences in those symptoms and disorders, including guilt. However, positive results for the offspring were found for lifetime prevalence disorders of the "direct transmission" (major and minor depression and anxiety disorders) but not for the "indirect transmission."

Study II

INHS (56) included offspring of both, Holocaust survivors and of European-born parents who had not resided in Nazi-occupied countries (57). The outcome variables included psychopathological domains explored in Study I, such as emotional distress and depressive and anxiety disorders, in addition to a number of new variables such as use of services, self-appraisal of health, self-reported physical health conditions and suicidal behavior.

The population sample of the total study, where this sub-study was part, was extracted from the National Population Register (NPR) and was comprised of non-institutionalized residents aged 21 and over. The index group included Israeli- or European-born respondents (except from the former Soviet republics) aged 30 and over whose parent or parents had lived in a Nazi-occupied country during WWII, only mother, n = 63; only father, n = 91; both parents, n = 276. This group of respondents was identified by answering these questions: "Did your father /mother live in a country that was under the Nazi regime or in a country that was under the direct influence of the Nazi regime?" Those who answered positively were further asked: "During the Holocaust, was your father/mother in a ghetto? In hiding? In a labor camp? In a death camp? Was forced to leave the place of residence because of the Nazi regime?" The comparison group included offspring of European-born parents who did not reside in Nazi-occupied countries (n = 417).

The Interview Schedule: It included sociodemographic information; the 12-item General Health Questionnaire (GHQ-12) (12); the World Mental Health Survey Composite International Diagnostic Interview (WMHS-CIDI) (56); general and mental health service utilization; general health (mental and physical); self-reported physical health conditions; smoking; and suicidal behaviors.

The GHQ-12 screens for psychiatric disorder and is a measure of emotional distress. Scores range between 12 and 48, where higher scores indicate increased distress. Cronbach's *alpha*, which measures internal reliability consistency, was .88 for the combined groups. The WMHS-CIDI assessed lifetime and 12-month prevalence of several mental disorders according to *ICD-10* and *DSM-IV*.

The following psychiatric disorders were included in Study II – anxiety disorders (panic disorder, generalized anxiety disorder, agoraphobia without panic disorder, and PTSD) and depressive disorders (major depressive disorder and dysthymia,). Twelve-month and/or lifetime prevalence rates of *DSM-IV* disorders were determined whenever respondents' current or past symptoms met diagnostic criteria. For each disorder, a screening section was administered to each respondent. Respondents were asked whether they had consulted with any one of a detailed list of health and community agents for problems related to their mental health during the preceding 12 months.

Respondents who did not use those services during the same period were asked whether they thought they needed mental health treatment. Respondents were asked to appraise their health using a 1 to 5 scale, from excellent to poor. Self-report of a number of health conditions with obvious psychological load was examined – sleep problems; hypertension and cardiovascular and cerebral-vascular disorders; asthma; diabetes; and body mass index (as an indicator of obesity). Smoking at the time of the study was measured at any level of the habit. Lastly, lifetime suicidal behavior (ideation, planning and attempt) was inquired.

One-way analysis of variance was used to assess differences in the means and standard errors of emotional distress among the offspring of Holocaust survivors and control group, adjusting for the confounding effect of education. A variable, AD, was created to include any anxiety or depressive disorder that was present during the last year and lifetime. Sleep disturbances included difficulties to fall and stay asleep and early-morning awakening. Suicidal behaviors, thinking, planning and attempts were collapsed into one measure. All other measures were analyzed singly. Chi-square statistics were applied to test significance of differences in the distributions between offspring of Holocaust survivors and the comparison group. Statistical significance was established at .05. Odds ratios (OR) and 95% confidence intervals (CIs) for the measures of psychopathology and other health dimensions adjusted for confounders were calculated using logistic regression analysis. CIs that excluded the unity were regarded as significant. Strata and cluster weights were assigned to each subject according to complex sampling design.

Results

Table 5 shows the sociodemographic features of offspring of both groups. No statistically significant differences were noted except for educational attainment ($p = .0007$), the offspring of survivors achieved more years of schooling than the comparison group. There were neither group differences with regard to separation from the biological parents before age 16 nor for placement outside the home before age 18.

Table 5. Offspring of Holocaust survivors and comparison group by sociodemographic features (raw numbers and weighted proportions) (57)

Variables	Holocaust group n = 430 n (%)	Comparison group n = 417 n (%)	Sig.
Gender			
Male	214 (48.1)	195 (45.9)	$x^2 = .46$, df = 1, $p = .50$
Female	216 (51.9)	222 (54.1)	
Age groups			
30–49	189 (45.8)	174 (45.2)	$x^2 = .03$, df = 1, $p = .86$
50+	241 (54.2)	243 (54.8)	
Marital status			
Married	346 (82.4)	317 (78.3)	$x^2 = 2.36$, df = 1, $p = .12$
Not married	84 (17.6)	100 (21.7)	
Years of education			
0–12	122 (28.0)	173 (40.8)	$x^2 = 14.47$, df = 2, $p = .0007$
13–15	118 (27.6)	98 (23.9)	
16+	189 (44.4)	248 (35.3)	
Place of origin			
Israeli born	275 (65.7)	248 (59.9)	$x^2 = 3.12$, df = 1, $p = .08$
European born	155 (34.3)	169 (40.1)	
Lived with both biological parents before age 16			
Yes	380 (88.3)	377 (91.1)	$x^2 = 1.85$, df = 1, $p = .17$
No	50 (11.7)	40 (8.9)	
Outside the home for more than 6 months before age 18			
Yes	45 (10.6)	40 (8.9)	$x^2 = .67$, df = 2, $p = .41$
No	384 (89.4)	377 (91.1)	

Neither of the groups differed statistically on emotional distress and anxiety and depressive disorders, for both lifetime and 12-month prevalence rates. Both groups did not differ in the age of onset of those disorders up to age 18, when almost all Jewish males and a sizeable proportion of Jewish females leave home for military service. Also, no differences were noted regarding suicidal behaviors, sleep disturbances or smoking. General health was self-assessed as excellent or very good by 67.2% of the children of Holocaust survivors and 59.2% by the comparison group. When this variable was adjusted for education, the difference did not reach statistical significance (OR = 1.3, 95% CI 1.0–1.7). No difference was found in the percentage of individuals who consulted health services for a mental condition either during the preceding year or in the past.

Table 6. Offspring of Holocaust survivors and comparison group by selected psychopathological measures (57)

Measures	Holocaust group n = 430	Comparison group n = 417	Holocaust vs. comparison group	Holocaust vs. comparison group, education adjusted
GHQ, M (SE)	17.4 (.3)	17.5 (.3)	F =.08, df = 1, p =.78	F =.03, df = 1, p =.86
	% (n)	% (n)	OR (95% CI)	OR (95% CI)
AD*, 12 months	6.7 (29)	4.2 (17)	1.6 (.9–3.0)	1.7 (.9–3.1)
AD, onset (before age 18)	3.8 (19)	2.9 (13)	1.2 (.9–1.7)	1.2 (.8–1.6)
AD, lifetime	12.6 (56)	11.2 (48)	1.2 (.8–1.8)	1.1 (.7–1.7)
Self-appraisal of mental and physical health	67.2 (281)	59.2 (232)	1.4 (1.1–1.9)	1.3 (1.0–1.7)
Suicidal behavior (ideation, planning or attempt) lifetime	3.6 (16)	2.4 (10)	1.5 (.7–3.5)	1.7 (.8–4.0)
Smoking	18.8 (81)	18.3 (76)	1.0 (.7–1.5)	1.1 (.8–1.6)
Sleep problems	26.2 (116)	24.9 (105)	1.1 (.8–1.5)	1.1 (.8–1.6)
Mental health treatment, last 12 months	13.6 (60)	12.1 (53)	1.1 (.8–1.7)	1.2 (.8–1.8)
Any health service treatment, lifetime	26.7 (120)	21.4 (91)	1.3 (1.0–1.9)	1.3 (.9–1.7)

* AD: *any anxiety or mood disorder.*

A similar lack of statistically significant difference was found in the physical health variables examined (table 7), including visits to the general health services in the preceding two weeks.

The above analysis was repeated for the sub-group of offspring of Holocaust survivors, where both of the parents were in extermination camps (n = 32) and where both parents went through the Holocaust (n = 276); there were no statistically significant differences with the comparison group.

Table 7. Offspring of Holocaust survivors and comparison group (%) by selected self-reported physical health measures (57)

Physical health measures	Holocaust group N = 430 (1)	Comparison group N = 417 (2)	(1) vs. (2) unadjusted	(1) vs. (2) education-adjusted
Body mass index (BMI) Mean (SE)	26.1 (.2)	25.8 (.2)	F =.79, df = 1, p =.37	F = 1.97, df = 1, p =.16
	% (n)	% (n)	OR (95% CI)	OR (95% CI)
BMI 30+	18.5 (76)	16.7 (65)	1.1 (.8–1.7)	1.2 (.8–1.8)
Physical problems for 6 months and over	34.5 (149)	33.5 (145)	1.0 (.8–1.4)	1.1 (.8–1.4)
Chronic pain, different locations	39.4 (173)	34.0 (143)	1.2 (.9–1.7)	1.3 (1.0–1.7)
Myocardial infarction, CVA or hypertension	25.6 (111)	28.6 (128)	.9 (.6–1.2)	.9 (.7–1.2)
Asthma	6.4 (28)	6.4 (28)	1.0 (.6–1.8)	1.0 (.6–1.8)
Diabetes	6.8 (31)	9.3 (43)	.7 (.4–1.2)	.8 (.5–1.2)
Use of health services, last 2 weeks	42.4 (179)	41.4 (179)	1.0 (.8–1.4)	1.0 (.8–1.4)

§ **Vulnerability with regard to life-threatening events**

The threat of war-related events

Solomon *et al.* (52) conducted a lab-like test on the vulnerability of soldiers diagnosed as suffering from combat stress reaction during the First Lebanon War in 1982 (see chapter 13). Their test answered several questions. They selected 44 soldiers whose mother or father or both parents survived the Holocaust and compared them with 52 soldiers equally affected whose parents were European born but did not go through the Holocaust. The two groups were asked to fill questionnaires by themselves, thus avoiding the lack of blindness on the part of interviewers. The questionnaire contained 13 items tapping the presence of *DSM-III* PTSD, including scales measuring the re-experiencing of the traumatic events, numbness and the presence of symptoms that did not exist before the war.

Both groups did not differ in sociodemographic variables or military features measured upon recruitment into the IDF. The soldiers completed the questionnaire after one, two and three years following the end of the war. PTSD rates of among the children of Holocaust survivors were 70%, 73% and 64% during years 1, 2 and 3 respectively. For the same years, the rates among the non-Holocaust group were 60%, 52%, and 39%, respectively. Careful multivariate analysis showed that at years 2 and 3, the group with survivor parents had a statistically higher PTSD score than the comparison group, while the slope of the decrease of the symptoms, although not statistically different, was steeper in the non-Holocaust group.

Contrary to those results, another study conducted by Solomon on the effect of parental Holocaust experience on captive soldiers of the 1973 Yom Kippur War yielded no increased risk in the subjects' mental health measures (53). Of the 240 prisoners of war (POW), 164 participated in the study. This group was matched with a group of 184 veterans who were not POW. Both groups were administered a battery of different scales including the Impact of Event Scale (13) and the Global Severity Index of the SCL-90 (11), which is a measure of emotional distress. The study was conducted 18 years after the war. While the mental health measures showed that the mental health of the former POWs was statistically more affected, previous parental experience with the Holocaust showed no effect.

The threat of a malignant disease

Baider *et al.* (51) studied the vulnerability to psychopathological and psychological dimensions among female offspring of Holocaust survivors who had breast cancer. Having identified a higher reactivity to the diagnosis of cancer among survivors (36), they assumed "that the offspring of Holocaust survivors might be as vulnerable as their parents are. Similar to their parents, many of their children function adequately in their daily activities but are unable to cope with the emotions of extreme stress or severe life-threatening situations" (51). Accordingly, they expected that the offspring of survivors would react more adversely than other breast cancer patients whose parents have not been in the Holocaust. In this study, the definition of the sample was clearest – the index group included offspring whose parents, one or both, had been in forced labor, concentration or extermination camps (n = 106) while the comparison group included patients with cancer whose parents, all European born, had not been in the Holocaust (n = 102). All respondents completed a self-report questionnaire that included the BSI (33), the IES (13), and the MAC (40). Medically, the subjects of the comparison group were in higher proportion treated with chemotherapy and in stages 3 and 4 of the illness. While the differences in the MAC, which measures coping, were absent, the offspring of the survivors had statistically significant higher scores of the IES and BSI (scales that measure symptoms).

Another study by the same research team (58) explored whether the level of distress among offspring of survivors affected by breast cancer was higher than "non-traumatized" parents and whether there was a synergistic action between the two variables – having a cancer diagnosis and being the daughter of a Holocaust survivor. As above, they studied patients with cancer whose parents were or were not traumatized in addition to two comparison groups of healthy individuals whose parents were and were not traumatized. Recruitment procedures, criteria for inclusion, measures and strategy of analysis were similar as above. In this component of their research, the authors showed that the two factors – cancer diagnosis and being an offspring of survivor – had a synergistic effect on two emotional distress subscales of the BSI, depression and psychoticism.

⚘ From research to data

Given the parents' ordeal during and immediately after WWII, the authors of Studies I and II (57) had expected that their offspring would be affected in terms of both their psychopathology as well as other related domains (59). Yet, all the domains investigated showed no differences between the group of Holocaust survivors' offspring and the comparison group. The agreement in the results between Study I and Study II is persuasive, since they used different diagnostic instruments and research strategies to produce them. Although both studies lack reliable information on the possible psychopathology of the respondents during their youth, when they were living in closer contact with the parents and at a time closer to the traumatic events of WWII, Study II did find no differences between the two groups with regard to the (early) age of onset of the anxiety and depressive disorders.

Those two epidemiological inquiries are not alone in their negative findings. Recently, in an ingenious laboratory-based study by Sagi *et al.* (48) found that attachment – a key psychological mechanism linking mothers with their offspring – was not more disrupted among a group of children of Holocaust survivors than in a suitable control group.

Thus, in contrast to epidemiological community-based inquiries that gather data from all community members whether healthy or sick, clinical studies based their observations on psychopathology actually diagnosed. Conceivably, offspring of Holocaust survivors who seek help from mental health services attribute the origin or the "coloring" of their problems to the family environment and parental behavior resulting from traumatic WWII experiences.

Study II would not seem to support a greater need of care among the offspring of the survivors, except for those seeking help. Results showed no evidence that the offspring of Holocaust survivors consulted in the past or planned to consult more frequently for mental health problems during the preceding year of the survey compared with their counterparts.

The disparity between the findings of Studies I and II with those obtained by all but one of those exploring the vulnerability of the offspring of Holocaust survivor facing major fateful stressors is difficult to reconcile – except for the fact that the criteria of inclusion implied selecting only individuals who had faced or were facing major fateful stressful events. Those individuals were carriers of a risk requiring triggers that are less ubiquitous in ordinary life to reach clinical expression.

These studies on the second generation would demand a modification in the research agenda. Rather than to limiting the studies to mental illness, the task that lies ahead is to add the exploration of factors that explain resilience. How is it that parents who underwent one of the cruelest human-made disasters in history and whose emotional scars could be elicited in community surveys long after their ordeal ended (2) were able to avoid transmitting to their offspring various expressions of trauma? It has been noted repeatedly that these survivors muted their personal dramas while striving to secure for their children a safer and better life (60). The mutual (over) protection inferred from the narratives of offspring in a study conducted in Israel (61) – construed by some observers as possibly pathogenic and a "conspiracy of silence" (43) and often decried – might have ultimately brought about the disorder-free outcomes that resulted. Importantly, Study II gathered some evidence of Holocaust survivors' ability to function as parents, while survivors were found to have a relatively low level of education than controls (2), the offspring of survivors achieved more years of education than the comparison group.

In conclusion, Studies I and II – in addition to their epidemiologic value – are testimony to a generation of parents who suffered maximum adversity in their lives but were able to grant protection to their children's mental health through adulthood.

❧ References

1. Bauer J. *History of the Holocaust*. New York: Franklin Watts, 1982.
2. Levav I. Individuals under conditions of maximum adversity: the Holocaust. In Dohrenwend BP, ed. *Adversity, stress, and psychopathology*. New York: Oxford University, 1998.
3. Eitinger L. *Concentration camp survivors in Norway and Israel*. London: Alen and Unwin, 1961.
4. Eitinger L, Krell R. *The psychological and medical affects of concentration camps and related persecutions on survivors of the Holocaust: a research bibliography*, Vancouver: University of British Columbia Press, 1985.
5. *Israel Journal of Psychiatry* 2001; 38: 1.
6. Solomon Z, Chaitin J, eds. *Childhood in the shadow of the Holocaust: survived children and second generation*. Tel Aviv: Hakibbutz Hameuhad, 2007 (Hebrew).
7. Sharon A, Levav I, Brodsky J, *et al*. Psychopathology among Holocaust survivors six decades thereafter. *British Journal of Psychiatry* (In press).
8. Helweg-Larssen P. Famine disease in German concentration camps. *Acta Psychiatrica* 1952; suppl 83.
9. Eitinger L. Pathology of the concentration camp syndrome. *Archives of General Psychiatry* 1961; 5: 371–379.
10. Levav I, Arnon A, Portnoy A. Two shortened versions of the CMI: a new test of their validity. *International Journal of Epidemiology* 1977; 6: 135–141.
11. Derogatis LR, Lipman RS, Covi L. SCL-90: an outpatient psychiatric rating scale; Preliminary report. *Psychopharmacology Bulletin* 1973; 9: 13–28.
12. Goldberg DP, Gater R, Sartorius N, *et al*. The validity of two versions of the GHQ in the WHO study of mental illness in general healthcare. *Psychological Medicine* 1997; 27: 191–197.
13. Horwitz MJ, Wilner N, Alvarez W. Impact of event scale: a measure of subjective stress. *Psychosomatic Medicine* 1979; 4: 209–218.
14. Antonovsky A. Maoz B, Dowty N, *et al*. Twenty-five years later: a limited study of the sequelae of the concentration camp experience. *Social Psychiatry* 1971; 6: 186–193.
15. Levav I, Abramson JH. Emotional distress among concentration camp survivors: a community study in Jerusalem. *Psychological Medicine* 1984; 14: 215–218.
16. Collins C, Burazeri G, Gofin J, *et al*. Health status and mortality in Holocaust survivors living in Jerusalem 40–50 years later. *Journal of Traumatic Stress* 2004; 17: 403–411.
17. Shrout PE, Dohrenwend BP, Levav I. A discriminant rule for screening cases of diverse diagnostic types: preliminary results. *Journal of Consulting and Clinical Psychology* 1986; 54: 314–319.
18. Carmil D, Carmel RS. Emotional distress and satisfaction in life among Holocaust survivors: a community study of survivors and controls. *Psychological Medicine* 1986; 16: 141–149.
19. Robinson S, Rapaport Bar-Sever M, Rapaport J. The present state of people who survived the Holocaust as children. *Acta Psychiatrica Scandinavica* 1994; 89: 242–245.
20. Landau R, Litwin H. The effects of extreme early stress in very old age. *Journal of Traumatic Stress* 2000; 13: 473–487.
21. Auslander GK, Litwin H. Social networks, social support and self-ratings of health. *Journal of Aging and Health* 1991; 3: 493–510.
22. Rotter J. Generalized expectations for internal versus external control of reinforcement. *Psychological Monographs* 1966; 80: 1–28.
23. Cochran M, Larner M, Riley D, *et al*. *Extended families: the social networks of parents and their children*. Cambridge: Cambridge University Press, 1990.
24. Shmotkin D, Blumstein T, Modan B, *et al*. Tracing long-term effects of early trauma: a broad scope view of Holocaust survivors of late life. *Journal of Consulting and Clinical Psychology* 2003; 71: 223–234.

25. Ben-Zur H, Zimmerman N. Aging holocaust survivors' well being and adjustment: associations with ambivalence over emotional expression. *Psychological Aging* 2005; 20: 710–713.

26. Amir M, Lev-Wisel R. Time does not heal all wounds: quality of life and psychological distress of people who survived the Holocaust as children 55 years later. *Journal of Traumatic Stress* 2003, 16: 295–299.

27. The WHOQOL Group. The World Health Organization QoL assessment, development and general psychometric properties. *Social Science and Medicine* 1998; 46: 1569–1585.

28. Shemesh AA, Levav I, Radomislensky I, et al. Emotional distress among elderly survivors of the *Shoa* living in the community. *Israel Journal of Psychiatry and Related Disciplines* 2008; 45: 230–238.

29. Shuval J. Some persistent effects of trauma: five years after the Nazi concentration camps. *Social Problems* 1957–58; 5: 230–243.

30. Rutter M. Psychosocial resilience and protective mechanisms. *American Journal of Orthopsychiatry* 1987; 57: 316–31.

31. Solomon Z, Prager E. Elderly Israeli Holocaust survivors during the Persian Gulf War: a study of psychological distress. *American Journal of Psychiatry* 1992; 12: 1707–1710.

32. Dekel R, Hobfoll SE. The impact of resource loss on Holocaust survivors facing war and terrorism in Israel. *Aging and Mental Health* 2007; 11:159–167.

33. Derogatis LR, Spencer P. *The Brief Symptom Inventory (BSI): administration, scoring, procedures manual*. Baltimore: Clinical Psychometric Research, Johns Hopkins University, 1982.

34. Gilbar O, Ben Zur H. Bereavement of spousal caregivers of cancer patients. *American Journal of Orthopsychiatry* 2002; 72: 422–432.

35. Baider L, Sarrel M. Coping with cancer among Holocaust survivors in Israel: an exploratory study. *Journal of Human Stress* 1984; 10: 121–127.

36. Baider L, Peretz T, Kaplan De-Nour A. Effect of the Holocaust on coping with cancer. *Social Science and Medicine* 1992; 34: 11–15.

37. Derogatis LR, Lopez MC. *PAIS and PAIS-SR. Administration, scoring and procedures manual*. Baltimore: Clinical Psychometric Research. Johns Hopkins University, 1983.

38. Baider L, Peretz T, Kaplan De-Nour A. Holocaust cancer patients: a comparative study. *Psychiatry* 1993; 56: 349–355.

39. Baider L, Goldzweig G, Ever-Hadani P, et al. Breast cancer and psychological distress: mothers' and daughters' traumatic experiences. *Supportive care in cancer* 2008; 16: 407–414.

40. Greer S, Moorey S, Watson M. Patients' adjustment to cancer: the mental adjustment to cancer (MAC) scale vs. clinical ratings. *Journal of Psychosomatic Research* 1989; 33: 373–377.

41. Procidiano ME, Heller K. Measures of perceived social support from friends and family: three validation studies. *American Journal of Community Psychology* 1983; 11: 1–24.

42. Hantman S, Solomon Z: Recurrent trauma: Holocaust survivors cope with aging and cancer. *Social Psychiatry and Psychiatric Epidemiology* 2007; 42: 396–402.

43. Danieli Y. Families of survivors of the Nazi Holocaust: some short- and long-term effects. In: Spielberger CD, Sarason IG, Milgram NA, eds. *Stress and Anxiety*, vol. 8. Washington, DC: Hemisphere, 1982.

44. Solomon Z, Benbenishty R, Neria Y, et al. Assessment of PTSD: validation of the revised PTSD inventory. *Israel Journal of Psychiatry and Related Sciences* 1993; 30: 110–115.

45. Fennig Sh, Levav I. Demoralization and social supports among Holocaust survivors. *Journal of Nervous and Mental Disease* 1991; 179: 167–172.

46. Kuch K, Cox BJ. Symptoms of PTSD in 124 survivors of the Holocaust. *American Journal of Psychiatry* 1992; 149: 337–340.

47. Freyberg JT. Difficulties in separation-individuation as experienced by the offspring of Nazi Holocaust survivors. *American Journal of Orthopsychiatry* 1980; 50: 87–95.

48. Sagi-Schwartz A, van Ijzendoorn M, Grossmann KE, et al. Attachment and traumatic stress in female Holocaust child survivors and their daughters. *American Journal of Psychiatry* 2003; 160: 1086–1092.

49. Kellerman NP. Psychopathology in children of Holocaust survivors: a review of the research literature. *Israel Journal of Psychiatry and Related Sciences* 2001; 38: 36–44.

50. Solkoff N. Children of survivors of the Nazi Holocaust: a critical review of the literature. *American Journal of Orthopsychiatry* 1992; 62: 342–358.

51. Baider L, Peretz T, Ever-Hadani P, et al. Transmission of response to trauma? Second-generation Holocaust survivors' reaction to cancer. *American Journal of Psychiatry* 2000; 157: 904–910.

52. Solomon Z, Mikulnicer M, Kotler M. Combat-related posttraumatic stress disorder among second-generation Holocaust survivors: preliminary findings. *American Journal of Psychiatry* 1988; 145: 865–868.

53. Solomon Z. The effect of prior stressful experience on coping with war trauma and captivity. *Psychological Medicine* 1995; 25: 1289–1294.

54. Schwartz S, Dohrenwend BP, Levav I. Non-genetic transmission of psychiatric disorders: evidence from children of the Holocaust. *Journal of Health and Social Behavior* 1994; 35: 385–402.

55. Levav I, Kohn R, Dohrenwend BP, et al. An epidemiological study of mental disorder in a 10-year cohort of young adults in Israel. *Psychological Medicine* 1993; 23: 691–708.

56. Levinson, D, Zilber N, Lerner Y, et al. Prevalence of mood and anxiety disorders: results from the Israel National Health Survey. *Israel Journal of Psychiatry and Related Sciences* 2007; 4: 94–103.

57. Levav I, Levinson D, Radomislensky I, et al. Psychopathology and other health dimensions among the offspring of Holocaust survivors: results of an epidemiological community study. *Israel Journal of Psychiatry and Related Sciences* 2007; 44: 144–151.

58. Baider L, Goldzweig G, Ever-Hadani P, et al. Psychological distress and coping in breast cancer patients and healthy women whose parents survived the Holocaust. *Psycho-Oncology* 2006; 15: 635–646.

59. Levav I, Kohn R, Schwartz S. The psychiatric after-effects of the Holocaust on the second generation. *Psychological Medicine* 1998; 28: 755–760.
60. Bar-On D, Eland J, Kleber RJ, *et al.* Multigenerational perspectives on coping with the Holocaust experience: an attachment perspective for understanding the developmental sequelae of trauma across generations. *International Journal of Behavioral Development* 1998; 22: 315–338.
61. Wiseman H, Metzl E, Barber JL. Anger, guilt, and intergenerational communication of trauma in the interpersonal narratives of second generation Holocaust survivors. *American Journal of Orthopsychiatry* 2006; 78: 176–184.

SECTION II

The Epidemiology of Psychiatric and Behavioral Disorders

Chapter 8

THE EPIDEMIOLOGY OF ALCOHOL USE AND DEPENDENCE IN ISRAEL

Yehuda D. Neumark and Hadar S. Schwartz

Alcohol misuse or abuse – especially among adolescents and young adults – is a widespread public health problem with severe adverse consequences. Alcohol-related violence, accidents, suicides and illness contribute in making alcoholism one of the major causes of preventable morbidity and mortality worldwide (1, 2).

The World Health Organization (who) has estimated that alcohol accounts for 3.5% of disability-adjusted life years (DALYs) lost globally, even allowing for putative cardio-protective effects (3). This is more than tobacco (2.6%) and far more than illegal drugs (.6%). In Europe and the Americas, alcohol is responsible for 5% to 6% of all deaths and 10% to 11% of DALYs (4, 5). These figures are considerably higher in a number of countries in Central and Eastern Europe such as Hungary, where alcohol accounts for 25% of deaths among adult men (6).

Anthony *et al.* have summarized the main contributions of epidemiology to alcohol and drug dependence research in relation to what they term the "five rubrics of epidemiology" (7). These are:

(a) Quantity – in terms of incidence and prevalence;

(b) Location – distribution of cases in time and space;

(c) Etiology – explanations as to why some people proceed further along the drug use continuum and others do not;

(d) Mechanisms – elucidation of biological and social processes that lead to the development of drug dependence; and

(e) Prevention and control – this rubric asks the question: what can be done to prevent, reduce or ameliorate the adverse impact of drug dependence? (7).

Earlier, Tomas and Kozel (9) posed four related sets of questions that define the foci of epidemiologic research in the area of substance use and abuse:

(a)   What is the magnitude of substance use and abuse in the general population? What are the characteristics of users? What are the trends in use?;
(b)   How many people require services as a consequence of substance use and abuse? What are their characteristics? What are the trends? What are the consequences?;
(c)   How are emerging problems identified? How are they characterized and monitored?; and
(d)   Which risk factors are associated with substance use and abuse? What consequences (health, family, social, etc.) are associated with use and abuse? (8).

It is important to keep in mind that much of what we know about drinking patterns and alcohol-related harms in any country comes from population-based surveys. While these provide the broadest window of information to address Anthony *et al.*'s five rubrics to answer the questions posed by Tomas and Kozel, they may miss certain groups at high risk for use and dependence, and thereby are likely to provide conservative estimates of the magnitude of use – as heavy drinkers tend to be under-represented in population-based surveys (9). Furthermore, sample sizes are seldom large enough to fully characterize subpopulation differences or subtle changes over time. In general, self reports by adolescents about their drinking habits have been shown to be reliable (10, 11), yet underestimation of point-prevalence rates of non-normative behaviors based on self-report data is a potential limitation of all health behavior surveys (12). For example, in Israel the degree of underreporting may be greater among Arab-Israeli respondents since they may be more reluctant to report religiously prohibited behaviors. Additionally, differences in methodology (including sampling techniques and questions or definitions) often hamper the ability to compare findings across surveys.

Bearing these limitations in mind, this chapter will attempt to answer the above questions regarding the situation in Israel. We aim to provide an overview of the epidemiological patterns of alcohol use and dependence nationally and in various age, gender and ethnic sub-populations, while exploring in some depth the influence of religion and culture on the prevalence of alcohol use and alcohol disorders.

Israeli society presents a rather unique and particularly informative environment in which to study the epidemiology of alcohol consumption, as it contains within a single small country three primary cultural groups or "nationalities" with differing attitudes toward alcohol consumption: Jewish Israelis (about five million people or 75% of the population), Arab Israelis (about 1.5 million or 20%), and immigrants from Russia and other former Soviet Union (FSU) states – the majority of whom are of Jewish ancestry (about one million). The Arab-Israeli population is predominantly Muslim (approximately 75%), while 17% are Christian and 8% Druze. Muslim tradition prohibits the drinking of alcohol, although historically this prohibition has been less than completely observed (12). The Jewish (and Christian) tradition tolerates and even advocates moderate and controlled alcohol consumption, at least within religious and ceremonial contexts (13). Since the late 1980s, Israel has witnessed an influx of about one million immigrants from the FSU, which has resulted in a population increase of approximately 15% and a substantial modification of the country's sociodemographic profile (14). In contrast to the traditionally low alcohol-drinking norms that have characterized mainstream Israeli society, Russia and other FSU states have some of the highest per-capita alcohol consumption levels in the world (15). Members of these three population groups often work and live in close geographic proximity, and the Arab community is increasingly being exposed to the predominating Western culture. This coexistence of disparate religious and cultural mores related to the drinking of alcohol within a changing social milieu, and the blending of traditional religion and religious observance with alcohol practices it has assimilated from Western society (16, 17) provides fertile ground for investigating patterns of alcohol consumption and the extent of alcohol-related mental disorders.

Throughout its 60-year history, Israel has lived in the shadow of war and terrorism, and this too has impacted on patterns of alcohol consumption. Schiff *et al.* (18) have shown that teenagers with more direct exposure to terrorism exhibit higher levels of alcohol consumption.

Traditionally, per-capita consumption of alcohol in Israel has been considerably lower than in most other Western countries (19) – even though alcohol is freely accessible in Jewish neighborhoods for purchase by adults in pubs/bars and supermarkets. Nearly 40 years ago, one researcher poignantly observed: "Israel has no alcoholism problem. On a visit [I made] there, the present writer nine years ago managed to unearth one old alcoholic" (20). While this observation clearly highlights the rarity of alcoholism in the country, it unquestionably underestimated the extent of the phenomenon even then. In 1966, for example, there were some 150 alcohol-related admissions to psychiatric hospitals in the country, for a prevalence of 7.4 alcoholics for every 100,000 inhabitants (21). While there is no definitive information on the number of Israeli alcoholics, estimates put the number between 50,000 (according to governmental sources) and 100,000 (according to the Israel Society for the Prevention of Alcoholism) (22).

The Israel National Health Survey (INHS), reviewed in other chapters as well, conducted in the years 2003–2004 on nearly 5,000 Israeli adults, found that 41% are lifetime abstainers (except for minor ritual use) and nearly half (48%) had not consumed any alcohol in the past year (23, 24). In comparison, according to the WHO Global Status Report on Alcohol 2004, the past-year abstinence rate in Luxembourg was 2.5%; 10% to 15%, in several Western European countries including the UK, Iceland and Sweden; about 20%, in Poland, Canada and Russia; and 30% to 40%, in the US, Spain and Mexico. Most countries with higher rates of abstention than Israel are Muslim countries such as Egypt, with a 99.5% rate of past-year abstention, as Islamic tenets prohibit the consumption of alcohol, as is more fully addressed below. Note here that the authors of the WHO report suggest caution in interpreting the results presented in the report due to the variability of the quality of the research among the studies:

"For many countries, the data are very limited, and the alcohol *per-capita* consumption estimates are clearly of varying quality…. The data are clearly only as reliable as the original data from the sources used…. The data for drinking patterns were obtained from surveys and other studies conducted in the respective countries, mainly from published peer-reviewed journal articles and official reports and in some cases grey literature such as conference papers and reports found on the Internet" (25).

Although Israel remains a relatively sober society by Western standards, alcohol misuse today poses significant social and public health consequences – predominantly among young adults – as drinking has become a form of entertainment with a concomitant growing number of drinking establishments (26). Recent years have also seen a rapid growth of the "fine wine" industry, which has created a local market and transformed the palate of many Israeli adults from sweet sacramental wine to internationally acclaimed fine wines. Average per capita consumption of wine has doubled in the past 15 years and is estimated (by the Ministry of Foreign Affairs) at six liters annually (compared with 60 to 70 per capita in France, Italy and Spain). Revenue from wine exports nearly doubled from US $8 million annually in 2001 to 14 million in 2005. Imports, which were virtually non-existent in 1990, now account for nearly one-quarter of all wine consumed in the country. Starting in the 1990s and continuing in the 2000s, there has been a growth explosion of new boutique wineries throughout Israel.

♪ Religion and alcohol

The Hebrew Bible as well as post-biblical Jewish teachings acknowledged the dual capacity of alcohol to provide pleasure in moderate amounts, yet, when drunk in excess, it can cause harm. Indeed, although the Prophet Isaiah warned against excessive drinking: "Woe to you who arise early in the morning to pursue liquor, who stay up late at night while wine inflames them" (Isaiah, 5: 11), King Solomon considered wine to be a source of happiness – "Wine makes life merry" (Ecclesiastes 10:19). He further alluded to the effects of alcohol on memory and cognition by advising: "Give strong drink to the woebegone and wine to those of embittered soul; let him drink and forget his poverty and not remember his travail any more" (Proverbs 31: 6–7). At the same time, King Solomon recommended abstinence for persons in positions of responsibility when he cautioned: "It is not proper for kings to drink wine and for princes to imbibe strong drink; lest he drinks and forgets the statutes and pervert the judgment of all of the children of the poor" (Proverbs 31: 4–5). And while wine held a prominent place as a libation in sacrificial ceremonies in the Holy Temple, priests doing service there were prohibited from drinking while performing their sacramental duties (Leviticus 10: 9; Ezekiel 44: 21). In post-Temple Judaism, wine was still considered an essential element in festive occasions: "Now that the Holy Temple does not stand and we cannot, therefore, offer any sacrificial animals, rejoicing is not fulfilled except with drinking wine – as it is stated 'and wine gladdens man's heart' (Psalms 104: 14)" (Babylonian Talmud, Tractate Pesachim 109a).

Keller suggested that the establishment of the Second Temple (500 to 400 BCE) brought an end to pagan (orgiastic) drinking practices, which were replaced with the integration of drinking into religious ceremonies (27). Moderate drinking practices became an established element of the emerging Jewish culture. Wine, in small amounts, is today present at Jewish ritual events including the circumcision ceremony, when the baby is given a symbolic drop of wine, and the Jewish wedding, when the bride and groom share from the same cup under the marriage canopy. It is also an essential part of every Sabbath and holiday meal.

Researchers have noted that this unique relationship between alcohol and ritual observance has created a model within Judaism of a normative pattern of drinking and produced a culture in which moderate alcohol consumption is encouraged within the context of religious celebration but is otherwise merely acceptable (28–30).

Interest in the phenomenon of low rates of alcoholism among Jews dates back to the late eighth century. In 1789, the philosopher Immanuel Kant commented that Jews "carefully avoid all appearance of it [drunkenness] because their civic position is weak, and they need to be reserved…they cannot relax in their self-control, for intoxication – which deprives one of cautiousness – would be a scandal for them" (31). Jews drank less, Kant proposed, because of a deep fear of the disruption of their tenuous relationship with Gentile society.

Beginning in the 1940s, researchers revisited this cultural practice and suggested alternative sociocultural reasons. Bales, for example, suggested a "ritual drinking" hypothesis whereby the low rates of heavy drinking are due to the integration of drinking into Jewish – especially Orthodox Jewish – culture and ritual (29). Glad, following Kant, conjectured that sanctions against drunkenness and Jews' conscious and unconscious avoidance of the public humiliation and punishment that often accompanies heavy drinking served as deterrents to excessive drinking (32).

More recently, Snyder largely supported Bales' basic claims while theorizing that Jews hold an unofficial but widely held stereotype that sobriety is a Jewish quality, while drunkenness is a non-Jewish problem (30).

Glassner and Berg (28) also supported Bales, further claiming that Jews internalize concepts of drinking through their connection with ritual ceremonies. They proposed four possibilities for the low rates of alcoholism among Jews, one of which – entitled "moderation practices from childhood" – emphasizes the integration of moderate drinking practices through ritual and symbolic Jewish – especially Orthodox Jewish – tradition.

Additionally, the study by Glassner and Berg (28) supports Snyder's claim that Jews perceive excessive drinking as somehow being "not Jewish" (30). As retold by Spiegel (33), one recovered alcoholic expressed the discordance between drunkenness and Jewish values and implied that since drunkenness is perceived as a violation of these values, whoever drinks excessively is "somehow not fully Jewish." This is why, she explained, "there are no Jewish alcoholics" (33). According to Glassner and Berg (28), the rarity of excessive drinking has created a (non-religious) tradition in which moderate drinking has been modeled and passed from generation to generation. Since Jews often consciously or unconsciously seek out Jewish friends, they strengthen this tradition by avoiding the integration of non-Jewish alcohol-related beliefs.

Snyder's main premise is that, since the low rates of alcohol-related disorders are inextricably tied to the Orthodox Jewish community, with the dissolution of traditional Judaism, the decline of Orthodoxy and the assimilation of Jews into mainstream Western culture, Jewish rates of these disorders would rise precipitously. He suggested that one could observe this phenomenon through the study of Jewish college students who, due to their integration and assimilation into a non-Jewish social environment, boast significantly higher levels of alcohol use than other Jews. This assumption has yet to be substantiated (30). Instead, Monteiro and Shuckit found lower rates of binge drinking in a small sample of Jewish male university students than among their Christian peers (34). In partial support of Snyder's claim, Engs *et al.* (35) reported that the rate of alcohol-related problems among American Jewish college students was comparable to those of Roman Catholics and non-abstinent Protestants. At the same time, the Jewish students exhibited lower consumption levels than these two comparison groups, and were comparable with their abstinence-oriented Protestant classmates. They acknowledged that their results could be due to the small sample. Of the 1526 Americans studied, only 21 were Jewish. In a recent study of drinking patterns among members of 22 religious denominations in the US, only 12.5% of Jewish drinkers reported episodic heavy drinking (or binge drinking, is commonly defined as consuming five or more standard alcoholic drinks – a bottle of beer, glass of wine or shot of whisky or other spirits – on a single drinking occasion or within a few hours), which is the lowest rate of such drinking among all other groups but one (8.5% of a small sample of members of the European Free Church reported heavy drinking) (3).

Adherence to religious traditions serves as a barrier against alcohol consumption or excessive drinking in different cultures (e.g., 37–40). Neumark *et al.* found religious lifestyle to be a stronger deterrent against drinking among Arab-Israeli respondents, particularly Arab-Israeli women, than among Jewish-Israeli respondents (41). Among Arab women, secular respondents were nearly seven times more likely to report alcohol drinking than religious women (Odds Ratio (OR) = 6.7, 95% CI 3.4–12.9), while among Jewish women, the difference was nearly three-fold (OR = 2.8, 95% CI 1.8–4.4). Furthermore, while the reported rate of binge drinking was considerably lower among secular Jewish women (6.3%) than secular Jewish men (19.2%), the rate among secular Arabs was identical in men and women – about 50% in both groups. Less than 7% of religious Arab women and 30.9% of religious Arab men reported binge drinking. Secular Jews in Israel were significantly more likely to report any alcohol consumption in the past month (OR = 2.1, 95% CI 1.8–2.5 for women, and OR = 1.6, 95% CI 1.3–1.9 for men), while religious Jews were more likely to report past-month episodic heavy drinking (i.e., binge drinking).

Many sources of evidence confirm the contribution of both environmental and genetic factors – and the interactions between them – in the development of an individual's drinking habits and the probability of transition across the drinking continuum from initiation to regular drinking to the development of alcohol dependence (42). The earlier stages of the drinking course seem to be influenced more by environmental determinants, while biological/genetic factors play a greater role in determining a person's likelihood to transition to chronic drinking and the development of alcohol-related disorders. It was suggested that, along with the influence of culture, a heightened biological sensitivity to the effects of ethanol among Jews might account for these reduced levels of alcohol consumption (43). It is estimated that 50% to 60% of observed variance in ethanol metabolism – individuals can vary two-to-three fold in their ability to eliminate alcohol – can be explained by hereditary factors (44).

The major alcohol metabolic pathway is a two-step oxidation of ethanol to acetyldehyde by alcohol dehydrogenase (ADH) and then to acetate by aldehyde dehydrogenase (ALDH). Of the seven known human genes that code for the alcohol dehydrogenases, four code for enzymes catalyzing the initial step in the pathway for the metabolism of ethanol: ADH1A (formerly known as ADH1), ADH1B (ADH2), ADH1C (ADH3) and ADH4. Polymorphic alleles at the ADH1B locus encode isozymes that differ strikingly (up to 20 fold) in their catalytic properties (45). Numerous studies, primarily amongst Asians (46–50) but also in Europeans (51, 52), have demonstrated an association between the *ADH1B*2* allele and reduced alcohol consumption and a lowered risk of alcoholism, even after accounting for the strong effect of ALDH polymorphisms. Among Caucasians, ALDH2 is not polymorphic. Neumark *et al.* have shown that inheritance of the *ADH1B*2* allele, which is prevalent in the Jewish population compared to other Caucasian groups, is associated with reduced frequency and quantity of alcohol intake (53) and also contributes to an increased rate of elimination of alcohol (54). The *ADH1B*2* association with drinking patterns has been subsequently confirmed in a number of studies of Jewish Israelis and American Jews (55–58). Accelerated metabolism would lower the exposure of the brain to alcohol for a given dose. This interpretation is consistent with our further observation that presence of the *ADH1B*2* allele is associated with an increased slope of the descending limb following equilibration of alcohol in the total body water (54). Another possibility is that the faster alcohol elimination attending the *ADH1B*2* status may increase the exposure of the genotype to relatively larger concentrations of acetaldehyde, known to be associated with aversive experiences, at least when achieved by slowing ALDH activity. Both factors may be at work, but it is clear that the influence of the *ADH1B*2* allele on reduced drinking patterns is mediated, at least in part, via its effect on alcohol elimination rate. Some support for a biological-genetic protective effect and/or a cultural transmission theory is found in the over-representation of non-Jewish immigrants from the former Soviet Union among Israeli patients with alcohol problems (59).

In his comparison of attitudes toward alcohol in the Hebrew Bible and the New Testament, Seller finds underlying similarities in their permissive attitude toward drinking in moderate amounts and their condemnation of excessive drinking or drunkenness (60). At the same time, a shift toward a more conservative approach to drinking is readily noticeable. For example, the New Testament contains no references to the divine origin of wine, as appear several times in the Hebrew Bible, and abstinence – which is not advocated in the Hebrew Bible – is, as described by Seller, "implicitly extolled through the exemplary role of John the Baptist in the New Testament" (60). Punishment for excessive drinking is described in the New Testament more elaborately than in the Hebrew Bible.

In contrast to the relative permissiveness within the Judeo-Christian tradition, Islam is a religion of abstinence. Careful reading of the three verses of the Koran that are most often quoted to illustrate the Muslim ban on drinking suggests that the prohibition evolved over time. "They ask you about intoxicants and games of chance. Say: in both of them there is a great sin and means of profit for men, and their sin is greater than their profit" (2: 219, Yusuf Ali translation). Rather than banning alcohol outright, the answer provided to the believers' question about whether alcohol is permitted weighs the potential harm and benefits of drinking (and gambling) and decrees that the sin outweighs the profit. Later, Muslims are warned that in moments of responsibility, alcohol is not permitted: "O you who believe! Approach not prayers with a mind befogged [by alcohol?], until ye can understand all that ye say, nor in a state of ceremonial impurity" (4: 43). This verse too, does not necessarily promulgate the complete prohibition of alcohol but rather forbids a person to pray while he/she is unable to concentrate, as may occur when under the influence of alcohol.

Finally, a strong warning against drinking wine appears in verse 5:90: "O ye who believe! Wine and the game of chance and idols, and divining arrows are only the abomination of Satan's handiwork. So shun each of them that you may prosper." It is in the later *hadith* (collection of oral traditions of the words and deeds of Muhammad) that the complete prohibition of alcohol is proclaimed. For example, *Hadith* No. 3392 (Sunan Ibn Majah, Book of Intoxicants, chapter 30) declares: "Anything that intoxicates in a large quantity is prohibited even in a small quantity," and *Hadith* No. 3380 warns that not only those who imbibe alcohol are cursed but also those who deal with them even indirectly.

From an alcohol research perspective, while this religious prohibition has not always been fully adhered to (13, 61), it does pose a challenge to researchers – as there may be strong pressure among Muslims to conceal this illicit behavior and its consequences.

৯ Youth and alcohol

Israeli media reports and anecdotal evidence in recent years suggest an enormous increase in alcohol consumption. For example, a Web site headline from January 3, 2008 announced: "Alcohol use amongst teenagers rising" (62). Findings from the latest national high school survey conducted in 2005 by the Israel Anti-Drug Authority reveal however that just under half (49.4%) of the nearly 6500 youth surveyed reported drinking alcohol of any kind (except for sacramental purposes) in the past year, and 37.2% in the past month. The past-year rate in 2005 remained virtually the same as that in 2001, when it was 47.3%. This current rate is 12.5% lower than the 1995 survey in which 61.9% reported drinking in the preceding year. A greater proportion of youth today are drinking "spirits" than a decade ago – 32.5% vs. 22.5% respectively – while the proportion that report beer-drinking went down by 10%, from 44.2% in 1995 to 34.2% in 2005.

One-quarter of the respondents surveyed in 2005 reported having gotten drunk at least once during the past year, and 20% reported at least one episode of binge drinking in the past month (63). Interestingly, while a higher percentage (65.6%) of adults who participated in the 2005 national household survey said they consumed alcohol, 22% reported at least one episode of having gotten drunk, and 18% reported binge drinking. A similar social-class gradient in drinking rates is noted among adults. For example, while 58.6% of those who report an income below the national average, nearly 80% of those with an above-average income reported drinking.

According to data from the 1998 national high school survey, binge drinking at least once in the past month was reported by 16.8% of young men and 5.8% of young women. Data from the WHO Global Status Report on Alcohol 2004 (15) revealed significant cross-national variation in youth binge-drinking rates ranging from less than 5% (e.g., Turkey, China, Mexico) to 30% or more (e.g., Hungary and Poland). It is noteworthy that the high rates in the UK and Ireland reflect three or more episodes of binge drinking in the past month, compared to one event or more in the other countries. There is equally wide variation in the gender differences in binge drinking, with many countries exhibiting similar rates in young men and women while in a few countries the rate is three to five times higher in males than females.

Youth that drink alcohol are significantly more likely to smoke – 36% of drinkers smoke compared with 4.9% of non-drinkers – and use illicit drugs (16.9% vs. 3.0%, respectively).

As expected, a greater proportion of young men report past-year drinking than young women – 59.1% and 41.1%, respectively. Among Arab-Israeli pupils, 13.4% reported drinking compared with 50% to 60% of the Jewish-Israeli youth. Interestingly, when asked about ever having gotten drunk, there was little difference between Arab and Jewish males (20.1% and 23.9%, respectively), while Jewish females were nearly four times more likely to answer affirmatively than Arab females (15.6% and 4.4%, respectively). Binge drinking was more frequently reported by Arab males (24.6%) than Jewish males (15.0%) while among females no difference was noted between Arabs (5.9%) and Jews (5.8).

There is a steep increase in the drinking rate with age, rising monotonically from 30.5% among seventh-grade pupils to 71.4% among twelfth graders (high school seniors). Pupils who defined themselves as secular were twice as likely to report drinking as "religious" pupils (60.4% and 31.9%, respectively). Victims of terror were significantly more likely to report drinking (59.3%) than others (48.8%), as were children of divorced parents (57.9%), compared with 48.3% among those with married parents. There is a clear social class gradient with regard to drinking, with a two-to-three-fold higher rate among those with more educated and employed parents and a lower household-crowding index. For example, while less than 30% of pupils with mothers with eight years or less of education reported drinking, 65% of those with academically educated mothers did so.

Israeli youth begin drinking, on average, at age 13.5. This is similar to the average age of initiation among American adolescents (64) and slightly older than European youth, among whom half are drinking by age 11 (66). Drinking at an early age carries elevated risk for a number of deleterious outcomes in later adolescence and young adulthood including alcohol-related injury and violence (66) and other alcohol-related problems (67–70).

For immigrant youth, the challenges of acculturation and integration into Israeli society, coupled with typical adolescent crises, contribute to a greater likelihood of social maladjustment and the development of risk-taking behavior patterns (71). This is reflected in the truancy and school dropout rates, which are more than double among immigrant youth. According to a recent report by the *Knesset* (Parliament), the use of psychoactive substances (alcohol, tobacco and illicit drugs) is considerably more prevalent among immigrant youth and offspring of immigrant parents than nonimmigrant youth (72).

Data from national surveys clearly show higher rates of self-reported alcohol drinking, binge drinking and inebriation among immigrant youth compared to Israeli-born youth. In a recent survey of 750 FSU immigrant youth aged 12 to 18 residing in eight cities, of whom ⅓ were not enrolled in school, nearly 90% reported drinking during the past year (73).

More than one-third (37%) of the immigrant drinking youth reported binge drinking at least once in the past year; one-third admitted to getting drunk at least four times in the year; and 17% did so six or more times.

These statistics are particularly worrisome given that FSU immigrants are reluctant to seek care and support from formal governmental agencies due to language and/or cultural barriers. Immigrants are also more likely to drop out of treatment or support programs once enrolled.

While the majority of immigrant youth are of FSU origin, a report by the Anti-Drug Authority (74) revealed particularly troubling symptoms among Ethiopian immigrant youth as well. In a survey of slightly over 500 Ethiopian, mostly male youth, 67% reported drinking alcohol in the year prior to the survey; of these, 43% had gotten drunk at least once. A quarter of Ethiopian youth admitted having used illegal drugs compared to nearly 15% of all school-attending immigrant youth and 10% of all school-attending youth in the country (72).

❧ Drinking patterns among adults

As mentioned above, 52% of adults surveyed in 2004 reported having drunk alcohol in the past year (22). The prevalence of past-year drinking was considerably higher in men (65.7%) than in women (38.9%) and among Jews (55.0%) than Arab respondents (22.7%). The rate of past-year drinking decreased monotonically with increasing age from 56.3% among 21- to 44-year-olds to 28.8% among those 75 years or older. The majority (60%) of Israeli adults drinks infrequently (three times per month or less) and 83.6% of drinkers consume fewer than three drinks on days when they drink. A small percentage of respondents (5.1%) reported "frequent" drinking (three or more times a week at least once in the past year), with this drinking pattern being more commonly reported by men, Jews, those 45 and older and those with more years of schooling. Frequent heavy drinking (three or more drinks three or more times a week at least once during the past year) was reported by 6.8% of men and less than 1% of women. Young adults were more likely to report frequent heavy drinking than older respondents – 4.6% among 21- to 44-year-olds compared with less than 2% among those 45 and older (75).

❧ Alcohol disorders

There is considerable heterogeneity in alcohol terminology in the published literature, and terms are used with multiple and sometimes unclear meanings. The WHO, for example, refers to "problem drinking" as "drinking that results in problems, individual or collective, health or social"; "harmful drinking" as a pattern of drinking that causes physical or mental damage to health, commonly but not invariably with adverse social consequences; and "hazardous drinking" as a level of consumption or pattern of drinking that increases the risk of harmful consequences for the user (76). The level of alcohol consumption that should be regarded as problematic, harmful or hazardous is not established, and this serves to compound the ambiguity. The WHO defines "heavy drinking" as "a pattern of drinking that exceeds some standard of moderate drinking" or – more equivocally – "social drinking," although this definition does little to clarify the ambiguity.

The nomenclature is considerably more standardized with regard to assessment of alcohol-related mental disorders, although there are important differences between the two consensus-based diagnostic classification schemes that evolved more or less simultaneously. The *International Classification of Diseases – Tenth Edition* (ICD-10) (77), defines the alcohol dependence syndrome as "a cluster of physiological, behavioral and cognitive phenomena in which the use of alcohol takes on a much higher priority for a given individual than other behaviors that once had greater value. A central descriptive characteristic of the dependence syndrome is the presence of a desire (often strong, sometimes overpowering) or sense of compulsion to take alcohol" (78).

ICD-10 diagnostic criteria for research purposes require three or more of the following manifestations to have occurred together for at least one month or, if persisting for periods of less than a month, should have occurred together repeatedly within a 12-month period:

(a) a strong desire or sense of compulsion to drink alcohol;
(b) impaired capacity to control drinking behavior in terms of its onset, termination or levels of use, as evidenced by alcohol often being consumed in larger amounts or over a longer period than intended or by a persistent desire or unsuccessful efforts to reduce or control drinking;
(c) a physiological withdrawal state when drinking is stopped or reduced; evidence of tolerance to the effects of alcohol, such that there is a need for significantly increased amounts of alcohol to achieve intoxication or the desired effect, or a markedly diminished effect with continued use of the same amount of alcohol;
(d) preoccupation with alcohol consumption, as manifested by important alternative pleasures or interests being given up or reduced because drinking;
(e) great deal of time being spent in activities necessary to obtain, take or recover from the effects of the alcohol;
(f) persistent drinking despite clear evidence of harmful consequences as evidenced by continued use when the individual is actually aware, or may be expected to be aware, of the nature and extent of harm. *ICD-10* criteria for a clinical diagnosis of alcohol dependence are slightly different.

The *Diagnostic and Statistical Manual of Mental Disorders – Fourth Edition* (DSM-IV) (79) also views alcohol dependence according to psychological and physiological symptoms and defines the disorder as "a maladaptive pattern of substance use, leading to clinically significant impairment or distress, as manifested by three (or more) of the following, occurring at any time in the same 12-month period:

(a) tolerance, as defined by either a need for markedly increased amounts of alcohol to achieve intoxication or desired effect or a markedly diminished effect with continued drinking;
(b) withdrawal syndrome or drinking to relieve or avoid withdrawal symptoms;
(c) drinking larger amounts or over a longer period than intended; persistent desire or unsuccessful efforts to cut down or control drinking;
(d) spending a great deal of time in activities to obtain alcohol, drink it or recover from the effects of drinking;
(e) giving up important social, occupational or recreational activities to drink; and
(f) continued drinking despite knowledge of having a persistent or recurrent physical or psychological problem caused or exacerbated by drinking."

Alcohol abuse, according to the DSM-IV, refers to repeated use despite recurrent adverse social consequences or injury: "A maladaptive pattern of drinking leading to clinically significant impairment or distress, as manifested by one (or more) of the following, occurring within a 12-month period:

(a) recurrent drinking resulting in a failure to fulfill major role obligations at work, school, home;
(b) recurrent drinking in physically hazardous situations; recurrent drinking-related legal problems; and
(c) continued drinking despite recurrent social or interpersonal problems caused or exacerbated by drinking."

According to the DSM-IV hierarchical diagnostic classification scheme, dependence takes precedence over abuse when applicable, so that a person who meets diagnostic criteria for abuse (which is considered to be a less severe problem) and dependence, will be diagnosed only as dependent.

This issue has recently generated considerable discussion. Using data from the US National Epidemiologic Survey on Alcohol and Related Conditions (NESARC, a national household survey of 42,392 adults 18 years and older), researchers (80) showed that a considerable proportion of respondents, (22% of women and 10% of men), who meet lifetime criteria for alcohol dependence did not meet abuse criteria. Analyzing the same data set, Degenhardt *et al.* (81) concluded that the "gated" approach to assessment of cocaine and other drug dependence (requiring at least one feature of DSM-IV drug abuse for a dependence diagnosis) produced no appreciable reduction of population prevalence estimates compared with the "ungated" approach.

Until findings from the 2004 Israel National Mental Health Survey became available, the prevalence of alcohol disorders in Israel was unknown. Data from this survey showed that 4.3% of the population met DSM-IV criteria for a lifetime diagnosis of an alcohol disorder (22). Nearly all (90.2%) of those with an alcohol disorder met criteria for alcohol abuse, 26.8% of whom with a past-year diagnosis. Of those with a diagnosis of dependence, 19.0% met past-year criteria.

Males were much more likely to meet criteria for an alcohol disorder than were females (OR adjusted = 7.3, 95% CI 4.8–11.1). A strong inverse relationship was found between the presence of an alcohol disorder and age – those in the youngest age group (21 to 34 years) were five times more likely to have an alcohol disorder than were those in the oldest (65 and over) age group (OR adjusted = 5.0, 95% CI 2.3–11.0). The likelihood of an alcohol disorder was also higher among immigrants from the former Soviet Union (OR adjusted = 2.0, 95% CI 1.4–2.9) compared with native Jewish Israelis, and respondents who had never married (OR adjusted = 1.6, 95% CI 1.1–2.4 compared with married respondents). The odds of having an alcohol disorder increased monotonically across the income quartiles, although only the difference between the fourth and the first quartile reached statistical significance (OR adjusted = 1.9, 95% CI 1.1–3.3). Upon adjustment for the effects of the other sociodemographic characteristics, no significant relationship was noted with education.

Respondents who met criteria for a past-year diagnosis tended to be younger than those with a lifetime (but not past-year) diagnosis. Of those with a past-year diagnosis, 69.4% were in the 21- to 34-year-old category compared with 48.2% of those with a lifetime diagnosis. Those with a past-year diagnosis were also more likely to never have been married (54.8%) compared with 30.5% among those with a lifetime, but not past-year diagnosis ($p = .01$). No other noteworthy sociodemographic differences were found between the two groups.

The lifetime Israeli prevalence of alcohol abuse (4%) is identical to the overall rate in other European countries (24), while drinking levels are considerably lower in Israel than in other European countries. For example, 11% of interviewed Europeans reported abstaining from drinking alcohol compared with 40% of Israelis, and the proportion of drinkers who report three or more drinking episodes weekly is 35% in Europe and 10% in Israel. Historically, Israel has had one of the lowest-per-capita alcohol consumption levels (19, 82). In the US, where overall lifetime alcohol abuse rates are estimated at 13.2% and the prevalence of dependence is 5.4% (83), Jews exhibit lower rates of alcohol abuse and dependence compared with other religious groups (84). Although other explanations (including selection and/or reporting biases) are likely, the putative inherited sensitivity to the effects of ethanol among Jews fits well with the observed low levels of alcohol consumption nationwide alongside relatively high rates of alcohol abuse. Specifically, the effects of even small quantities of alcohol among ADH1B*2 carriers may be sufficiently powerful to cause respondents to endorse subjective DSM-IV criteria for alcohol abuse (e.g., "hangover interfered with daily activities").

§ Alcohol-related accidents, injury and violence

In industrialized countries, drunk driving is one of the major causes of driving fatalities (85), and crashes are the main cause of alcohol-related mortality (64). In Israel over the past decade, 500 Israelis have died annually, on average, from motor vehicle accidents (86); in the year 2003, the death rate for automobile-related mortality was 8.4 per 100,000 (87). Recent data from the Trauma Research Center at the Gertner Institute for Epidemiology and Health Policy Research revealed that in the five-year period from 2000 to 2004, the prevalence of driver casualties with breath-alcohol concentration (BrAC) levels above the legal limit soared by nearly 200% – from 5.0% to 14.7% (88).

In a recent study of some 6,000 college/university students, more than a third (35%) of those surveyed admitted to driving under the influence of alcohol, and 20% admitted that they had driven while they knew they were too drunk to do so (89). At the same time, these students generally considered the risks associated with alcohol consumption to be quite modest. Approximately 45% of those surveyed felt that only minor harm may result from drinking beer or wine, while about 26% saw no harm in consuming these beverages. Nearly one-quarter (22%)

of Israeli high school pupils believe there is little or no danger in drinking alcohol several times a week (63). In a 1995 study of drinking and driving among pub patrons in Israel, Shinar found no relationship between willingness/readiness to drive and breath alcohol concentrations or the legal driving limit of 50 mg/100 ml. The author concluded that there was alarming ignorance regarding the harmful effects of alcohol and the risks associated with drunk-driving (90). This was confirmed in a survey of 500 young adults (17 to 24 years of age) carried out by the National Road Safety Authority in 2004, in which 36% of respondents maintained that two to three drinks did not affect driving ability; a full 10% felt that even four to five drinks did not impact on fitness to drive (91). Compounding this lack of awareness of the dangers of drinking and driving among young adults is an alarming ignorance among parents as to the drinking habits of their children. In a parallel survey of 500 parents of young adults, 60% thought their child did not drink alcohol, while only 21% of the young adults reported abstinence. Whereas more than half (54%) of the young adults reported consuming more than two drinks the last time they went out, only 19% of the parents thought that their child did so. As a result of this unawareness, while three-quarters of the young Israeli adults surveyed felt that driving under the influence of alcohol is a major problem, a similar proportion of parents (78%) expressed no concern about drinking and driving among their children – and half of all parents had no intention of intervening with their children to reduce the risk associated with possible drinking and driving.

Alcohol is a powerful central nervous system (CNS) depressant that is rapidly absorbed into the bloodstream from the gastrointestinal tract; the average adult metabolizes 10 to 15 ml of absolute alcohol (about the amount of alcohol in a bottle of beer, glass of wine or shot of whisky) per hour. However, there are marked inter-individual differences resulting from complex interactions between numerous physiological, biological, genetic and behavioral factors. Some of these include gender, age, weight, liver size, acquired tolerance, recent food intake and various genetic polymorphisms (92, 93).

As a central nervous system (CNS) depressant, alcohol initially depresses inhibitory and behavioral control centers of the brain on the ascending limb often leading to heightened activity and disinhibition, thereby increasing the risk for accidents, injuries and violence (94). Young adults experience alcohol-related violence more than other age groups, with much of the violence occurring in bars and clubs (95, 96) although the precise mechanism by which alcohol induces violent behavior remains to be fully explained. The "alcohol myopia" theory, for example, suggests that alcohol diminishes attention to those cues that would normally inhibit aggression, while the "anxiolysis-disinhibition" model suggests that alcohol-induced cognitive disruption impacts on the perception of anxiety-eliciting cues, resulting in suppression of socially unacceptable behaviors such as aggression (97).

It is well known that alcohol impairs cognition, behavior and motor skills even at low BrAC levels (i.e., under the accepted legal driving limit of .05 g/dl), and chronic drinking can lead to permanent memory loss, inability to concentrate, immunodeficiency and brain damage (94). Adolescence is a critical phase in brain development – and alcohol's deleterious effects on brain development and function are particularly acute among youth who are episodic heavy drinkers (98, 99).

Numerous studies have demonstrated detrimental effects of alcohol on visual special attention (100), eye movement responses (101, 102), word discrimination (103), spatial and learning capacity (104, 105), memory, logic (106) and executive function (107). The effects of alcohol on cognition are modified by numerous factors, including past exposure to alcohol, dose consumed, age, gender, educational attainment, culture and genetic makeup (108, 109); however, much of the inter-individual differences in alcohol-induced cognitive changes are yet to be described (106, 110). Furthermore, it remains unclear as to whether these effects result from a global impairment on the CNS rather than specific changes in certain brain systems (110, 108).

ৡ From epidemiology to mental health action

Harmful patterns of drinking, particularly among young adults, pose a potential serious social threat and a real challenge for public health practitioners, health service providers and public policy makers. The consequences of dependence on these substances are increasingly felt in many spheres of life at the level of the individual, the family and society as a whole. The 2006 Communication of the Commission of the European Communities to the European Union summarized the vast social costs associated with alcohol: "Harmful and hazardous alcohol consumption has a major impact on public health and also generates costs related to healthcare, health insurance, law enforcement and public order and workplaces, and thus has a negative impact on economic development and on society as a whole" (111).

The 1995 European Charter on Alcohol (112) articulates five ethical principles to guide public policy regarding alcohol:

(a) All people have the right to a family, community and working life protected from accidents, violence and other negative consequences of alcohol consumption;
(b) All people have the right to valid impartial information and education, starting early in life, on the consequences of alcohol consumption on health, the family and society;
(c) All children and adolescents have the right to grow up in an environment protected from the negative consequences of alcohol consumption and, to the extent possible, from the promotion of alcoholic beverages;
(d) All people with hazardous or harmful alcohol consumption and members of their families have the right to accessible treatment and care; and
(e) All people who do not wish to consume alcohol or who cannot do so for health or other reasons have the right to be safeguarded from pressures to drink and be supported in their non-drinking behavior.

We have attempted to address as thoroughly as possible the five epidemiological rubrics set out by Anthony *et al.* (7) with regard to the epidemiology of alcohol use and dependence in Israel. Relatively little information is available regarding the issues of prevention and control, and considerable more research work needs to be done in order to answer the question: "What can be done to prevent, reduce or ameliorate the adverse impact of alcohol dependence?"

Through a greater understanding of the role of alcohol in society and the deleterious effects associated with harmful drinking habits, efforts can be made to improve people's knowledge about alcohol and its effects, reduce the frequency of harmful drinking and provide accessible and useful prevention and treatment opportunities. While the phenomenon of harmful alcohol consumption is not as widespread in Israel as in most Western countries, the growth of the pub/club culture, and the greater acceptance of alcohol into the social fabric of young Israelis suggests the need for vigilance.

§ References

1. Wechsler H, Dowdall GW, Davenport A, *et al.* A gender-specific measure of binge drinking among college students. *American Journal of Public Health* 1995; 85: 982–985.

2. Oei TP, Morawska A. A cognitive model of binge drinking: the influence of alcohol expectancies and drinking refusal self-efficacy. *Addictive Behavior* 2004; 29:159–179.

3. Jernigan DH, Monteiro M, Room R, *et al.* Towards a global alcohol policy: alcohol, public health and the role of WHO. *Bulletin of the World Health Organization* 2000; 78: 491–499.

4. Rehm J, Taylor B, Patra J. Volume of alcohol consumption, patterns of drinking and burden of disease in the European region 2002. *Addiction* 2006; 101: 1086–1095.

5. Rehm J, Monteiro M. Alcohol consumption and burden of disease in the Americas: implications for alcohol policy. *PanAmerican Journal of Public Health* 2005; 18: 241–248.

6 Rehm J, Sulkowska U, Mańczuk M, *et al.* Alcohol accounts for a high proportion of premature mortality in central and Eastern Europe. *International Journal of Epidemiology* 2007; 36: 458–467.

7. Anthony JC, Chen CY, Storr CL. Drug dependence epidemiology. *Clinical Neuroscience Research* 2005; 5: 55–68.

8. Tomas JN, Kozel NG. National substance abuse epidemiology initiatives in the United States: what works for what? *Journal of Addictive Diseases* 1991; 11: 5–21.

9 Pothos EM, Cox WM. Cognitive bias for alcohol-related information in inferential processes. *Drug and Alcohol Dependence* 2002; 66: 235–241.

10. Lintonen T, Ahlström S, Metso L. The reliability of self-reported drinking in adolescence. *Alcohol and Alcoholism* 2004; 39: 362–368.

11. Shannon EE, Mathias CW, Marsh DM, *et al.* Teenagers do not always lie: characteristics and correspondence of telephone and in-person reports of adolescent drug use. *Drug and Alcohol Dependence* 2007; 90: 288–291.

12. Bales RF. Cultural differences in rates of alcoholism. *Quarterly Journal of Studies on Alcohol* 1946; 6: 480–499.

13. Kotek SS. "Do not drink wine or strong drink": alcohol and responsibility in ancient Jewish sources. *Medicine and Law* 1989; 8: 255–259.

14. Sicron M. Demography of the wave of immigration. In: Sicron M and Leshem E, eds. *Profile of an immigration wave: the absorption process of immigrants from the former Soviet Union, 1990–1995.* Jerusalem: Magnes Press, 1998.

15. WHO Global Status Report on Alcohol 2004 [online]. 2004 [cited November 15, 2007]. Available from URL: http://www.who.int/substance_abuse/publications/global_status_report_2004_overview.pdf.

16. Weiss S, Sawa GH, Abdeen Z, *et al.* Alcohol use among Muslims and Druze in Israel, Jordan and the Palestinian Authority: theoretical aspects and trends. In: Isralowitz R, Afifi M, Rawson R, eds. *Drug problems: cross-cultural policy and program development.* London: Auburn House, 2002.

17. Barnea Z, Teichman M, Rahav G. Substance use and abuse among deviant and non-deviant adolescents in Israel. *Journal of Drug Education* 1993; 23: 223–236.

18. Schiff M, Rahav G, Teichman M. Israel 2000: immigration and gender differences in alcohol consumption. *American Journal of Addiction* 2005; 14: 234–247.

19 Harkin AM, Anderson P, Goos C. *Smoking, drinking and drug taking in the European region.* Copenhagen: World Health Organization Regional Office for Europe, 1997.

20. Glatt MM. Alcoholism and drug dependence among Jews. *British Journal of Addictions* 1970; 64: 297–304.

21. Miller L. The epidemiology of drug abuse in Israel. *Israel Journal of Psychiatry and Related Disciplines* 1971; 9: 3–10.

22. Neumark YD, Lopez-Quintero C, Grinshpoon A, *et al.* Alcohol drinking patterns and prevalence of alcohol-abuse and dependence in the Israel National Health Survey. *Israel Journal of Psychiatry and Related Sciences* 2007; 44: 126–135.

23. Levinson D, Paltiel A, Nir M, *et al.* The Israel National Health Survey: issues and methods. *Israel Journal of Psychiatry and Related Sciences* 2007; 44: 85–93.

24. Alonso J, Angemeyer MC, Bernert S. ESEMeD/MHEDEA 2000 Investigators. Prevalence of mental disorders in Europe: results from the European study of the epidemiology of mental disorders (ESEMeD) Project. *Acta Psychiatrica Scandinavica* 2004; 109: 21–27.

25. World Health Organization. WHO Global Status Report on Alcohol 2004 [online]. 2004 [cited November 15, 2007]. Available from URL: http://www.who.int/substance_abuse/publications/global_status_report_2004_overview.pdf.

26. Isralowitz RE, Peleg A. Israeli college student alcohol use: the association of background characteristics and regular drinking pattern. *Drug and Alcohol Dependence* 1996; 42: 147–153.

27. Keller M. The great Jewish drink mystery. *British Journal of Addictions* 1970; 64: 287–296.

28. Glassner B, Berg B. How Jews avoid alcohol problems. *American Sociological Review* 1980; 45: 647–664.

29. Bales RF. Cultural differences in rates of alcoholism. *Quarterly Journal of Studies on Alcohol* 1946; 6: 480–499.

30. Snyder, CR. Alcoholism: its rarity among Jews. In: Goodman RM, Motulsky AG, ed. *Genetic diseases among Ashkenazi Jews.* New York: Raven Press, 1979.

31. Jellinek EM. Immanuel Kant on drinking. *Quarterly Journal of Studies on Alcohol* 1941; 4: 778.

32. Glad DD. Attitudes and experiences of American-Jewish and American-Irish male youths. *Quarterly Journal of Studies on Alcohol* 1947; 8: 406–472.

33. Spiegel MC. Profile of the alcoholic Jew. *British Journal of Alcohol and Alcoholism* 1981; 16: 141–149.

34. Monteiro MG. Schuckit MA. Alcohol, drug, and mental health problems among Jewish and Christian men at an American university. *Journal of Drug and Alcohol Abuse* 1989; 15: 403–412.

35. Engs RC, Hanson DJ, Gliksman L, *et al.* Influence of religion and culture on drinking behaviours: a test of hypotheses between Canada and the USA. *Addiction* 1990; 85: 1475–1482.

36. Michalak L, Trocki K, Bond J. Religion and alcohol in the US National Alcohol Survey: how important is religion for abstention and drinking? *Drug and Alcohol Dependence* 2007; 87: 268–280.

37. Maselko J, Buka S. Religious activity and lifetime prevalence of psychiatric disorder. *Social Psychiatry and Psychiatric Epidemiology* 2008; 43: 18–24.

38. Kendler KS, Liu x-Q, Gardner CO, et al. Dimensions of religiosity and their relationship to lifetime psychiatric and substance use disorders. *American Journal of Psychiatry* 2003; 160: 496–503.

39. Francis LJ. Attitudes towards alcohol, church attendance and denominational identity. *Drug and Alcohol Dependence* 1992; 31: 45–50.

40. Clark L, Beeghley L, Cochran JK. Religiosity, social class and alcohol use: an application of reference group theory. *Sociological Perspectives* 1990; 33: 201–218.

41. Neumark YD, Rahav G, Teichman M, et al. Alcohol drinking patterns among Jewish and Arab men and women in Israel. *Journal of Studies on Alcohol* 2001; 62: 443–447.

42. Rose RJ, Dick DM. Gene-environment interplay in adolescent drinking behavior. *Alcohol Research and Health* 2005; 28: 223–229.

43. Monteiro MG, Klein JL, Schuckit MA. High levels of sensitivity to alcohol in young adult Jewish men: a pilot study. *Journal of Studies on Alcohol* 1991; 52: 464–469.

44. Schuckit MA. Genetics of the risk for alcoholism. *American Journal of Addiction* 2000; 9: 103–112.

45. Bosron WF, Li TK. Genetic polymorphisms of human liver alcohol and aldehyde dehydrogenases, and their relationship to alcohol metabolism and alcoholism. *Hepatology* 1986; 6: 502–510.

46. Chao YC, Young TH, Tang HS, et al. Alcoholism and alcoholic organ damage and genetic polymorphisms of alcohol metabolizing enzymes in Chinese patients. *Hepatology* 1997; 25: 112–117.

47. Chen CC, Lu RB, Chen YC, et al. Interaction between the functional polymorphisms of the alcohol-metabolism genes in protection against alcoholism. *American Journal of Human Genetics* 1999; 65: 795–807.

48. Maezawa Y, Yamauchi M, Toda G, et al. Alcohol-metabolizing enzyme polymorphisms and alcoholism in Japan. *Alcoholism: clinical and experimental research* 1995; 19: 951–954.

49. Shen YC, Fan JH, Edenberg HJ, et al. Polymorphism of ADH and ALDH genes among four ethnic groups in China and effects upon the risk for alcoholism. *Alcoholism: Clinical and Experimental Research* 1997; 21: 1272–1277.

50. Thomasson HR, Crabb DW, Edenberg HJ, et al. Low frequency of the ADH2*2 allele among Atayal natives of Taiwan with alcohol use disorders. *Alcoholism: Clinical and Experimental Research* 1994; 18: 640–643.

51. Borras E, Coutelle C, Rosell A, et al. Genetic polymorphism of alcohol dehydrogenase in Europeans: the ADH2*2 allele decreases the risk for alcoholism and is associated with ADH3*1. *Hepatology* 2000; 31: 984–989.

52. Whitfield JB, Nightingale BN, Bucholz KK, et al. ADH genotypes and alcohol use and dependence in Europeans. *Alcoholism: Clinical and Experimental Research* 1998; 22: 1463–1469.

53. Neumark YD, Friedlander Y, Thomasson HR, et al. Association of the ADH2*2 allele with reduced ethanol consumption in Jewish men in Israel: a pilot study. *Journal of Studies on Alcohol* 1998; 59: 133–139.

54. Neumark YD, Friedlander Y, Durst R, et al. Alcohol dehydrogenase polymorphisms influence alcohol-elimination rates in a male Jewish population. *Alcoholism: Clinical and Experimental Research* 2004; 28:10–14.

55. Hasin D, Aharonovich E, Liu x, et al. Alcohol dependence symptoms and alcohol dehydrogenase 2 polymorphism: Israeli Ashkenazis, Sephardics, and recent Russian immigrants. *Alcoholism: Clinical and Experimental Research* 2002; 26: 1315–1321.

56. Shea SH, Wall TL, Carr LG. ADH2 and alcohol-related phenotypes in Ashkenazi Jewish American college students. *Behavioral Genetics* 2001; 31: 231–239.

57. Carr LG, Foroud T, Stewart T, et al. Influence of ADH1B polymorphism on alcohol use and its subjective effects in a Jewish population. *American Journal of Medical Genetics* 2002; 112: 138–143.

58. Luczak SE, Shea SH, Carr LG, et al. Binge drinking in Jewish and non-Jewish white college students. *Alcoholism: Clinical and Experimental Research* 2002; 26: 1773–1778.

59. Kaptsan A, Telias D, Bersudsky Y, et al. Ethnic origin of alcoholics admitted to an Israeli treatment center. *American Journal of Drug and Alcohol Abuse* 2006; 32: 549–553.

60. Seller SC. Alcohol abuse in the New Testament. *Alcohol and Alcoholism* 1987; 22: 83–90.

61. Weiss S. Trends of alcohol consumption in Israel in 1990–1998. *Alcolgia* 2000; 12: 27–30.

62. Trabelsi-Hadad T. Alcohol use amongst teenagers rising [online]. 2008 [cited January 9, 2008]. Available from URL: http://www.ynetnews.com/articles/0,7340,L-3489902,00.html.

63. Anti-Drug Authority (Israel). The use of psychoactive substances among Israeli residents, 2005 [online]. 2005 [cited January 10, 2008]. Available from URL: http://www.antidrugs.org.il/template/default.asp?maincat=14.

64. Ahlstrom SK, Osterberg EL. International perspectives on adolescent and young adult drinking. *Alcohol Research & Health* 2005; 28: 258–268.

65. Jernigan DH. *Global status report: alcohol and young people*. Geneva: World Health Organization, 2005.

66. Hingson RW, Heeren T, Jamanka A, et al. Age of drinking onset and unintentional injury involvement after drinking. *Journal of the American Medical Association* 2000; 284: 1527–1533.

67. Chou SP, Pickering RP. Early onset of drinking as a risk factor for lifetime alcohol-related problems. *British Journal of Addictions* 192; 87: 1199–1204.

68. Grant BF, Dawson DA. Age at onset of alcohol use and its association with DSM-IV alcohol abuse and dependence: results from the National Longitudinal Alcohol Epidemiologic Survey. *Journal of Substance Abuse* 1997; 9: 103–110.

69. Hingson RW, Heeren T, Winter MR. Age at drinking onset and alcohol dependence: age at onset, duration, and severity. *Archives of Pediatric and Adolescent Medicine* 2006; 160: 739–746.

70. Kraus L, Bloomfield K, Augustin R, *et al.* Prevalence of alcohol use and the association between onset of use and alcohol-related problems in a general population sample in Germany. *Addiction* 2000; 95: 1389–1401.

71. Tartakovsky E. A longitudinal study of acculturative stress and homesickness: high-school adolescents immigrating from Russia and Ukraine to Israel without parents. *Social Psychiatry and Psychiatric Epidemiology* 2007; 42: 485–494.

72. Mi-Ami N. Drug and Alcohol Addiction among Immigrant Youth (Hebrew) [online]. 2006 [cited December 20, 2007]. Available from URL: http://www.knesset.gov.il/MMM/data/pdf/m01647.pdf.

73. Edelstein O. Substance use and related delinquency among former Russian youth in Israel (Hebrew) [online]. 2007 [cited December 20, 2007]. Available from URL: http://www.antidrugs.gov.il/download/files/microsoft_word_-_.

74. Bar-Hamburger R. Patterns of psychoactive-drug use among Ethiopian immigrant youth in Israel, Jerusalem: National Anti-Drug Authority, 2003 (Hebrew).

75. Alonso J, Ferrer M, Romero B, *et al.* The European study of the epidemiology of mental disorders (ESEMeD/MHEDEA 2000) project: rationale and methods. *International Journal of Methods in Psychiatric Research* 2002; 11: 55–67.

76. World Health Organization. Lexicon of alcohol and drug terms [online]. 2008 [cited January 7, 2008]. Available from URL: http://www.who.int/substance_abuse/terminology/who_lexicon/en.

77. World Health Organization. *Mental and behavioral disorders. International classification of diseases – Tenth edition. Diagnosis criteria for research.* Geneva: World Health Organization, 1992.

78. World Health Organization. Dependence Syndrome [online]. 2008 [cited January 7, 2008]. Available from URL: http://www.who.int/substance_abuse/terminology/definition1/en/index.html.

79. American Psychiatric Association. *Diagnostic and statistical manual of mental disorders – Fourth edition.* Washington, DC: American Psychiatric Association, 1994.

80. Hasin DS, Grant BF. The co-occurrence of DSM-IV alcohol abuse in DSM-IV alcohol dependence: results of the National Epidemiologic Survey on Alcohol and Related Conditions on heterogeneity that differ by population subgroup. *Archives of General Psychiatry* 2004; 61: 891–896.

81. Degenhardt L, Bohnert KM, Anthony JC. Assessment of cocaine and other drug dependence in the general population: "gated" versus "ungated" approaches. *Drug and Alcohol Dependence* 2008; 93: 227–232.

82. Verhoek J. *World drink trends.* Oxfordshire, UK: NTC Publications, 1995.

83. Kessler RC, Berglund P, Demler O, *et al.* Lifetime prevalence and age-of-onset distributions of DSM-IV disorders in the National Comorbidity Survey Replication. *Archives of General Psychiatry* 2005; 62:593–602.

84. Yeung PP, Greenwald S. Jewish Americans and mental health: results of the NIMH Epidemiologic Catchment Area Study. *Social Psychiatry and Psychiatric Epidemiology* 1992; 27: 292–297.

85. Hingson R, Winter M. Epidemiology and consequences of drinking and driving. *Alcohol Research & Health* 2003; 27: 63–78.

86. Central Bureau of Statistics. Road accidents/casualties in road accidents by type of casualty and severity (Hebrew) [online]. 2004 [cited December 15, 2007]. Available from URL: http://www.cbs.gov.il/data/E1050103001034.csv.

87. Central Bureau of Statistics. Road accidents rates of road accidents with casualties, casualties and motor vehicles involved in road accidents (Hebrew) [online]. 2004 [cited December 15, 2007]. Available from URL: http://www.cbs.gov.il/data/E1050103001656.csv.

88. Peleg K, Aharonson-Daniel L, Savitsky B. Israel is on the way to captivate peak in the list of countries with high proportion of drunk drivers among road fatalities [online]. 2007 [cited January 3, 2008]. Available from URL: http://www.isrjem.org/IAEM2007a.pdf.

89. Bar-Hamburger R, Lederman S. A survey of the use of psychoactive substances among students in institutions of higher learning, 1996. Jerusalem: The Israel Anti-Drug Authority, 1997 (Hebrew).

90. Shinar D. Drinking and driving of pub patrons in Israel. *Accident Analysis & Prevention.* 1995; 27: 65–71.

91. The National Road Safety Authority of Israel. Available from URL: http://pasimlev.mot.gov.il/RoadSafety/Downloads/Research/researches.htm.

92. Edenberg HJ. The genetics of alcohol metabolism: role of alcohol dehydrogenase and aldehyde dehydrogenase variants. *Alcohol Research in Health* 2007; 30: 5–13.

93. Li TK, Yin SJ, Crabb DW, *et al.* Genetic and environmental influences on alcohol metabolism in humans. *Alcoholism: clinical and experimental research* 2001; 25: 136–144.

94. World Health Organization. *Expert committee on problems related to alcohol consumption, Second report.* WHO Technical Support Series, No. 944; Geneva: World Health Organization, 2007.

95. Buddie AM, Parks KA. The role of the bar context and social behaviors on women's risk for aggression. *Journal of Interpersonal Violence* 2003; 18: 1378–1393.

96. Quigley BM, Leonard KE. Alcohol use and violence among young adults. *Alcohol Research & Health* 2005; 28: 191–194.

97. Abrams D, Hopthrow T, Hulbert L, *et al.* The effect of alcohol on risk attraction among groups versus individuals. *Journal of Studies on Alcohol* 2006; 67: 628–636.

98. Monti PM, Miranda R Jr, Nixon K, *et al.* Adolescence: booze, brains, and behavior. *Alcoholism: Clinical and Experimental Research* 2005; 29: 207–220.

99. Hiller-Strumhofel S, Swartzwelder HS. Alcohol's effects on the adolescent brain: what can be learned from animal models. *Alcohol Research & Health* 2005; 28: 213–221.

100. Post RB, Lott LA, Maddock RJ, *et al.* An effect of alcohol on the distribution of spatial attention. *Journal of Studies on Alcohol* 1996; 57: 260–266.

101. Blekher T, Beard JD, O'Connor S, *et al.* Response of saccadic eye movements to alcohol in African American and non-Hispanic white college students. *Alcoholism: Clinical and Experimental Research* 2002; 26: 232–238.

102. Holdstock L, De Wit H. Ethanol impairs saccadic and smooth pursuit eye movements without producing self-reports of sedation. *Alcoholism: Clinical and Experimental Research* 1999; 23: 664–672.

103. Ross DF, Pihl RO. Alcohol, self-focus and complex reaction-time performance. *Journal of Studies on Alcohol* 1988; 49: 115–125.

104. Mungas D, Ehlers CL, Wall TL. Effects of acute alcohol administration on verbal and spatial learning. *Alcohol and Alcoholism* 1994; 29: 163–169.

105. Pearson P, Timney B. Effects of moderate blood alcohol concentrations on spatial and temporal contrast sensitivity. *Journal of Studies on Alcohol* 1998; 59: 163–173.

106. Williams CM, Skinner AEG. The cognitive effects of alcohol abuse: a controlled study. *British Journal of Addiction* 1990; 85: 911–917.

107. Pihl RO, Paylan SS, Gentes-Hawn A, *et al.* Alcohol affects executive cognitive functioning differentially on the ascending versus descending limb of the blood alcohol concentration curve. *Alcoholism: Clinical and Experiment Research* 2003; 27: 773–779.

108. Krahn D, Freese J, Hauser R, *et al.* Alcohol use and cognition at mid-life: the importance of adjusting for baseline cognitive ability and educational attainment. *Alcoholism: Clinical and Experimental Research* 2003; 27: 1162–1166.

109. Tapert SF, Cladwell L, Burke C. Alcohol and the adolescent brain. *Alcohol Research & Health* 2005; 28: 205–212.

110. Bartholow BD, Pearson M, Sher KJ, *et al.* Effects of alcohol consumption and alcohol susceptibility on cognition: a psychophysiological examination. *Biological Psychology* 2003; 64: 167–190.

111. Commission of the European Community (Brussels). An EU strategy to support Member States in reducing alcohol related harm [online]. 2006 [cited March 20, 2008]. Available from URL: http://ec.europa.eu/health/ph_determinants/life_style/alcohol/documents/alcohol_com_625_en.pdf.

112. World Health Organization. Framework for alcohol policy in the WHO European Region [online]. 2006 [cited March 20, 2008]. Available from URL: http://www.euro.who.int/document/e88335.pdf.

Chapter 9

THE EPIDEMIOLOGY OF DRUG USE AND DEPENDENCE IN ISRAEL

Yehuda D. Neumark and Hadar S. Schwartz

The use of psychotropic drugs – marijuana, inhalants, cocaine, steroids, heroin, lysergic acid diethyl amide (LSD) and 3, 4-methylenedioxymethamphetamine (MDMA-Ecstasy) – particularly among adolescents, is a major public health problem worldwide (1). Early initiation of drug use is correlated with an increased risk for adverse social outcomes (2–4), psychiatric and drug use disorders (5) and acute and chronic medical conditions (3, 6, 7). According to the World Health Organization (WHO), nearly 10% of total years-of-life are lost globally due to drug-related disability (DALYs), and 12% of all deaths are attributable to the use of drugs (8). This places drug use as the eighth leading risk factor for disease burden in developed countries. Unfortunately, while the prevalence of drug use has stabilized or even declined in recent years in some high-income countries, it is increasing in a number of low- and middle-income countries, especially among young people and women (8, 9).

Biomedical, behavioral and sociological theoretical perspectives have been used to explain the factors that induce individuals to adopt high-risk (or protective) behaviors (10–24). A wide range of predictors of drug use during adolescence have been identified using theoretical models (10) that consider one's relationship to self (e.g., ethnicity [11], early aggressive behaviors [12], impulse-control behaviors [13], poor emotional control [14] and prior use of tobacco and alcohol [15]), to others (e.g., peers and siblings with problem behaviors including drug abuse [16], lack of parental monitoring [17–19]), to nature (e.g., genetic factors [17, 20]) and to society (culture, social class [11]). Such risk factors often interact with one another, thereby increasing risk in an additive (11) or even a multiplicative manner. For example, some of these risk factors may be particularly potent, but only in the presence of certain "contextual" factors (21, 22) such as neighborhood characteristics (23), levels of social cohesion in the community (24), family and school climate (25), community delinquency rates and drug trafficking (24).

In addition to the above factors, there are at least two rather specific factors that influence the pattern of drug use in Israel and stem directly from the sociopolitical climates that have defined the past two decades. The 1990s saw the largest-ever immigration to Israel, while the beginning of this decade saw a marked increase in acts of terrorism and their horrendous consequences to individuals and society. Local research has clearly demonstrated that drug use is more common among immigrant youth and offspring of immigrant parents than non-immigrant youth (26). Though immigrant youth comprise only 13% of Israeli youth, they are responsible for almost 40% of drug-related police records among minors. These statistics are especially alarming – as with alcohol treatment, immigrants may be reluctant to seek treatment for drug abuse – because of cultural and language barriers or societal stigma (27). Also, the prevalence of drug use of all types is higher among terror-attack victims and children of families directly victimized by terror (28).

The identification of individual and contextual risk factors for drug use and the understanding of the complex interactions between them are fundamental for the development of both effective health promotion activities and comprehensive policy strategies. For these measures to prevent and control drug use successfully, an examination of the interactions between risk factors and protective factors at the different levels of influence is also essential (29).

Traditionally, researchers begin the investigation of the drug use continuum at the point of drug use initiation and then follow subsequent transitions from experimental use to established use, misuse and chronic addiction. Within the last decade, an earlier stage – the *opportunity* to use drugs – has received increased attention predominantly among researchers in the US and Latin America (14, 30–38). Estimates of opportunity for using drugs by non-institutionalized US residents 12 years or older ranged from 45% to 50%, for marijuana (30, 31); 23%, for cocaine; 14%, for hallucinogens; and 5% for heroin (31).

This earlier stage describes passive or active opportunities to try a drug prior to initiation of actual use (34–37). This is a critical stage in the drug use pathway and has considerable implications for intervention, as earlier age at first opportunity to try marijuana is associated with an increased likelihood of its later use (30). Also, first use before mid-adolescence has been shown to cascade into an increased risk of later drug problems (39). Furthermore, among those who reported an opportunity to use drugs, a considerable proportion of them make the transition to first use within one year (marijuana, 43% to 66%; hallucinogens, 50%; cocaine, 36%; and heroin, 17%) (30, 31). Hence, delaying initial opportunity to try drugs may decrease the likelihood of use and the subsequent transitions to further drug involvement (15).

Data from the US (40) clearly demonstrated that gender differences in drug use can be traced to differences in opportunities to use drugs, but once an opportunity arises, men and women are equally likely to initiate drug use. This suggests that the well-established male/female differential in drug use can be attributed mostly to differences in their exposure and opportunity experiences (30, 31, 35, 36, 40).

Data from 1995 and 1998, obtained in combined nationally representative surveys conducted by the Israel Anti-Drug Authority among adults, revealed a similar phenomenon (unpublished report). Focusing on adult Jewish respondents aged 18 to 24, researchers noted a considerable gender difference in reported lifetime use of illicit drugs – 12.3% of men reported having ever used drugs compared with 7.7% of women. Similarly, a higher proportion of men (63.3%) than women (46.1%) reported having had the opportunity to obtain drugs if they had wanted to. Restricting the analysis to those who reported an opportunity, the gender difference in lifetime use disappears completely – 29% of men and women reported having used drugs at least once in their lifetime. Preliminary analyses of the still unpublished data from the most recent national high school survey conducted in 2005 (41) suggested that although boys are nearly twice as likely as girls to report having ever used cannabis, the likelihood of use among those who had been offered the drug is identical. Little is known, however, about the factors that influence the outcomes of initial and subsequent opportunities of youths and adults to try drugs.

Research studies on the prevalence of drug use in Israel date back to more than 40 years ago. In 1966, Drapkin and Landau surveyed the population of drug offenders to understand the relatively small number of drug offences (42). At that time, only seven of every 1 million cases of suspected criminal offence in Israel were drug-related, and some 300 drug addicts were registered with the health authorities (43). Less than a decade later, researchers were struck by a dramatic increase in drug use. Researchers proposed that post-1967, that is, after the Six Day War, drug abuse – which had once been confined to "marginal deviant and criminal groups" – had become more popular among "show-business people, bohemians, pseudo-bohemians and their camp followers, and their camp followers, considerable segments of high school and university students" (44, 45). Today, the use of illicit drugs can be found in all segments of society, and 10% to 15% of adolescents and adults report having used drugs.

❧ Drug use among the young

Drug use among adolescents

The most recent national high-school drug survey (N=6410) was conducted in 2005 by the Anti-Drug Authority (41). The prevalence of illicit drug use in the past year remained virtually unchanged among high school pupils over the past decade. In 2005, 9.9% of pupils (12.1% of boys and 7.6% of girls) reported having used an illicit drug in the past year compared with 9.3% in 1995 (41). These data showed, furthermore, that the reported use of "hard" drugs (such as cocaine/crack or LSD but excluding cannabis) declined from 5.3% in 1995 to 3.9% in 2005 (6.0% of boys and 1.4% of girls). On the other hand, self-reported past-year inhalant drug use doubled from 7.4% in 2001 (the first year in which this class of drugs was included in the survey) to 15.8% in 2005, making inhalants the most widely used drug class – except for alcohol and tobacco – among Israeli schoolchildren. For example, while 6.0% of tenth grade pupils reported having used cannabis in the past year, 16.0% used inhalant drugs. Inhalants tend to be the first drug tried by Israeli youth, with an average age at first use of 12.2 years compared with 14.6 for cannabis. Unlike cannabis, there is no gender difference in the use of inhalants nor does the rate of inhalant use differ by degree of religiosity, as seen with other drugs.

Similar to Israeli findings, the peak age of inhalant use in the US is 14 to 15 years of age, with use typically declining by age 17 to 19 (46). According to data from the 2006 Monitoring the Future (MTF) survey (47), 9.1% of eighth graders in the US reported having used inhalant drugs in the past year, compared with 4.5% among American twelfth graders. This may reflect transient behavior as older adolescents move on to other drugs or stop using them. However, data do not necessarily support the conclusion that inhalant use is transitory – a large proportion of those who use inhalants take multiple inhalant drugs and do so repeatedly for long periods or both (48).

The percentage of pupils who reported any past-year drug use increased from 6.9% of seventh graders to 14.3% of twelfth graders. The prevalence of "hard drug" use did not vary much or consistently across the grades (3.8%, in seventh grade; 5.5%, in eighth grade; and 2.5%, in twelfth grade), while the rate of cannabis use showed a steep increase across the grades (from 2.4% in seventh grade to 11.0% in twelfth grade). While pupils who described themselves as "secular" were much more likely to report having used cannabis in the past year (8.1%) than "religious" students (3.9%), observant youth were more likely than secular youth to report the use of "hard" drugs (5.4% and 3.7%, respectively). There was no difference between the groups with regard to inhalant drug use with 16% of both groups reporting past-year use of inhalants.

Drug use among detached youth

Drug use is much more prevalent among non-school-attending (detached) youth. In a parallel survey of nearly 800 detached adolescents (41), about 20% of them reported using an illicit drug in the past year – twice as high as among high school pupils. The use of medications without a doctor's prescription was also considerably higher among detached youth (8.3%) compared with those who attended school (5.8%). A very troubling finding is that 4% of detached youth reported having used drugs intravenously.

Drug use among immigrant youth

Immigrant youth from the former Soviet Union (FSU) (who immigrated to Israel since 1991 or were born to parents who immigrated since 1991) are considerably more likely to report illicit drug use than their non-immigrant peers. In a survey of 750 immigrant youth aged 12 to 18 years old – of whom two-thirds were pupils and one-third detached youth no longer attending school – 35% admitted to using an illicit drug in the past year and 16% in the past month (49). The prevalence rates of past-year drug use was nearly twice as high among detached immigrant youth (48%) as among those who were at schools (26%).

Past-year use of medications (stimulants or tranquilizers) without a doctor's prescription was reported by 12% of respondents – 15% and 7% among detached youth and pupils, respectively. The use of "hard" drugs (LSD, opiates, cocaine/crack, and Ecstasy) was three times higher among detached youth (15%) as school-attending youth (5%). Youth who used cannabis or other illicit drugs were also significantly more likely to smoke and drink alcohol.

Studies showed that 30% of the youth reported committing violent crimes and 20% committed property crimes while under the influence of drugs. In addition, about 15% committed criminal acts in order to obtain drugs. Furthermore, over half (55%) of the respondents were victimized by youths who were under the influence of drugs. Youths who lived in institutional settings such as a boarding school, school dropouts before seventh grade and those who reported feeling alienated from mainstream society were more likely to use drugs and be involved in drug-related criminal offences.

In the national high-school survey (41), teenagers from families who immigrated after 1990 were significantly more likely to report past-year drug use than non-immigrant pupils – 14.6% and 9.0%, respectively.

Drug use among Arab-Israeli youth

A countrywide survey was conducted in 2004 among some 3000 Arab high school pupils. The researchers concluded that the Arab sector in Israel is "undergoing a process of social and cultural transformation. This process of moving from a traditional society to an open one has brought with it social phenomena such as risky behaviors; one such phenomenon is drug abuse" (50). They found that 6% of respondents reported past-year cannabis use, and 5% reported using other drugs including opiates, LSD, cocaine/crack, Ecstasy, and phencyclidine (PCP). Slightly lower rates were noted for all drugs among Druze school pupils. The prevalence of all drug use was higher among boys than girls. Inverse relationships were found between drug use and degree of family harmony and religiosity. The inverse relationship between drug use and religious affiliation is observed in many cultures and populations (51–53).

The use of multiple illicit drugs by Arab drug users has been noted; only 2.3% of 350 Palestinian drug users located by social services, physicians, and treatment centers reported the use of a single drug type (54). In a study of 100 Arab secondary school pupils in Jaffa, 13 had reported using at least one type of illicit drug in the previous month; 5, had used marijuana/hashish in the previous month; 7, LSD or opiates; 6, Ecstasy; and 4, cocaine (55). Particularly high rates of use were noted among 603 Christians Arab adolescents aged 11 to 17 living in east Jerusalem. The use of hashish 25 times or more in the past year was reported by 5.2% of respondents, and 2.6% reported this frequent use of LSD. The authors concluded that Arab adolescents were more knowledgeable about drugs and were more involved in drugs than were Jewish adolescents (56).

Drug use among university students

In 2003, the Anti-Drug Authority surveyed nearly 7,000 students in 12 universities and colleges in the country (57). Almost half of all respondents (42%) reported having ever used drugs and nearly one-third (30%) did so within the year prior to the survey. These rates were about 35% higher than those observed in a similar survey conducted in 1996 in which the lifetime rate was 31%, while 22% reported past-year use. Interestingly, past-month use of any illicit drug was slightly higher in 1996 (10.9%) than in 2003 (9.3%).

The prevalence rates of past-year use of any illicit drug varied considerably across institutions – from 14% to 40%.

As with adolescents, the vast majority (90%) of reported use involved cannabis. The use of "hard" drugs (cocaine/crack, heroin, hallucinogens or MDMA) was reported by 9% of respondents, and 4.5% reported using one or more of these drugs in the past year. The comparative rates in 1996 were 5.6% and 3%, respectively, for lifetime and past-year use of "hard" drugs. The reported past-year use of cocaine increased most dramatically from .6% in 1996 to 2.4% in 2003, while the prevalence of LSD, Ecstasy, heroin and amphetamines showed little or no change.

Men were more likely to report use of all drug classes than women, as were single compared with married students. A strong positive relationship was noted between cannabis use and parental education. For example, compared with students whose mothers had completed only their primary school education, students whose mothers had a university education were two-and-a-half times more likely to report cannabis use (31.7% vs. 12.4%) and the use of "hard" drugs (5.7% vs. 2.4%).

Illicit drug use was also strongly associated with alcohol drinking. Among students who did not drink, 8.4% reported having used drugs in the past year compared to 66.3% of students who consumed several alcoholic drinks a day, and 66.6% of those who reported getting drunk more than once a month. Similarly, students who smoke cigarettes were more likely to use drugs; 56.6% of smokers reported past-year drug use compared with 15.2% of nonsmokers.

Three-quarters of the respondents had "backpacked" in other countries; of these, 32% had used drugs while abroad. More than half of those who had traveled to the Far East or South America used drugs during their travels, compared with 32.0% and 28.0% among those who traveled to Europe or Africa.

Nearly all respondents (87.5%) reported exposure to anti-drug campaigns at some point, mostly within elementary or high-school school (76.5%), but also in the army (48.5%), university (17.2%), workplace (10.4%) and media community (9.6%). Interestingly, the prevalence of drug use was actually slightly higher among those who had been exposed to some anti-drug messages. Only among those who reported exposure in all five settings was the use of drugs less common than among those not exposed to any anti-drug campaigns. However, willingness to try drugs was not influenced by exposure to anti-drug messages. One-third (36%) of the students indicated that they would or might be willing to try an illicit drug if it were offered to them, and nearly half (46.6%) felt the same about cannabis. Men were more likely to express a liberal attitude towards trying drugs than were women (25.1% and 17.4% respectively). Nearly 30% of those who expressed unwillingness to take drugs had used them in the past.

One-quarter of respondents were in favor of legalizing marijuana/hashish, and 42% were against such a move, while the rest were undecided.

Drugs in the Israel Defense Forces

The Israel Defense Forces (IDF) maintains a strict, zero-tolerance drug policy and prohibits the use or sale of any illicit drug among military personnel – at the risk of stiff punishment for offenders. The IDF's drug-deterrence program relies heavily upon random and non-random urine testing as well as ongoing drug awareness information campaigns. According to a report submitted to the *Knesset* (Parliament) Committee on Psychoactive Drugs (58), nearly 2,000 soldiers were investigated by the military police for suspicion of drug use or drug trafficking in 2004, 11% of whom were women. In 2007, the military police carried out over 12,000 urine tests and opened investigations against almost 1600 soldiers (59).

Israeli youth entering the high-risk period for drug use also face their impending induction into military service at age 18. Serving in the IDF has strong social implications, and those who do not serve often find themselves outside of mainstream society (more so in the past than in recent years). It is possible that this serves as a deterrent, as illicit drug use may lead to rejection by the IDF. This may partially account for the low prevalence of drug use among mainstream young adults as compared with developed countries elsewhere (60, 61).

Since 1982, the IDF Medical Corps' Public Health Branch has conducted a continuous sample survey of drug use among army personnel on the day of discharge from compulsory military service. During the period of study, the population of military recruits in Israel accounted for about 80% of the entire 18-year-old Jewish-Israeli male cohort in any given year and about two-thirds of the female population of this age. For the entire 20-year survey period from 1982 to 2001, 6.9% of men and 3.9% of women reported having used drugs at least once in their lives (62). Marijuana accounted for ⅔ to ¾ of all drug use in this population. The percentage of respondents who said they had used drugs one or more times (lifetime prevalence) was consistently higher among men than women.

Overall, there was a steady monotonic decrease in the rate of lifetime drug use in both genders during the 1980s – dropping from 14% in 1982 to 4% in 1989 among men and from 8% in 1982 to 1% in 1990 in women. From 1990 onward, the rate among men remained fairly constant until 1998 when a relatively sharp increase was evident, while among women a gradual increase in drug use was noted during the 1990s, with a similar steep upturn in the late 1990s. The proportion of men who reported the recent use of drugs (in the six months prior to discharge) ranged from 1.3%–6.1% during the 1982–2001 period. Among women, this rate was lower throughout, and ranged from .4% to 3.0%. In both genders, the rate of recent drug use declined .during the 1980s followed by an increase in the 1990s, with a steeper increase among men particularly in the last few years.

An inverse relationship between lifetime drug use and education was evident in both genders. The average rate of drug use in men with 0 to 8 years of schooling (15.7%) was twice the rate in men with 9 to 11 years (6.9%, $p < .001$) and three times higher than the rate among those with 12 or more years of schooling (5.0%, $p < .001$). The rate of drug use among female respondents with 12 or more years of schooling (3.0%) was 60% that of the males with similar schooling, while the rates were similar in women and men with 9–11 years of schooling (7.7 and 6.9, respectively).

ꙮ Drug use among adults

The Israel National Health Survey (INHS), comprising nearly 5000 adults aged 21 and over, was conducted in 2003 to 2004 as part of the WHO/World Mental Health Survey initiative (63). The use of any illicit drug ever (lifetime prevalence) was reported by 12.8% of all respondents (Y. Neumark *et al.*, unpublished). Cannabis accounted for nearly all of the reported drug use, 11.5% reported ever having used cannabis and 3.6% having ever used other illicit drugs. As expected, lifetime use of cannabis was more commonly reported by younger adults, as shown in the table below. Disappointingly, despite intensive anti-smoking campaigns and legislation, the prevalence of tobacco smoking is not lower, and the prevalence of alcohol drinking is higher in the younger cohorts.

Table 1. At least one-time use of alcohol, tobacco, cannabis and cocaine (%) in a national sample of Israeli adults, ages 21 and above. Years 2003–2004

Age group	Alcohol	Tobacco	Cannabis	Cocaine
21–34	62.9	47.0	19.3	.3
35–49	59.6	49.6	11.6	.3
50–64	57.6	51.5	6.0	.2
65+	46.4	41.8	.6	.0
All ages	58.3	47.9	11.5	.1

Focusing on respondents aged 21–44, the lifetime prevalence rate of any drug use was higher among men than women (23.0% and 13.8%, respectively), and considerably higher among Jewish- (20.7%) than Arab-Israeli respondents (5.0%). Educational differences were greater for women than for men, with women who completed high school and those holding an academic degree being about twice as likely as others to report the use of drugs. In a recently published multi-national comparison of drug use based on data from the WHO/World Mental Health surveys in 17 countries (64), Israel ranked seventh in terms of adult cannabis use, eleventh for cocaine use, and fourth and fifth for tobacco and alcohol use.

About 1% of the adult population meets DSM-IV criteria for drug abuse or dependence (65), which is similar to the rate in the US (66). Official government estimates suggest there are 12,500–15,000 drug- (mostly heroin) dependent persons (41), and some 12,000 Israelis were treated for drug problems in 2006 (9). Approximately one-quarter of heroin addicts in the country are immigrants from the FSU. The percentage that use heroin by intravenous injection in this group is upwards of 90% (67). From a public health perspective, perhaps the most pressing issue with regard to the drug-dependent community is hepatitis C infection (HCV). HCV is highly prevalent in this community with an average national rate of 45.8% (68), and about 70% among drug-treatment patients from the FSU (67). Effective HCV-treatment is offered virtually free-of-charge since 2005, within the government-subsidized basket of health services available to all insured residents of the country. However, very few of the estimated 7000 HCV-infected drug-dependent individuals in the country are treated.

⸹ Treatment services and prevention programs

Drug treatment services and prevention programs are operated by a number of national state and local government and quasi-governmental agencies. The multitude of agencies involved in the provision of these services makes it difficult to provide an accurate and current estimate of the number of drug users and drug-dependent persons who benefit from the various services. Several ambulatory and in-patient drug treatment facilities and programs operate throughout the country under the auspices of the Ministry of Health –the national state agency that assumes the main responsibility for the treatment of drug dependency. In addition, this agency is responsible for 11 clinics in six cities throughout the country that provide methadone maintenance therapy to some 3000 opiate-dependent persons. The Ministry of Welfare and Social Services also operates ambulatory day care centers for recovering drug addicts and several "therapeutic communities" (long-term residential programs), as well as community-based programs specifically for drug-using youth. Prevention and treatment programs designed specifically for immigrant youth and adults have been established by the Ministry of Immigrant Absorption, sometimes in conjunction with other national or local agencies. The Ministry of Education is responsible for the development, delivery and evaluation of the numerous school-based drug prevention programs and activities offered in hundreds of elementary and high schools.

Treatment gap has been defined as the difference between the number of persons who need treatment for the use of illicit drugs and the number receiving treatment in a given year (69). Reducing the treatment gap is one of the objectives (Objective 26–18) of the US program called *Healthy People 2010* (70). There seems to be a consensus in Israel that current treatment needs are not being met. As an example, a law has just recently been tabled to expand the network of methadone clinics throughout the country.

⸹ Legislation and law enforcement

The Dangerous Drugs Ordinance (Revised Version) 1973 defines the legislative parameters of the use, possession, sale, import and export of psychotropic chemicals. The drug-related offences as established under this law broadly include the use or possession of drugs for personal use, production, trade, import and export of banned chemicals without a permit and the possession of drugs or utensils for the purposes of committing one of these offences (71). An amendement to the Dangerous Drug Ordinance adopted in 1990 (Amendment No. 3, Law 1989) stiffened the penalties for drug dealing, and a person convicted for this crime is subject to seizure of all personal property and may be disqualified from holding a passport or a driver's license or operating a vehicle or business. The law was further amended in 2007 and 2008 to include a number of synthetically prepared drugs not previously covered under the existing legislation but commonly used by Israeli youth. One example of these newly-banned substances is cathinone (*hagigat*, in Hebrew jargon) which is an alkaloid found in the *khat* plant (*Catha edulis*) – a traditional and legal stimulant (72).

Israel has signed and ratified all of the international conventions related to narcotics including the UN 1961 Single Convention on Narcotic Drugs (73), the Convention on Psychotropic Substances of 1971 (74) and the 1988 Convention Against the Illicit Traffic in Narcotic Drugs and Psychotropic Substances (75); it has been a member of the Commission on Narcotic Drugs in the UN Office on Drugs and Crime (UNODC) since 2003.

It is worth citing here the opening sentences of Drapkin and Landau's 1966 article: "There is some controversy as to whether it is justifiable to regard drug addiction as a crime and whether arrest and court punishment are able to deter people from using drugs. However, as long as the Israeli law sees activities associated with drugs as an offence, all those who deal with criminological research must also consider this aspect of deviant behavior. Similarly, knowledge on all aspects of the problem provides a basis for reform in attitudes as well as in the treatment of the problem" (42).

The main goals of law enforcement agencies regarding illicit drugs are the prevention of drugs from being imported into the country and the identification of those who import these drugs or finance their import, and identification of sellers and users of illicit drugs. According to their own estimates, though, the police seize less than 10% of all drugs smuggled into the country and admit that "Israel's borders with Egypt and Jordan are completely open to smugglers," allowing more than 100 tons of marijuana and hashish to be brought into Israel from the Egyptian Sinai Peninsula in 2007 (76). The data presented in table 2 (culled from a number of official Internet sources that are listed in a footnote to the table) suggest that well under 10% of the estimated 100 tons were seized in 2007. Indeed, there has been a drastic decline in the quantity of marijuana and hashish seized since 2004. The quantities of cocaine and heroin seized have been fairly constant over the years and have not changed dramatically since 1999. A large drop in the number of LSD blotters ("*tabs*") was also seen in 2007 compared to previous years. Of the nearly 900,000 Ecstasy tablets seized in 2007, 777,000 were seized from one container in the port of Haifa arriving from Europe. According to the UN Office on Drugs and Crime (9), a slight decline in seizures from 2005 to 2006 was noted globally – from 32.5 billion units in 2005 to 31 billion in 2006. According to the report, this was likely due to the stabilization in global drug production and consumption rather than reduced law enforcement activity.

Table 2. Time-trends in quantities of drugs seized by the Israel Police. Years 1999–2007

Drugs	1999	2004	2005	2006	2007
Marijuana/hashish (kg)	3,400	16,000	10,000	6,000	2,200
Cocaine (kg)	28	32	169	44	35
Heroin (kg)	110	69	140	70? 92?	94
Ecstasy (pills)	460,000	313,800	138,000? 267,000?	113,000? 270,000?	891,300*
LSD (tabs)	7,000	75,750	3,000	12,000	1,900

** Data for January – November, 2007.*
Data sources: 1999 data are from the Israel Police website (77);
2005–2007 data (78, 79); International Narcotics Control Strategy Report (80).

The annual number of criminal charges filed by the Israel Police for drug use, possession and/or trafficking doubled from 14,264 in 1997 to 28,352 in 2003 (81). The question remains open as to whether this represents an increase in the magnitude of drug availability and use in Israel or an intensification of efforts on the part of the law enforcement agencies in their battle against drugs. During this period, the proportion of drug offence charges filed against minors rose from 7.8% to 16.5%, an increase that likely reflects a policy adopted by the police in the late 1990s to focus on drug use among youth. Indeed, one of the stated parameters of success of this policy is the ability to identify groups of young drug users and their drug suppliers. In 2006, 25,732 drug offence charges were filed (15% against minors), representing a 10% decrease since 2003 (79). A further reduction was noted in 2007, when 22,830 drug offence charges were filed -14,750 for use, just over 3000 for trafficking, and nearly 4800 for possession (80). While Israel is not a significant producer or trafficking point for drugs, Israeli nationals have been heavily and repeatedly implicated in global drug trafficking networks, particularly those involving Ecstasy (80).

The Israel Prison Service (IPS) is responsible for the supervision of prisoners and for the identification of drug-using and drug-dependent prisoners (it carries out some 15,000 urine tests annually) and their subsequent treatment and rehabilitation (82).

৶ From epidemiology to mental health action

The decision to use or not use drugs when presented with an opportunity to do so is the product of numerous personal, familial, social and cultural forces (83). Once drug use is initiated, it is associated with adverse personal, academic and social outcomes, especially during the formative years of adolescence. Interventions therefore, if they are to be successful, must address individuals' risk factors including psychosocial, behavioral and even genetic influences (84), community norms and their interaction with local law enforcement, and drug availability (85). As stated in *Healthy people 2010* (70), strategies for preventing drug abuse among youth should include raising awareness, educating and training parents and others, strengthening families, providing alternative activities, building skills and confidence, mobilizing and empowering communities and employing environmental approaches.

The use of illicit drugs among Israeli youth and adults is no longer a rare event, as it once was. About 10% of youth and adults reported using illicit drugs – and this proportion is considerably higher in high-risk populations, such as immigrant youth and school-age teenagers who are not currently attending school. It is particularly worrisome that there has been a steep increase in recent years in the use by adolescents of inhalant drugs. Numerous reports suggest that early use of inhalants increases the likelihood of progression to more severe drug-taking behaviors (such as injection drug use) or other problem behaviors, including delinquency and suicidal behavior (86–94). In their study of 178 Israeli adolescent inpatients diagnosed with schizophrenia or schizoaffective disorder, Shoval *et al.* (95) found that those who had attempted suicide were nearly six times more likely to have reported inhalant drug use (OR = 5.5, 95% CI 1.6–19.3). Inhalant use also poses a risk of sudden death and of an array of mental and physical health hazards including neurological dysfunction, depression, renal and hepatic failure, and arrhythmia (88, 92, 96–98) as well as social dysfunction (99). Despite these risks, many youth do not view experimentation with inhalant drugs as dangerous (47). Given the increasing use of inhalant drugs by Israeli adolescents and the lack of awareness of the potential deleterious effects of such use, further research and prevention efforts are warranted in this area, including increasing the knowledge and awareness of the dangers of inhalant drug use among parents, teachers and healthcare providers.

The aims of Israel's national strategy against drugs should be to reduce the prevalence and incidence of drug use particularly among young people, cut the magnitude of drug-related harm to the individual (truancy, cognitive deficit, HIV) and to society (crime) and maintain a network of drug treatment services in keeping with the demand. Achievement of these aims requires the development, successful implementation and evaluation of effective and integrated comprehensive knowledge-based measures. These include a reduction in drug supply, prevention, early intervention, treatment, harm reduction, rehabilitation and social reintegration measures for drug-dependent individuals (100, 101). The national strategy must also encourage the expansion of research in the field of drug use and misuse and the regular collection of reliable and comparable data on key epidemiological indicators. It is hoped that by providing a comprehensive system of drug prevention and treatment services, Israel can stem the spread of drug use among youth and effectively care for its drug users, their families and society at large.

❧ References

1. World Health Organization. Neuroscience of psychoactive substance use and dependence [online]. 2004 [cited July 25, 2008]. Available from URL: http://www.who.int/substance_abuse/publications/en/Neuroscience.pdf.

2. Ellickson PL, Tucker JS, Klein DJ. Ten-year prospective study of public health problems associated with early drinking. *Journal of Pediatrics* 2003; 111: 949–955.

3. Centers for Disease Control and Prevention. Alcohol-attributable deaths and years of potential life lost – United States, 2001. *Morbidity and Mortality Weekly Report* 2004; 53: 8668–8670.

4. Brook JS, Brook DW, Rosen Z, *et al.* Earlier marijuana use and later problem behavior in Colombian youths. *Journal of the American Academy of Child and Adolescent Psychiatry* 2003; 42: 485–492.

5. Brook DW, Brook JS, Zhang C, *et al.* Drug use and the risk of major depressive disorder, alcohol dependence, and substance use disorders. *Archives of General Psychiatry* 2002; 59: 1039–1044.

6. Frishman WH, Del Vecchio A, Sanal S, *et al.* Cardiovascular manifestations of substance abuse. Part 1: Cocaine. *Heart Disease* 2003; 5: 187–201.

7. American Heart Association. *Heart Disease and Stroke Statistics –2004 Update.* Dallas, TX: American Heart Association, 2003.

8. World Health Organization's World Health Report 2002 [online]. 2002 [cited July 25, 2008]. Available from URL: http://www.who.int/whr/2002/en/whr02_en.pdf.

9. United Nations (United States). 2008 World Drug Report [online]. 2008 [cited July 28, 2008]. Available from URL: http://www.unodc.org/documents/wdr/WDR_2008/WDR_2008_eng_web.pdf.

10. Lettieri DJ, Sayers M, Wallenstein-Pearson H, eds. *Theories on drug abuse: selected contemporary perspectives.* NIDA Research Monographs 1980; 30: 1–488.

11. National Institute on Drug Abuse (US). *Preventing drug use among children and adolescents: a research-based guide for parents, educators, and community leaders.* Second edition. National Institute on Drug Abuse. Washington, DC: US Government Printing Office, 2003.

12. Knyazev GG. Behavioral activation as predictor of substance use: mediating and moderating role of attitudes and social relationship. *Drug and Alcohol Dependence* 2004; 75: 309–321.

13. Neumark YD, Anthony JC. Childhood misbehavior and the risk of injecting drug use. *Drug and Alcohol Dependence* 1997; 48: 193–197.

14. Stenbacka M, Allebeck P, Romelsjo A. Initiation into drug abuse: the pathway from being offered drugs to trying cannabis and progression to intravenous drug abuse. *Scandinavian Journal of Social Medicine* 1993; 21: 31–39.

15. Kandel D, Yamguchi K, Chen K. Stages of progression in drug involvement from adolescence to adulthood: further evidence for the gateway theory. *Journal of Studies on Alcohol* 1992; 53: 447–457.

16. Latimer W, Floyd LJ, Kariis T, *et al.* Peer and sibling substance use: predictors of substance use among adolescents in Mexico. *Pan-American Journal of Public Health* 2004; 15: 225–232.

17. Neumark Y, Friedlander Y, Bar-Hamburger R. Family history and other characteristics of heroin-dependent Jewish males in Israel: results of a case-control study. *Israel Medical Association Journal* 2002; 4: 766–771.

18. Griffin KW, Botvin GJ, Scheier LM, *et al.* Factors associated with regular marijuana use among high school students: a long-term follow-up study. *Substance Use and Misuse* 2002; 37: 225–238.

19. Wood MD, Read JP, Mitchell RE, *et al.* Do parents still matter? Parent and peer influences on alcohol involvement among recent high school graduates. *Psychology of Addictive Behaviors* 2004; 18: 19–30.

20. Miles DR, Van Den Bree MB, Gupman AE, *et al*. A twin study on sensation seeking, risk taking behavior and marijuana use. *Drug and Alcohol Dependence* 2001; 62: 57–68.

21. Wilcox P. An ecological approach to understanding youth smoking trajectories: problems and prospects. *Addiction* 2003; 98 (Suppl 1): 57–77.

22. Duncan C, Jones K, Moon G. Health-related behaviour in context: a multilevel modelling approach. *Social Science and Medicine* 1996; 42: 817–830.

23. Duncan SC, Duncan TE, Strycker LA. A multilevel analysis of neighborhood context and youth alcohol and drug problems. *Preventive Sciences* 2002; 3: 125–133.

24. Storr CL, Arria AM, Workman ZR, *et al*. Neighborhood environment and opportunity to try methamphetamine ("ice") and marijuana: evidence from Guam in the Western Pacific region of Micronesia. *Substance Use and Misuse* 2004; 39: 253–276.

25. Kumpfer KL, Turner CW. The social ecology model of adolescent substance abuse: implications for prevention. *International Journal of Addictions* 1990–1991; 25: 435–463.

26. Mi-Ami N. Drug and alcohol addiction among immigrant youth (Hebrew) [online]. 2006 [cited December 20, 2007]. Available from URL: http://www.knesset.gov.il/MMM/data/pdf/m01647.pdf.

27. Edelstein O. Substance use and related delinquency among former Russian youth in Israel (Hebrew) [online]. 2007 [cited December 20, 2007]. Available from URL: http://www.antidrugs.gov.il/download/files/microsoft_word_-_ -2007.pdf.

28. Schiff M, Zweig HH, Benbenishty R, *et al*. Exposure to terrorism and Israeli youths' cigarette, alcohol, and cannabis use. *American Journal of Public Health* 2007; 97: 1852–1858.

29. Biglan A. Contextualism and the development of effective prevention practices. *Prevention Science* 2004; 5: 15–21.

30. Van Etten ML, Neumark YD, Anthony JC. Initial opportunity to use marijuana and the transition to first use: United States, 1979–1994. *Drug and Alcohol Dependence* 1997; 49: 1–7.

31. Van Etten ML, Anthony JC. Comparative epidemiology of initial drug opportunities and transitions to first use: marijuana, cocaine, hallucinogens and heroin. *Drug and Alcohol Dependence* 1999; 54: 117–125.

32. Storr CL, Chen CY, Anthony JC. "Unequal opportunity": neighbourhood disadvantage and the chance to buy illegal drugs. *Journal of Epidemiology and Community Health* 2004; 58: 231–237.

33. Wagner FA, Anthony JC. Into the world of illegal drug use: exposure opportunity and other mechanisms linking the use of alcohol, tobacco, marijuana and cocaine. *American Journal of Epidemiology* 2002; 155: 918–925.

34. Department of Health and Human Services (US). Substance Abuse and Mental Health Services Administration (SAMHSA). *National household survey on drug abuse, main findings: 1995* (DHHS Pub. No. 3085). Rockville, MD, 1996.

35. Van Etten ML, Neumark YD, Anthony JC. Male-female differences in the earliest stages of drug involvement. *Addiction* 1999; 94: 1413–1419.

36. Crum RM, Lillie-Blanton M, Anthony JC. Neighborhood environment and opportunity to use cocaine and other drugs in late childhood and early adolescence. *Drug and Alcohol Dependence* 1996; 43: 155–161.

37. Delva J, Van Etten ML, Gonzalez GB, *et al*. First opportunities to try drugs and the transition to first drug use: evidence from a national school survey in Panama. *Substance Use and Misuse* 1999; 34: 1451–1467.

38. Dormitzer CM, Gonzalez GB, Penna M, *et al*. The PACARDO research project: youthful drug involvement in Central America and the Dominican Republic. *Pan-American Journal of Public Health* 2004; 15: 400–416.

39. Anthony JC, Petronis KR. Early-onset drug use and risk of later drug problems. *Drug and Alcohol Dependence* 1995; 40: 9–15.

40. Van Etten ML, Anthony JC. Male-female differences in transitions from first drug opportunity to first use: searching for subgroup variation by age, race, region, and urban status. *Journal of Women's Health and Gender-Based Medicine* 2001; 10: 797–804.

41. Anti-Drug Authority (Israel). The use of psychoactive substances among Israeli residents, 2005 [online]. 2005 [cited January 10, 2008]. Available from URL: http://www.antidrugs.org.il/template/default.asp?maincat=14.

42. Drapkin I, Landau SF. Drug offenders in Israel: a survey. *British Journal of Criminology* 1966; 6: 376–390.

43. Jermulowicz ZW. Control and treatment of drug addicts in Israel. *Bulletin of Narcotics* 1962; 2: 11–18.

44. Peled T, Schimmerling H. The drug culture among the youth of Israel: the case of high school students. In: Shoham S, ed. *Israel studies in criminology, 1972–1973*. Vol. 2. Jerusalem: Academic Press, 1973.

45. Shoham SG, Geva N, Kliger D, *et al*. Drug abuse among Israeli youth: epidemiological pilot study. *Bulletin of Narcotics* 1974; 26: 9–28.

46. Williams JF, Storck M. The Committee on Substance Abuse and Committee on Native American Child Health. Inhalant Abuse. *Pediatrics* 2007; 119: 1009–1017.

47. Johnston LD, O'Malley PM, Bachman JG, *et al*. *Monitoring the future national results on adolescent drug use: overview of key findings, 2006* (NIH Publication No. 07-6202). Bethesda, MD: National Institute on Drug Abuse, 2007.

48. Neumark YD, Delva J, Anthony JC. The epidemiology of adolescent inhalant drug involvement. *Archives of Pediatrics and Adolescent Medicine* 1998; 152: 781–786.

49. Edelstein A, Bar-Hamburger R. Substance use and related delinquency among former Russian youth in Israel (Hebrew, English abstract) [online]. 2007 [cited August 6, 2008]. Available from URL: http://www.antidrugs.gov.il/template/default.asp?maincat=12&catId=41&pageId=91&parentId=224.

50. Azaiza F, Abu-Asbah K. Psychoactive substance use among Arab and Druze high school students in Israel-2004 (Hebrew) [online]. 2004 [cited July 25, 2008]. Available from URL: http://www.antidrugs.gov.il/template/default.asp?maincat=12&catId=41&pageId=805.

51. Benjet C, Borges G, Medina-Mora ME, *et al*. Drug use opportunities and the transition to drug use among adolescents from the Mexico City Metropolitan Area. *Drug and Alcohol Dependence* 2007; 90: 128–134.

52. Degenhardt L, Chiu WT, Sampson N, *et al.* Epidemiological patterns of extra-medical drug use in the United States: evidence from the National Comorbidity Survey Replication, 2001–2003. *Drug and Alcohol Dependence* 2007; 90: 210–223.

53. Van der Meer Sanchez Z, de Oliveira LG, Nappo SA. Religiosity as a protective factor against the use of drugs. *Substance Use and Misuse* 2008; 43: 1476–1486.

54. Khamis V, Habash A. Drug addiction among Palestinians in the West Bank. Bethlehem University, 1995. Cited in Weiss S, Sawa GH, Abdeen Z, *et al.* Substance abuse studies and prevention efforts among Arabs in the 1990s in Israel, Jordan and the Palestinian Authority: a literature review. *Addiction* 1999; 94: 177–198.

55. Dgani A. *Drug use in Tel Aviv-Jaffa* (Hebrew). Tel Aviv, Geocartography Institute, 1992. Cited in Weiss S, Sawa GH, Abdeen Z, *et al.* Substance abuse studies and prevention efforts among Arabs in the 1990s in Israel, Jordan and the Palestinian Authority: a literature review. *Addiction* 1999; 94: 177–198.

56. Abdeen Z. *Substance abuse among Palestinian youth in 1996.* East Jerusalem, Jerusalem: Al-Quds University, 1996. Cited in Weiss S, Sawa GH, Abdeen Z, *et al.* Substance abuse studies and prevention efforts among Arabs in the 1990s in Israel, Jordan and the Palestinian Authority: a literature review. *Addiction* 1999; 94: 177–198.

57. Bar-Hamburger R. Survey of attitudes and use of psychoactive drugs among students in institutes of higher learning in Israel – 2003 (Hebrew) [online]. 2004 [cited July 20, 2008]. Available from URL: http://www.antidrugs.gov.il/download/files/ -2003.

58. Tikvah R. Addressing the phenomenon of drug use in the Israeli Defense Forces: enforcement, prevention and treatment (Hebrew) [online]. 2005 [cited July 18, 2008]. Available from URL: http://www.knesset.gov.il/mmm/data/docs/m01269.doc.

59. Israel Defense Forces. Drugs targeted (Hebrew) [online]. 2007 [cited January 20, 2008]. Available from URL: http://dover.idf.il/IDF/News_Channels/bamahana/07/47/01.htm.

60. Harkin, AM, Anderson P, Goos C. *Smoking, drinking and drug taking in the European Region.* Copenhagen: WHO Regional Office for Europe, 1997.

61. Kandel D, Adler DBI, Sudit M. The epidemiology of adolescent drug use in France and in Israel. *American Journal of Public Health* 1981; 71: 256–265.

62. Neumark YD, Grotto I, Kark JD. Twenty-year trends in illicit drug use among young Israelis completing military duty. *Addiction* 2004; 99: 641–648.

63. Levinson D, Paltiel A, Nir M, *et al.* The Israel National Health Survey: issues and methods. *Israel Journal of Psychiatry and Related Sciences* 2007; 44: 85–93.

64. Degenhardt L, Chiu WT, Sampson N, *et al.* Toward a global view of alcohol, tobacco, cannabis, and cocaine use: findings from the WHO World Mental Health Surveys. *PLoS Medicine* 2008; 5 (7): e141 DOI: 10.1371/journal.pmed.0050141.

65. American Psychiatric Association. *Diagnostic and statistical manual of mental disorders – Fourth edition.* Washington, DC: American Psychiatric Association, 1994.

66. Compton WM, Grant BF, Colliver JD, *et al.* Prevalence of marijuana use disorders in the United States: 1991–1992 and 2001–2002. *Journal of the American Medical Association* 2004; 291: 2114–2121.

67. Isralowitz R, Reznik A, Spear SE, *et al.* Severity of heroin use in Israel: comparisons between native Israelis and former Soviet Union immigrants. *Addiction* 2007; 102: 630–637.

68. Cohen-Moreno R, Schiff M, Levitt S, *et al.* Knowledge about hepatitis-C among methadone maintenance treatment patients in Israel *Substance Use and Misuse.* (In press).

69. Woodward A, Epstein J, Gfroerer J, *et al.* The drug abuse treatment gap: recent estimates. *Health Care and Finance Review* 1997; 18: 5–17.

70. Healthy People 2010. Risk of substance use and abuse [online]. 2002 [cited July 25, 2008]. Available from URL: http://www.healthypeople.gov/Document/HTML/Volume2/26Substance.htm#_Toc489757841.

71. Ben-Gurion University of the Negev as a Drug-Free Environment [online]. [cited July 27, 2008]. Available from URL: http://web2.bgu.ac.il/global/General/documents/drugs.doc.

72. Bentur Y, Bloom-Krasik A, Raikhlin-Eisenkraft B. Illicit cathinone (*Hagigat*) poisoning. *Clinical Toxicology* 2008; 46: 206–210.

73. United Nations Office on Drugs and Crime. Single Convention on Narcotic Drugs [online]. 1961 [cited July 20, 2008]. Available from URL: http://www.unodc.org/unodc/en/treaties/single-convention.html.

74. United Nations Office on Drugs and Crime. Convention on Psychotropic Substances [online]. 1971 [cited July 20, 2008]. Available from URL: http://www.unodc.org/unodc/en/treaties/psychotropics.html.

75. United Nations Office on Drugs and Crime. Convention against the illicit traffic in narcotic drugs and psychotropic substances [online]. 1988 [cited July 20, 2008]. Available from URL: http://www.unodc.org/unodc/en/treaties/illicit-trafficking.html

76. Ravid B. Police: less than 10% of illegal drugs smuggled into Israel are caught [online]. 2007 [cited July 20, 2008]. Available from URL: http://www.haaretz.com/hasen/spages/884796.html.

77. Israel Police. Criminal negligence in Israel – 1999: sale and use of dangerous drugs (Hebrew) [online]. 1999 [cited July 20, 2008]. Available from URL: http://www.police.gov.il/statistica_umipui/statistica/xx01b_13bd_stat.asp.

78. United Nations Office on Drugs and Crime. World Drug Report 2008: Seizures [online]. [cited July 20, 2008]. Available from URL: http://www.unodc.org/documents/wdr/WDR_2008/SEIZURE_Tables.pdf.

79. The Anti-Drug Authority. The sale of drugs in Israel (Hebrew) [online]. 2008 [cited July 20, 2008]. Available from URL: http://www.antidrugs.gov.il/template/default.asp?maincat=3&catid=47.

80. United States Department of State (United States). International narcotics control strategy report (INCSR) 2008, vol. 1 [online]. 2008 [cited July 25, 2008]. Available from URL: http://www.state.gov/documents/organization/102583.pdf.

81. Zwebner S, Bar-Natan R. Drugs In Israel: magnitude of use and treatment and prevention programs. Report submitted to the Committee on Psychoactive Drugs of the Israeli Knesset (Hebrew) [online]. 2004 [cited July 20, 2008]. Available from URL: http://www.knesset.gov.il/mmm/data/docs/m01269.doc.

82. Israel Ministry of Foreign Affairs. Israel Prison Service [online]. 2003 [cited July 20, 2008]. Available from URL: http://www.mfa. gov.il/MFA/MFAArchive/2000_2009/2003/3/Ministry%20of%20Public%20Security.

83. Winfred W, Khan AJ. Adolescent illicit drug use: understanding and addressing the problem. *Medscape Public Health & Prevention* 2005; 3 (2). Available from URL: http://www.acpm.org/Khan&Wu_AdolescentDrugUse.pdf.

84. Fishbein D. The importance of neurobiological research to the prevention of psychopathology. *Preventive Sciences* 2000; 2: 89–106.

85. US Department of Health and Human Services (HHS) (USA). National Institute on Drug Abuse. New research-based guide now available to help prevent teen drug use. HHS Press Release [online]. 1997 [cited August 20, 2008]. Available from URL: http://www. hhs.gov/news/press/1997pres/970306.html.

86. Dinwiddie SH, Reich T, Cloninger CR. Solvent abuse as a precursor to intravenous drug abuse. *Comprehensive Psychiatry* 1991; 32: 133–140.

87. Beauvais F. Volatile solvent abuse: trends and patterns. In: Sharp CM, Beauvais F, Spence R, eds. *Inhalant abuse: a volatile research agenda* (NIDA Research Monograph 129; DHHS publication (ADM) 93-3475). Washington, DC: Superintendent of Documents, US Government Printing Office, 1992.

88. Compton WM, Cottler LB, Dinwiddie SH, *et al.* Inhalant use: characteristics and predictors. *American Journal of Addictions* 1994; 3: 263–272.

89. Schütz CG, Chilcoat HD, Anthony JC. The association between sniffing inhalants and injecting drugs. *Comprehensive Psychiatry* 1994; 35: 99–105.

90. Johnson EO, Schütz CG, Anthony JC, *et al.* Inhalants to heroin: a prospective analysis from adolescence to adulthood. *Drug and Alcohol Dependence* 1995; 40: 159–164.

91. Borges G, Walters EE, Kessler RC. Associations of substance use, abuse, and dependence with subsequent suicidal behavior. *American Journal of Epidemiology* 2000; 151: 781–789.

92. Kelder SH, Murray NG, Orpinas P, *et al.* Depression and substance use in minority middle-school students. *American Journal of Public Health* 2001; 91: 761–766.

93. Mackesy-Amiti ME, Fendrich M. Inhalant use and delinquent behavior among adolescents: a comparison of inhalant users and other drug users. *Addiction* 1999; 94: 555–564.

94. Wu L-T, Pilowsky DJ, Schlenger WE. Inhalant abuse and dependence among adolescents in the United States. *Journal of the American Academy of Child and Adolescent Psychiatry* 2004; 43: 1206–1214.

95. Shoval G, Sever J, Sher L, *et al.* Substance use, suicidality, and adolescent-onset schizophrenia: an Israeli 10-year retrospective study. *Journal of Child and Adolescent Psychopharmacology* 2006; 16: 767–775.

96. Bowen SE, Daniel J, Balster RL. Deaths associated with inhalant abuse in Virginia from 1987 to 1996. *Drug and Alcohol Dependence* 1999; 53: 239–245.

97. American Academy of Pediatrics (United States). Inhalant abuse. *Pediatrics* 1996; 97: 420–423.

98. Anderson CE, Loomis GA. Recognition and prevention of inhalant abuse. *American Family Physician* 2003; 68: 869–874.

99. Howard MO, Jenson JM. Inhalant use among antisocial youth: prevalence and correlates. *Addictive Behavior* 1999; 24: 59–74.

100. The European Union (Europe). The EU action plan on drugs (2000–2004) [online]. 2008 [cited August 21, 2008]. Available from URL: http://www.emcdda.europa.eu/html.cfm/index1338EN.html

101. The European Union (Europe). EU Drugs Action Plan (2005–2008). Official Journal of the European Union [online]. 2008 [cited August 21, 2008]. Available from URL: http://www.emcdda.europa.eu/attachements.cfm/att_10512_EN_en.pdf.

Chapter 10

The epidemiology of tobacco addiction in Israel

Lital Keinan-Boker and Orna Baron-Epel

Tobacco is an agricultural product processed from the fresh leaves of plants in the genus *Nicotiana*. Commercially available in both dried and cured forms, it is often smoked in the form of a cigar or cigarette – or in a stem pipe, water pipe or hookah. Tobacco can also be chewed (*bidi*), "dipped" (placed between the cheek and gum), or sniffed into the nose as finely powdered snuff.

All means of consumption result in the absorption of nicotine, in varying amounts, into the user's bloodstream. Over time, tolerance and dependence develop. The amount absorbed at each exposure to tobacco, the frequency of exposure and the absorption speed seem to have a direct relationship with how strong dependence develops and tolerance is formed.

As smoking is associated with considerable morbidity and mortality, many countries have developed policies and interventions aimed at regulating the purchase and use of tobacco products aimed at decreasing tobacco use. Global efforts are being invested into lowering smoking rates and smoking dependency, creating tobacco-free environments and reducing the health effects imposed by active and secondhand smoking.

Smoking status in Israel and the problems associated with it reflect those of other developed countries. This chapter will describe the epidemiology of tobacco addiction in the world and particularly in Israel, from data to policy.

§ A short history

Tobacco, processed from the leaves of annual plants in the genus *Nicotiana*, mostly *Nicotiana tabacum*, grows natively in North and South America and belongs to the nightshade (*Solanaceae*) family, just like potato, pepper and tomato plants (1). In medieval times, the historian Oviedo documented the history of Native American Indians and claimed that the word "tobacco" originated from the name of a device employed by the pre-Columbian inhabitants of America for making use of the weed. The device – which was called *tabaco* – was a small tube in the shape of the letter Y. The stem was thrust into the smoke of the burning weed while the branches were put into the nostrils (2).

The tobacco plant, as we know it today, could be found in the Americas since about 6000 before the Common Era (BCE). Around 1 BCE, the Mayas – a highly cultured people in Central America – had begun using tobacco in sacred and religious ceremonies. The Mayan term for smoking was *sik'ar* (3). When the Europeans first arrived in the Americas in 1492, cultivation and use of tobacco for pleasure and medicinal purposes were common among the natives. Christopher Columbus brought a few tobacco leaves and seeds with him back to Europe. Most Europeans, however, did not get their first taste of tobacco until the mid-sixth century, when adventurers and diplomats like Jean Nicot de Villemain, the French ambassador to Portugal, began to popularize its use. Interestingly, the plant is dubbed *Nicotiana* in Jean Nicot's honor, and ninth century scientists borrowed his name to label the chemical known as nicotine. The major reason for its growing popularity in Europe was its presumed healing properties: people believed that tobacco could cure almost anything from bad breath to cancer.

In 1612, the first successful commercial crop was cultivated in Virginia (today a US state). Within seven years, it was the colony's largest export. In the next decades and centuries, the global tobacco industry grew enormously and became dominating and powerful (4).

Initially, tobacco was produced mainly for clay-pipe smoking, chewing and snuffing (sixth and seventh centuries). Cigars became popular around the early 1800s during the Napoleonic wars. Cigarettes, which existed in crude form since the early 1600s, did not become widely popular until the late nineteenth century, when introduction of patented, efficient cigarette-making machines enabled mass production of cigarettes. Consequently, production costs plummeted, and with the invention of the safety match a few decades later, cigarette smoking began its explosive growth. Cigarettes are the predominant type of smoking nowadays (4).

§ Tobacco use: prevalence and trends in the world

Almost one billion men in the world smoke – about 35% of men in developed countries and 50% of men in developing countries. About 250 million women in the world are daily smokers – respectively about 22% and 9% of women in developed and developing countries. In addition, many women in southern Asia chew tobacco. At the current rate, the number of smokers around the world will rise from approximately 1.3 billion today to 1.7 billion by 2025 (5).

Current smoking rates in developed countries in 2005 were around 20 to 25% – 24% in the UK (25%, in men; 23%, in women) (6); 23%, in Australia (26%, in men; 20%, in women) (7); 22%, in Canada (25%, in men, 19%, in women) (8); and 21%, in the US (24% in men; 18%, in women) (9). In developing countries, the rates were much higher; for example, in China, almost two-thirds of the men smoke (10).

Data regarding smoking rates in Arab countries are scarcer. However, according to the WHO regional data, in 1998 to 2000, current smoking was reported by 35.0% and 1.6% of Egyptian men and women respectively. Corresponding rates in Morocco were 34.5% and 1.6%; in Syria, 50.6% and 9.9%; in Jordan, 48.0% and 10.0%; in Lebanon, 46.0% and 35.0%; and in Yemen, 77.0% and 29.0% (11).

Trends in both developed and developing countries show that men's smoking rates have now peaked and started to decline. However, this is an extremely slow trend over decades. In general, the educated man gives up the habit first, so that smoking is becoming a habit of poorer, less educated men. Cigarette smoking among women is declining in many developed countries, notably Australia, Canada, the UK and the US (5). For example, current smoking rates for the UK were 61% and 42% for men and women, respectively, in 1960; 55% and 44%, in 1970; 38% and 37%, in 1980; 31% and 29%, in 1990; 28% and 26%, in 1998; and 24% and 23%, in 2005 (5, 6). In the US, the corresponding rates were 52% and 34% for men and women, respectively in

1960; 44% and 32%, in 1970; 44% and 30%, in 1980; 38% and 23%, in 1990; 28% and 22%, in 1998; and 21% and 19%, in 2005 (5, 9). Current smoking trends for the years 1994 to 2004 in selected European countries are presented in table 1. However, this trend is not evident in all developed countries. In several southern, central and eastern European countries, cigarette smoking is either still increasing among women or has not shown any decline (5).

Table 1. Smoking prevalence rates (%) over time in European adults by gender. Years 1994–1998, 1999–2001 and 2002–2005

Country	Men			Women			Total		
	1994–1998	*1999–2001*	*2002–2005*	*1994–1998*	*1999–2001*	*2002–2005*	*1994–1998*	*1999–2001*	*2002–2005*
Croatia	34	34	34	32	27	22	33	30	27
Denmark	39	32	28	35	29	23	37	30	25
France	35	33	30	21	21	21	28	27	25
Germany	43	39	37	30	31	30	37	35	34
Greece	46	47		28	29		37	38	
Hungary	46	41	40	28	26	28	37	33	34
Israel	33	30	32	25	24	18	29	27	18
Italy	33	32	31	17	17	17	25	24	24
Netherlands	38	39	31	31	30	25	35	34	28
Norway	33	29	27	32	30	25	33	30	26
Poland	44	42	38	24	23	26	34	32	32
Slovenia	33	28		20	20		26	24	28
Sweden	17	18	14	21	20	19	19	19	16
UK	29	29	28	28	25	24	28	27	26

World Health Organization, Regional Office for Europe, The European Report on Tobacco and Control Policy, Copenhagen: 2001

A conceptual framework was developed linking four stages of the cigarette epidemic as a continuum. The power of this model is that it allows virtually all communities to place themselves in relation to the larger pandemic. In stage one, less than 20% of men smoke, and minimal smoking in women is measured. Stage two is characterized by increases in smoking prevalence rate of men to above 50% and a small increase in smoking in women. In these communities and societies, it is not socially acceptable for women to smoke. Stage three is characterized by a marked downturn in smoking prevalence rates among men and a more gradual decline in women. In stage four, there is a further decline in both women and men. The US, UK and Canada are in stage four, whereas China and Japan, for example, are in stage two (12).

Exposure to secondhand smoke is high; many millions of Americans, both children and adults, are still exposed to secondhand smoke in their homes and workplaces despite substantial progress in tobacco control (13). This reflects, in fact, the situation all around the world. Tobacco claims 4.9 million lives a year, and if the present consumption patterns continue, the number of deaths will increase by 2020 to 10 million, 70% of which will occur in developing countries (5).

꩜ Tobacco use: prevalence and trends in Israel

Adult smoking

The Ministry of Health collects periodical data on smoking trends based on self-reported data. The survey participants, usually a representative sample of the Israeli population, are interviewed (face to face or by telephone) and asked (among other questions) about their smoking habits. Based on the results of the Knowledge, Attitudes and Practices National Health Survey which was carried out in 2004 and 2005 on a sample of approximately 3000 Israelis aged 21 and over, the smoking prevalence in the Israeli adult population was estimated at 25.5%. The highest smoking rate was reported in Arab men (41.2%), followed by Jewish men (30.3%); Jewish women (21.3%); and Arab women (8.3%). In numbers, these rates translate into a total of 1,179,400 smokers (14). (figure 1).

Figure 1. Smoking rates (%) in Israel by gender and population group (14)

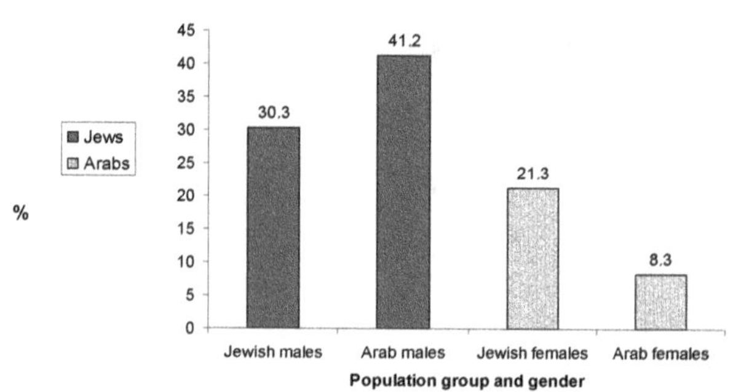

Figure 2a. Smoking rates (%) by population group and age group – men (14)

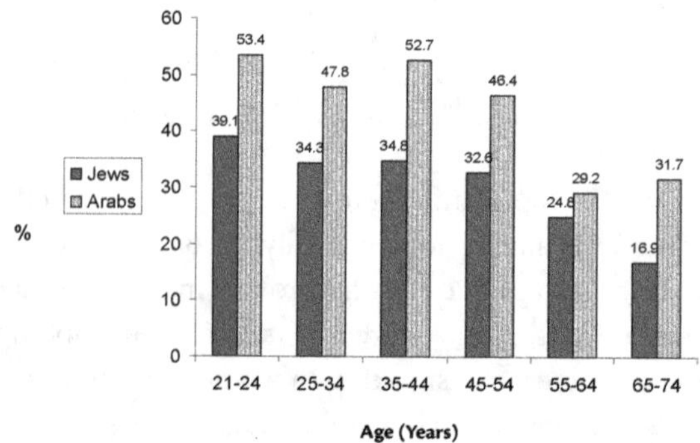

Figure 2b. Smoking rates (%) by population group and age group – women (14)

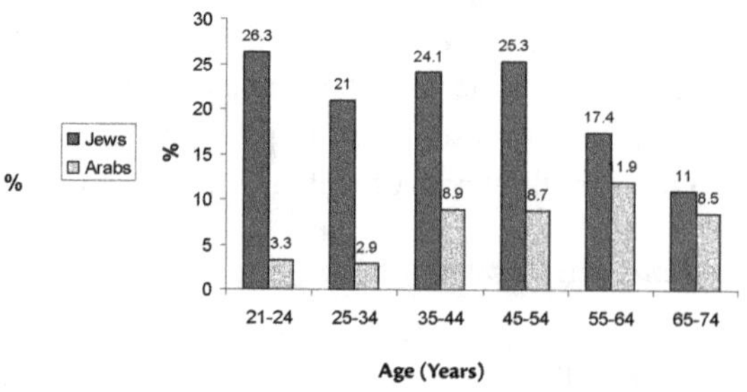

Smoking rates are age-dependent and found to be higher in the younger age groups (21 to 54 years old) in Jewish and Arab men as well as in Jewish women. In Arab women, however, smoking rates were generally very low, but higher in the older age groups. The distribution of smokers by gender, population group and age group is presented in figures 2a and 2b.

A pooled analysis was conducted on smoking data gathered from three national health surveys conducted between 1999 and 2001. The results indicated that smoking prevalence was associated with population group, gender, education attained and level of religiosity (tables 2 and 3). Marital status was associated with smoking prevalence only in women: single, separated or divorced women smoked significantly more than married women. In logistic regression models, higher smoking prevalence in men was significantly associated with population group (Arabs); immigration status in Jews (immigrants from the former Soviet Union [FSU]); age (younger); level of religiosity (being secular or traditional); and education (lower).

Table 2. Rates (%) of current Jewish smokers, immigrant smokers1 and Arab smokers by gender and education level (15)

Smokers	Education level	%	n	Sig.
Jews, nonimmigrants				
Men	Nonacademic	34.6	1,087	
	Academic	23.9	282	< .0001
Women	Nonacademic	26.1	960	
	Academic	19.9	266	< .0001
Jews, immigrants[1]				
Men	Nonacademic	42.4	128	
	Academic	28.9	90	.002
Women	Nonacademic	17.6	74	
	Academic	18.6	83	.350
Arabs				
Men	Nonacademic	51.5	343	
	Academic	41.0	75	.011
Women	Nonacademic	8.9	76	
	Academic	3.0	3	.110

[1] *Immigrating to Israel after 1989 from the former Soviet Union*

Table 3. Rates (%) of current Jewish smokers, immigrant smokers and Arab smokers by gender and degree of religious observance (15)

Smokers	Religious observance	%	n	Sig.
Jews, nonimmigrants				
Men	Secular/traditional	33.4	1252	
	Orthodox	21.8	133	< .0001
Women	Secular/traditional	27.9	1180	
	Orthodox	6.6	56	< .0001
Jews, immigrants[1]				
Men	Secular/traditional	36.2	217	
	Orthodox	11.7	2	.110
Women	Secular/traditional	18.6	154	
	Orthodox	8.1	3	.260
Arabs				
Men	Secular/traditional	51.6	313	
	Orthodox	42.8	89	.033
Women	Secular/traditional	7.4	35	
	Orthodox	7.6	34	.860

[1] *Immigrating to Israel after 1989 from the former Soviet Union*
Sig.: Statistical significance

In women, factors significantly associated with higher smoking prevalence were slightly different and included population group (Jews); immigration status in Jews (*not* being an immigrant from the FSU); age (younger); level of religiosity (being secular or traditional); and education (lower). The authors concluded that several specific high-risk groups for smoking may be thus identified, such as younger people, less educated men, Arab and immigrant men, as well as single, secular, less educated Jewish women (15). Lifestyle habits were also found to be associated with smoking prevalence; higher smoking rates were reported for those being engaged with physical activity at low compared to high frequency (odds ratio (OR)=1.3, 95% (confidence interval) CI 1.2–1.5); for those reporting ever compared to never alcohol consumption (OR=1.6, 95% CI 1.4–1.8, for Jews; OR=1.6, 95% CI 1.1–2.3, for Arabs) and for those reporting being stressed all or most of the time as compared to feeling stressed less often (OR=1.7, 95% 1.4–2.0, for Jews) (14).

℘ Adolescent smoking

Data on smoking in Israeli adolescents are derived from periodical epidemiologic surveys. One of the most important sources is the ongoing multinational project of the WHO, the Health Behavior in School-Aged Children (HBSC), of which Israel has been a member since 1994. This information source provides valuable data on smoking, alcohol consumption and violence in school-aged children (sixth, eighth and tenth graders) and enables the assessment of trends.

Results of the HBSC survey carried out in 2006 on a representative sample of 6,613 Jewish and Arab sixth, eighth and tenth graders indicated that 28.6% and 17.2% of the participating boys and girls, respectively, reported having ever smoked at least one cigarette. As for more regular smoking, a total of 5.8% of Israeli adolescents have smoked at least one cigarette per week (Jewish men, 6.8%; Arab men, 12.6%; Jewish women, 4.1%; and Arab women, 2.6%). Weekly smoking was most frequent among older adolescents and highest for Arabs in the tenth grade males (47.0%) (figure 3).

Figure 3. At least one-time incidence of smoking (%) in adolescents
by population group, gender and school grade (16)

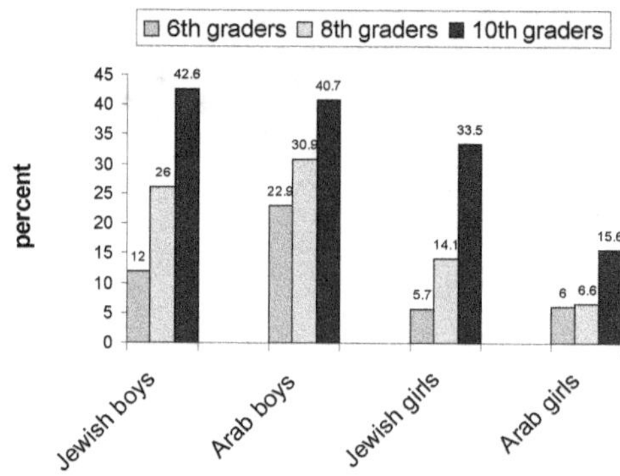

Daily smoking of at least one cigarette was reported by 3.6% in total – Jewish boys, 4.3%; Arab boys, 7.0%; Jewish girls, 2.8%; and 1.3% in Arab girls (16). Adolescent smoking was associated with parental and sibling smoking. Smoking prevalence rates were 75% and 83% for adolescents reporting paternal and maternal smoking, respectively, and 2.9-fold higher when sibling smoking was reported, as compared to adolescents reporting no parental or sibling smoking (14). When compared to adolescents in other member countries of the HBSC international survey, Israeli adolescents smoking rates seem to be among the lowest reported (figure 4) (14).

Figure 4. Smoking rates (%) by gender among 15-year-olds in selected countries (14)
Smoking at least one cigarette per week

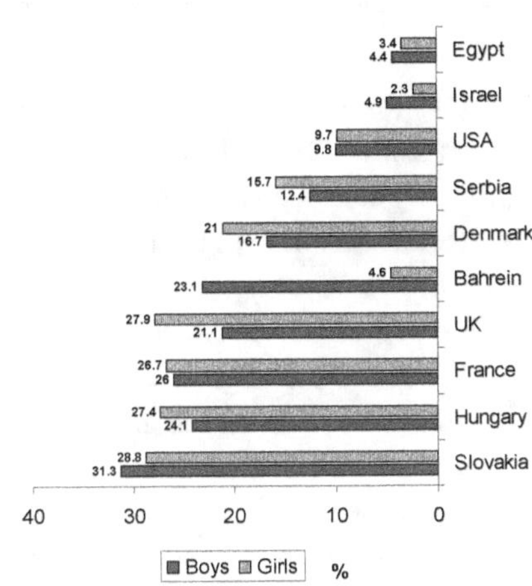

Smoking rates of Israeli adolescents, according to the HBSC survey, are validated by other national surveys. In reply to the survey question: "Do you smoke cigarettes?" 3.6% of 10, 942 eighth graders (13 to 14 years old) in Israel, interviewed in 2003 to 2004 through a self-administered questionnaire in the National Survey on Asthma Prevalence, said that they do. Smoking was more prevalent in boys as opposed to girls (4.9% and 2.3%, respectively) and more frequent in Jewish adolescents (3.6%) compared to Arab adolescents (3.1%). Among Jews, the highest and the lowest smoking rates were reported for participants of FSU and American origin, 4.1% and 2.4%, respectively. Among Arabs, the highest and the lowest smoking rates were reported for Bedouins (5.6%) and for Druze (.7%), respectively (14). Smoking rates among 18-year-old Israel Defense Force (IDF) enlistees in 2006 were 41.6%, for men and 28.9%, for women (14).

ẞ Smoking trends

Smoking trends in Israel for the period 1980 to 2004 indicate a mild decrease. Smoking rates in 1980 and 2004 were 45% and 30.3%, respectively, among Jewish men; 30.0% and 21.3%, respectively, in Jewish women; and 50.0% and 41.2%, respectively, in Arab men. In Arab women, smoking rates in 1996 and 2004 were 12.0% and 8.0% respectively (14) (figure 5).

Figure 5. Trends in smoking rates (%) among 18 years of age and older in
Israel by gender and population group. Years 1980–2004 (14)

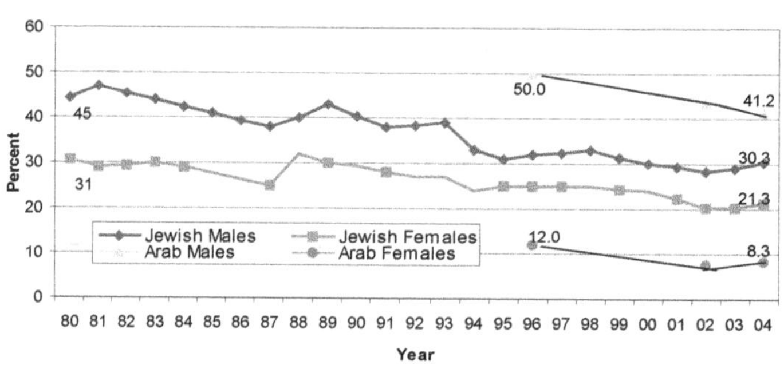

Regarding adolescents, smoking rates (at least one cigarette per week) seem to have declined
between 1998 and 2006 for Jewish (12.4% and 6.8%, respectively) and Arab (17.1% and 12.6%,
respectively) boys. For Jewish girls, the rates decreased only since 2004 (6.9% in 2004 and 4.1%
in 2006). For Arab girls, the rates declined from 1998 to 2004 (5.6% and 2.0%, respectively) and
have remained stable ever since (16).

Despite the decline in smoking prevalence in Israel since 1980, the number of cigarettes
consumed annually has continued to rise. Total cigarette consumption grew from 6.0 billion
cigarettes in 1980 to 8.1 billion in 2002 (10). The overall growth in cigarette consumption can
be explained largely by a population increase in each of these decades. Another factor that may
contribute to this increase is an average rise in the daily smoking rate by Israelis who continued
to smoke regularly (17). Of the current smokers in 2003, 62.7% among Jewish men, 67.1%, among
Arab men, 49.0% among Jewish women and 20.5% among Arab women reported consuming
more than 10 cigarettes daily. Smoking more than 20 cigarettes per day was reported by 19.6%,
30.3%, 14.3%, and 8.9% of the Jewish men, Arab men, Jewish women and Arab women who
were current smokers respectively (18).

§ Physical effects of tobacco use and related morbidity, mortality and costs

Tobacco smoke contains more than 4000 chemicals. At least 400 are known to be hazardous
to health, and more than 50 cause cancer. This is why smoking harms nearly every organ of the
body, causing many diseases and affecting the general health of anyone inhaling smoke, either
actively or passively.

A cautionary word regarding the potential adverse health effects of tobacco use was published as early as 1586 in Germany, calling the tobacco plant a "violent herb" (4). Sixteen years
later an anonymous British physician published a document called *Worke of Chimny Sweepers* [sic] (also referenced as *Chimny-Sweepers* or *A Warning for Tobacconists* [sic]). The author
stated that illness of chimney sweepers is caused by soot and that tobacco may have similar effects and discussed many of the health risks related to tobacco use – which were later proven
to be correct (19). However, the first edition of the medical *Merck Manual*, published in 1899,
recommended smoking tobacco for the treatment of bronchitis and asthma (4).

Several epidemiological studies conducted in the first half of the twentieth century suggested an association between tobacco use and lung cancer (20) as well as cardiovascular disease
(21). The publication in 1950 of three important epidemiological studies that provided powerful

links between smoking and lung cancer (22–24) was, in fact, an important cornerstone in this regard. In 1964, the first *US Surgeon General's Report on Smoking and Health* was issued. It received widespread media and public attention which, together with the former publications, have initiated and promoted extensive comparative and controlled research into smoking health effects and outcomes, and this continues today.

In 1981, Doll and Peto (25) published a comprehensive quantitative analysis on the avoidable causes of cancer in the US. According to their review, smoking was responsible for around 35% of total cancer mortality globally (25). These estimates are correct today as well. The *US Surgeon General's Report*, 2004 (26) included a comprehensive list of diseases and adverse health effects for which smoking is identified as a cause, based on the scientific data available.

The report stated that the evidence is sufficient to infer a causal relationship between active smoking and cancer of the lung, oral cavity and pharynx, larynx, esophagus, stomach, pancreas, bladder, renal cell carcinoma and renal pelvis cancer, cervical cancer and leukemia. It also indicated that the evidence is sufficient to infer a causal relationship between active smoking and cardiovascular diseases such as coronary heart disease, cerebrovascular disease, atherosclerosis and abdominal aortic aneurysm.

Regarding respiratory diseases, the report claimed that the evidence is sufficient to infer a causal relationship between active smoking and chronic obstructive pulmonary disease, acute respiratory infections including pneumonia, premature onset of and an accelerated age-related decline in lung function, asthma-like symptoms and poor asthma control.

Smoking-related respiratory effects are also seen in-utero and include reduction in the lung function of fetuses of smoking mothers. In childhood, adolescence and early adulthood, smoking-related respiratory effects include impaired lung growth, respiratory symptoms (such as coughing, phlegm, wheezing, dyspnea and asthma-related symptoms) and early onset of lung function decline.

According to the report, evidence is sufficient to infer a causal relationship between active smoking and reproductive effects, such as reduced fertility in women, pregnancy complications (placenta previa, placental abruption, premature rupture of the membranes, preterm delivery and shortened gestation), fetal growth restriction and low birth weight, and sudden infant death syndrome (SIDS). Other smoking-related health effects that were listed in the report included (among others) low bone density, hip fractures and nuclear cataracts, as well as increased absenteeism from work and increased use of medical care services (26).

With time, data accumulated on the serious and deadly health effects of involuntary exposure to tobacco smoke (secondhand smoking) in healthy nonsmokers. More than 50 carcinogens have been identified in sidestream and secondhand smoke. The *US Surgeon-General's Report*, 2006 (13) summarized the accumulated evidence. According to this report, secondhand smoke causes premature death and disease in nonsmoking children and adults. Children exposed to secondhand smoke are at increased risk for sudden infant death syndrome (SIDS), acute respiratory infections, ear problems and more severe asthma. Smoking by parents causes respiratory symptoms and slows lung growth in their children. Exposure of adults to secondhand smoke has immediate adverse effects on the cardiovascular system and causes coronary heart disease and lung cancer. The scientific evidence indicates that there is no risk-free level of exposure to secondhand smoke (13).

Smoking-related mortality is a major concern throughout the world. In the US, cigarette smoking is the single most preventable cause of premature death. Each year, more than 400,000 Americans die from cigarette smoking, and approximately 38,000 die from secondhand smoke exposure. In fact, one in every five deaths in the US is smoking related –and more deaths are caused each year by tobacco use than by all deaths from human immunodeficiency virus (HIV), illegal drug use, alcohol use, motor vehicle injuries, suicides and murders combined. On average, adults who smoke cigarettes die 14 years earlier than nonsmokers.

Premature deaths from smoking annually rob more than five million years from the potential lifespan of those who die in the US (9). Similar statistics are reported from the United Kingdom, where in 1997, cigarette smoking accounted for an estimated 117,400 of the total of 628,000 deaths in that country. Cigarette smoking was thus responsible for approximately one in every five deaths (27). In a cohort of male British doctors that was followed up for 50 years, smoking was associated with excess mortality that chiefly involved vascular, neoplastic and respiratory diseases. Men born between 1900 and 1930 who smoked cigarettes and continued to smoke died on average about 10 years younger than lifelong nonsmokers. The cigarette smoker vs. nonsmoker probabilities of dying in middle age (35 to 69 years) were 42% vs. 24% (a twofold death rate ratio) for those born between 1900 and 1909, and 43% vs. 15% (a threefold death rate ratio) for those born in the 1920s (28).

The morbidity and mortality associated with smoking result in a considerable economical burden. It is estimated that cigarette smoking is responsible for $167 billion in annual health-related economic losses in the US ($75 billion in direct medical costs and $92 billion in lost productivity) – or about $3561 per adult smoker. The total economic burden of cigarette smoking is estimated at $7.18 per pack of cigarettes sold in the US in the years 1997 to 2001. Furthermore, cigarette smoking annually results in 5.5 million years of potential life lost in that country (29).

In the UK, the West Midlands Public Health Steering Group (WMPHSG) commissioned a study to model the economic costs of smoking on the regional economy. The report found that the total cost of treating smokers and the effects of premature death, ill health and loss of productivity amounted to more than £1.25 billion in 2001 alone (30). In 1997, cigarette smoking in the UK was estimated to account for the loss of 205,000 years of life under age 65 and 551,000 years of life under 75, based on the distribution of deaths from smoking by age and mortality risks in neversmokers (27). In Canada, smoking-attributable healthcare costs were Can$ 2.5 billion in 1991 (31).

In view of the smoking rates and trends and the lack of accurate data on costs of cancer-associated mortality and morbidity, similar impact is expected to be found in Israel as well.

§ Tobacco addiction

An important aspect of tobacco use is the physical dependence associated with it. "Addiction" and "dependence" are terms whose definition has a social as well as a scientific dimension. In principle, they may be distinguished, but in practice such a distinction serves little purpose and the terms are used interchangeably. The terms refer to a situation in which a drug or stimulus has unreasonably come to control behavior. This definition is very different from that used in the past and to which the general public mostly subscribe.

The earlier and popular view is that addiction refers to a state in which an individual needs to continue to take a drug in order to stave off unpleasant or dangerous physical withdrawal effects. The main shortcoming of this approach to defining addiction is that it addresses just one aspect of a wider problem. For example, individuals given morphine for pain relief may experience withdrawal symptoms when it is withdrawn but do not become compulsive users, yet individuals attempting to stop using drugs – including nicotine – continue to relapse at a high rate long after withdrawal symptoms have resolved. Moreover, controlling withdrawal symptoms alone is not necessarily sufficient to prevent relapse to drug use.

Another outmoded feature of the definition of addiction is inclusion of the concept of intoxication. Under this view, addictive drugs lead to changes in users' psychological state, leaving some degree of impairment. This feature no longer appears in any official definition of "addiction" or "dependence" because it clearly is neither a necessary nor a sufficient condition for compulsive, harmful drug seeking. Many cannabis and alcohol users become intoxicated but do not develop dependence, while cocaine and amphetamine use can be compulsive without a noticeable impairment of the performance (32).

Nicotine metabolism

Cigarette smoke is composed of volatile and particulate phases. Some 500 gaseous compounds including nitrogen, carbon monoxide (CO), carbon dioxide, ammonia, hydrogen cyanide and benzene have been identified in the volatile phase, which accounts for about 95% of the weight of cigarette smoke; the other 5% is accounted for by particulates which contain about 3500 different compounds, of them the major one is the alkaloid nicotine (32).

The particulate matter without its alkaloid and water content is called tar. While smoking, small droplets of tar containing nicotine are inhaled and deposited in the small airways and alveoli. The nicotine is rapidly absorbed into the pulmonary alveolar capillary and venous circulation and hence directly into systemic arterial blood. It takes about 10 to 19 seconds for nicotine to reach the brain. In those who typically do not inhale the smoke –such as cigar and pipe smokers and smokeless tobacco users – nicotine is absorbed through the mucosal membranes of the upper airways and reaches peak blood levels and the brain more slowly (33).

Following cigarette smoking, the arterial blood perfusing the brain contains levels of nicotine that exceed venous levels by a factor of two- to six-fold (32). Nicotine levels in the plasma as well as the brain decline rapidly as a result of distribution to peripheral tissues and of excretion and elimination. When smokers smoke multiple cigarettes during the day, there are oscillations between peak and trough plasma nicotine levels. However, because of its half-life of two hours, nicotine accumulates over six to eight hours, reaching levels in the plasma typically ranging from 20 to 40 mg/ml, which then fall progressively during the night when the person does not smoke (32). The rapid absorption of nicotine from cigarette smoking and the high arterial levels that reach the brain as a result, allow for rapid behavioral reinforcement from smoking. Falling nicotine levels in-between smoking of individual cigarettes allow time for the brain nicotinic receptors to become somewhat re-sensitized after each cigarette. While tolerance to the toxic effects of nicotine such as nausea rapidly develops and persists, the reinforcing effects of nicotine are renewed with each cigarette. Thus, the typically noxious pharmacological experience of the novice smoker becomes an addictive pharmacological experience for the experienced smoker.

Possible mechanisms of nicotine addiction and dependence

Most smokers use tobacco regularly because they are addicted to nicotine. Studies of the mechanisms underlying the positive reinforcing properties of addictive drugs have been significantly influenced by experiments with psycho-stimulant drugs such as amphetamine and cocaine. These compounds have been shown to act as locomotor stimulants and reinforce self admin-istration in experimental animals, due to their ability to enhance neurotransmission at dopa-mine synapses in the mesolimbic system of the brain. The fact that lesions of the mesolimbic pathway cause a marked attenuation of these drugs' locomotor stimulant properties – and their ability to serve as a reinforcer in a self-administration paradigm – support this mechanism (32).

The locomotor stimulant properties of nicotine and its ability to act as a reward in a self-administration paradigm also seem to depend upon the ability of nicotine to stimulate the dopamine-secreting neurons in the nucleus accumbens in the mesolimbic system. Indeed, the fact that mesolimbic dopamine neurons express nicotinic receptors is well established (32). These data are almost entirely derived from studies with animal models (34, 35). However, there is circumstantial evidence that suggests that this mechanism is also valid in humans. The ad-ministration of a drug called haloperidol, which blocks the dopamine receptors in the brain, increases smoking in habitual smokers. If nicotine reward depends upon increased dopamine release in the brain, this is the anticipated response, since it reflects an attempt to overcome the blockade produced by the antagonist, haloperidol (32). In another human study, smokers were shown to have a significantly greater dopamine activity in the basal ganglia as compared to nonsmokers (36).

The influence of nicotine on the brain is not limited to dopaminergic pathways. Many neu-rons in the brain express the neuronal nicotinic receptors and, as a result, the drug stimulates other pathways which may be important to the development of addiction. These pathways in-clude noradrenalin-secreting neurons, acetylcholine-secreting neurons and terminals that se-crete the excitatory amino acid, glutamic acid and the inhibitory amino acid, g-aminobutyric acid (32, 37).

Tobacco smoking habits are heterogeneous, and people smoke cigarettes at varying fre-quencies and in different ways. The plasma nicotine concentration is likely to remain fairly stable throughout the day for people who smoke frequently, whereas for those who smoke less frequently, significant peaks and troughs of nicotine may be observed. For the non-frequent smokers, the trough experienced may be sufficient to avoid nicotinic receptor desensitization, and thus each cigarette is "rewarded" with increased dopamine release. The recurrent stimulation of dopamine release in this group is probably the predominant mechanism underlying addiction to nicotine. In contrast, in frequent or heavy smokers who experience desensitization of dopa-mine release, the addiction mechanism may be different; for example, the nicotinic receptors located in noradrenalin-secreting neurons may also be desensitized by nicotine concentrations similar to those found in the plasma of many smokers. This may contribute to the "tranquilliz-ing" properties of tobacco smoke often reported by smokers exposed to environmental stressors and promote tobacco addiction (32). Since nicotine exerts its effects in the brain by acting as a family of nicotine receptors, it is possible that other neural responses – mediated by recep-tors more resistant to desensitization – may also play an important role in nicotine addiction.

Nicotine's psychoactive impact may be enhanced by other ingredients in tobacco smoke; currently, more than 600 additives can legally be added to tobacco products to enrich flavor and improve taste. These include coffee extract, sugar, vanilla, cocoa, menthol, oil from clove stems, caramel, chlorophyll, ammonia compounds and many more. Some of these additives, however, may also have more sinister effects. For example, cocoa, when burned in a cigarette, produces bromine gas that dilates the airways of the lung and increases the body's ability to absorb nicotine. Menthol is also suspected of enabling the smoker to inhale more easily by numbing the throat. Other additives may manipulate the delivery of nicotine; the addition of ammonia compounds, for example, speed the delivery of nicotine to smokers by raising the alkalinity of tobacco smoke, which enhances its absorption in the airways. Addition of acetaldehyde and pyridine strengthen nicotine's impact on the brain and central nervous system (38).

The chemical dependency of the brain on nicotine is not the only aspect of tobacco dependence; other physiological aspects include a general slowdown of body functions' regulation due to the noradrenergic influence of nicotine, accompanied by a decrease in sugar, blood pressure and body temperature levels. Additionally, the strong alkaline properties of nicotine affect the body homeostasis, thus tobacco withdrawal shifts the body's pH into a more acidic one and necessitates adjustments.

Furthermore, behavioral responses are an important component as well. Most smokers respond to certain social conditioning and smoke automatically at certain circumstances, such as after a meal, during coffee drinking, while waiting or watching the television and so on. Individual beliefs regarding smoking may also play a role in developing psychological tobacco dependence. Many smokers strongly believe that smoking facilitates their ability to cope with anxiety, stress, boredom, loneliness and frustration (39). In fact, tobacco dependence can be summarized as a complex brain-body-behavior-belief interaction.

Nicotine withdrawal signs and symptoms

Tolerance and withdrawal symptoms are two important features of nicotine addiction. Tolerance is the reduction in drug response that occurs after chronic exposure. Withdrawal symptoms are the adverse side effects that occur after chronic drug exposure ends. The development of nicotine tolerance forces smokers to increase their nicotine intake to compensate for the reduced chemical and psychological effects of the drug. It also contributes to habitual smoking by reducing the adverse physiological effects of nicotine. Nicotine withdrawal symptoms include anxiety, irritability, craving, sleep disturbances, cognitive and attention deficits and increased appetite, which may be attributable to either compensating for the bodily pH fluctuations or for the behavioral and psychological needs associated with tobacco addiction.

These symptoms may begin within a few hours after the last cigarette, quickly driving people back to tobacco use. Symptoms peak within the first few days of smoking cessation and may subside within a few weeks. For some people, however, symptoms may persist for months. While withdrawal is related to the pharmacological effects of nicotine, many behavioral factors can also affect the severity of withdrawal symptoms (33). A recent study examined the extent to which the habitual abstinence of Orthodox Jews during the Sabbath is associated with craving to smoke and with other reactions to smoking abstinence. Twenty heavy smokers in the Orthodox Jewish community were assessed on a workday when smoking as usual, on a Sabbath when not smoking and on a forced abstinence workday. Craving, irritability and other commonly reported smoking withdrawal symptoms were assessed retrospectively. The results indicated that craving to smoke and – to a lesser extent – irritability was lower during the Sabbath than during the two other test days. Self-reported difficulty in abstaining was also lower on the Sabbath than on the workday. Craving in the evening preceding the test day was always significantly higher than in the next morning, despite the overnight abstinence before the morning assessment. The authors concluded that craving to smoke is determined to a large extent by smoking-related habits, cues and expectations – and not solely by biological factors (40).

Factors associated with nicotine addiction and dependence
Addiction to tobacco is individual; the question is what factors determine this effect. The considerable variation between people both in their plasma nicotine levels and intake of nicotine from a cigarette may serve as a partial explanation for varying levels of addiction:

(a) Ethnic differences in nicotine metabolism have recently been demonstrated. African-Americans have been shown in several studies to have higher levels of cotinine (a metabolite of nicotine), adjusted for cigarettes smoked per day. They were also shown to take in 20% more nicotine per cigarette, that is, an intake of 20% more tobacco smoke per cigarette. This may be related to the fact that the majority of African-Americans smoke mentholated cigarettes – whereas relatively few Caucasians smoke such cigarettes. Menthol cools the airways and might be associated with a greater volume or depth of inhalation. These factors – greater smoke intake per cigarette and slower nicotine metabolism – explain the higher cotinine levels per cigarette and possibly also the higher lung cancer risks (adjusted for cigarette consumption) in African-Americans compared to Caucasians. Genetic polymorphism, which may be associated with individual metabolism of nicotine, may be involved (32).
(b) Gender (women) may affect tobacco addiction as well. In women, menstrual-cycle variation and the associated changes in steroid hormones have been related to cigarette craving. Furthermore, there is also evidence that women have significantly higher rates of nicotine metabolism than men, particularly when using oral contraceptives (41), which may enhance tobacco addiction.
(c) Age (younger) may also be an important determinant in tobacco addiction. In animal studies, adolescent rats were found to be more susceptible to the reinforcing effects of nicotine than adult rats and to take more nicotine when it is available than do adult animals. Furthermore, adolescent rats may also be more sensitive to the reinforcing effects of nicotine in combination with other chemicals found in cigarettes, thus increasing susceptibility to tobacco addiction.

Acetaldehyde, a tobacco additive, increases nicotine's addictive properties in adolescent (but not adult) animals. In other words, adolescent animals performing a task to receive nicotine showed greater response rates to nicotine when combined with acetaldehyde (33). A recent study in humans reported that a young cigarette smoker (sixth grader) can begin to feel powerful craving for nicotine within two days of first inhaling. About half of children who become addicted report symptoms of dependence by the time they are smoking only seven cigarettes a month; the appearance of tobacco withdrawal symptoms and failed attempts at cessation sometimes preceded daily smoking (42).

(d) A sub-population at a special risk for tobacco addiction is the group of patients hospitalized in psychiatric wards. An Israeli study from 1993 reported a very high prevalence of smoking among both the staff (48.1%) and the patients (76.0%) of three psychiatric hospitals in the country. Apparently, nurses generously had used cigarettes in order to appease the patients and encouraged them to smoke (43). A more recent study from Switzerland indicated that smoking prevalence was still very high among psychiatric inpatients (72%) as opposed to 31% among the staff and that smoking habits were affected by the hospitalization itself: 74% of the heavy smokers decreased cigarette consumption while 80% of light and 57% of moderate smokers increased their consumption upon hospitalization. Compared to the staff, the psychiatric inpatients were also more nicotine dependent (44).

Patients diagnosed with schizophrenic and bipolar disorders may present a specific high risk group. A study from Scotland reported a smoking rate as high as 58% among patients diagnosed with schizophrenia, compared to 28% in healthy controls. Smoking volume was also significantly higher among those diagnosed with schizophrenia compared to healthy controls, but the age for starting to smoke was usually similar, and preceded the diagnosis of schizophrenia. The study indicated that the rate of smoking and level of nicotine addiction are greater in patients diagnosed with schizophrenia than in the general population (45). Similar results were reported from Turkey (46). Equally high rates of smoking were also reported for patients diagnosed with bipolar disorder. In an Israeli study, the prevalence rate in those patients was similar to that of patients diagnosed with schizophrenia (43% and 45% respectively) and higher than expected for the general population (27.5%) (47). Thus, schizophrenia, bipolar disorder and smoking may all be related to dopamine transmission and therefore dopaminergic interactions may provide an explanation for the results (47).

Attention-deficit hyperactivity disorder (ADHD) alone and combined with other psychopathology was also reported to be a risk factor for the development of substance use disorders in general and tobacco addiction in particular. It is estimated that approximately one-fifth of adults with substance use disorders have ADHD. Pharmaco-therapeutic treatment of ADHD in children reduces the risk for later cigarette smoking and substance use disorders in adulthood (48).

♠ From epidemiology to tobacco control programs worldwide

Millions of people throughout the world could be spared disease and early death if effective policies for tobacco control were widely adopted and well implemented. Since tobacco addiction is considered to be a brain-body-behavior-belief interaction and since it impacts the public as well as the smoking individual, strategies for tobacco control are targeting the biochemical aspect of the addiction, as well as the psychological, social and public ones. These strategies are often multidisciplinary and tailored to address specific high risk groups and individuals.

The Health Evidence Network (HEN) Synthesis Report on Tobacco Control was published in 2003 by the World Health Organization (WHO) Regional Office for Europe (49). It included a synthesis of the best available evidence, including a summary of the main findings and policy options related to tobacco control.

There are two main arms for tobacco control – community interventions aimed at lowering rates of smoking (which may be further divided into educational interventions and policy interventions) and individual smoking cessation interventions.

Policy interventions include (a) raising prices of tobacco products via tax increases; (b) smoking restrictions in work places and public spaces; and (c) bans on advertising and promotion. Educational intervention includes (d) consumer education, including multimedia and counter-advertising campaigns, widespread dissemination of tobacco-risk evidence and improved warning labels. Individual smoking cessation interventions include (e) nicotine replacement treatment (NRT) and other smoking-cessation therapies (49).

Interventions should be aimed at two distinct targets – first, to reduce smoking initiation that occurs mainly at adolescence, and second, to encourage smoking cessation among current smokers, which may be the key to averting consequent deaths and diseases. There is a general consensus that a combination of these strategies will yield the best overall results in slowing the tobacco epidemic. However, specific population groups may benefit from different combinations of tobacco control strategies. Therefore, tobacco control programs should be specifically tailored to defined population groups and adequately evaluated for their effectiveness, to enhance the use of the best practice strategy for each population group and for each target (49).

§ Community interventions aimed at lowering rates of smoking

Policy interventions

These strategies mostly address the public and the social aspect of smoking, and also target potential barriers such as lack of knowledge regarding the health impact of smoking:

(a) Raising prices on tobacco products. Price increases on tobacco products are one of the most productive and cost-effective means for reducing the demand for tobacco with very little administrative burden. A price increase of 10% is estimated to result in a decrease of 2.5% to 5% in cigarette consumption. Given the addictive nature of smoking, the response is expected to be more pronounced in the long run, when the influence of addiction is relatively more diffuse. There is a strong rationale for governments to intervene with tobacco tax increases. However, in order to be effective, the tax should constitute approximately 70% to 80% of the total price and should increase regularly to keep pace with inflation. Optimally, a portion of the tobacco tax revenues is consequently earmarked for publicly funded tobacco interventions.

Teenagers and young adults have been shown to be especially responsive to cigarette price increases. Likewise, adult women appear to be more sensitive to price increases than adult men, and the same is true for lower socioeconomic groups (as compared to higher socioeconomic groups) (49–51).

(b) Smoking restriction. Environmental restrictions on smoking appear to be effective in reducing both demand and consumption of tobacco, although it is difficult to quantify these benefits. Carefully planned restrictions on smoking in public areas, as components of a comprehensive strategy, were shown to be effective in reducing public smoking. As to restrictions at work settings, there is evidence that the prevalence of smoking is reduced by almost 4% at smoke-free workplaces and may yield reductions of up to 10% (49, 50).

(c) Bans on advertising and promotion of tobacco products. Advertising bans impose essential limits on the sophisticated and cunning strategies of the tobacco industry for encouraging adults and even children to use its products. Among countries that have instituted comprehensive advertising bans, there has been an associated 6.3% reduction in smoking per adult. In contrast, partial bans were found to have little or no effect on smoking, as the tobacco industry in these cases simply redirects marketing to other mediums. It is, however, difficult to achieve public and political support for a complete ban because the tobacco industry enlists the support and influence of other stakeholders like the media, sports industry and cultural activity planners – many of whom rely, in some cases heavily, on tobacco advertising revenue (49, 50).

Educational interventions

Consumer education. The available evidence for the effectiveness of various forms of consumers' education as a tobacco control suggests that this should be included as a component of a comprehensive program against tobacco. Mass media campaigns can raise awareness and change attitudes about the risks of using tobacco and the benefits of quitting. There is evidence that multimedia campaigns can actually prevent young people from starting to smoke (primary prevention) and increase smoking cessation among youth and adults who are current smokers when combined with other interventions.

"Information shocks" – for example, widespread dissemination of research findings showing the harmful effects of tobacco use on health – are particularly effective among populations in which knowledge of the health consequences of tobacco use is low. Warning labels on tobacco products should be as effective as possible; to increase the potential for effectiveness, it has been recommended that warning labels be prominent, placed on the largest surfaces (front and back) of the packages and be very distinct graphically from the rest of the package design (49, 50).

However, raising the knowledge and the awareness of the population in itself is not enough to promote a behavior change, and such an intervention should be implemented together with other strategies. A good example for that is the classical health education programs used in the school system, which were shown to be effective in regard to smoking reduction only when implemented as a comprehensive approach, together with other strategies such as cigarette taxing, media educational programs and environmental restrictions on smoking (49, 50).

⑨ Individual smoking-cessation interventions

These strategies mostly address the biological and psychological aspects of smoking.

Nicotine replacement and other therapies

Nicotine replacement treatment (NRT) includes nicotine-containing preparations such as nicotine gum, nicotine skin patches, nicotine nasal spray and nicotine inhaler. The rational for using NRT is to relieve nicotine withdrawal symptoms and urges to smoke while not exposing the user to the carbon monoxide, tar and carcinogens in cigarette smoke. Another medication which is used in this context is bupropion, a non-nicotine anti-depressant that reduces the withdrawal symptoms associated with smoking quitting. Bupropion appears to act on pathways in the brain that are involved in nicotine addiction (48, 51). The characteristics of the currently available NRT are summarized in table 4 (49).

Table 4. FDA-approved smoking-cessation medications (49)

Name	Form	Dosage	Length of use	Precautions/ contraindications	Side effects
Nicotine gum	Nicorette[2] Nicorette DS[2] Nicorette Mint[2] Nicorette Orange[2]	Up to 24 pieces/ day; <25 cigs/day = 2 mg; ≥25 cigs/day = 4 mg	Up to 12 wks		Sore mouth, dyspepsia
Nicotine inhaler	Nicotrol inhaler[1]	6–16 cartridges/day	Up to 6 mo		Mouth/throat irritation
Nicotine nasal spray	Nicotrol NS[1]	8–40 doses/day	3–6 mo	Dependency	Nasal irritation
Nicotine skin patch	Nicoderm CQ[2] generic/house brand Patches[1,2] Nicotrol[2]	21 mg/24 h; 14 mg/24 h; 7 mg/24 h; 15 mg/16 h	4 wks; then 2 wks; then 2 wks 8 wks		Local skin reaction
Bupropion, sustained-release	Zyban[1]	150 mg in morning for 3 days, then 150 mg twice a day	Begin 1–2 wks before quit date, then 7–12 wks	Seizure, eating disorder	Insomnia, dry mouth

1 *Prescription only*
2 *Over the counter (OTC) only*

Physician advice to patients to quit smoking has been demonstrated to have a significant effect on reducing smoking. NRT has been shown to double the chances of successfully quitting smoking when used in conjunction with physician advice (49). In fact, nicotine replacement treatment prescribed after general practitioners' brief advice against smoking can result in up to 10% of smokers stopping, but NRT together with support from specialist counselors can result in up to 20% of smokers quitting. NRT is generally well tolerated, and most side effects arise from the irritant effect of nicotine (such as rashes with nicotine patches).

Regarding bupropion, experience from many years of use in the US indicates that in the dose used for smoking cessation, it causes seizures in about one in 1000 users, and figures from initial use in the UK are consistent with this. The most common side effects, however, are relatively minor; insomnia and dry mouth are the commonest. Data suggest that non-nicotine pharmacotherapy such as bupropion has equivalent efficacy for women and men (41). It is important, though, to individually adapt the right cessation approach, since nicotine replacement therapy and bupropion are suitable only for heavier smokers (10 to 15 cigarettes a day or more) who clearly want to stop and are ready to try. Indiscriminate prescribing to unselected smokers is unlikely to be effective (53). NRT effectiveness does not appear to decrease when they are available over the counter. These therapies seem to be cost-effective compared to other common medical interventions for secondary prevention, such as drug therapies for hypertension and high blood cholesterol (49).

Individual and group counseling

There is evidence that individual counseling by a cessation specialist as well as group therapy programs are effective in helping smokers quit. However, the effectiveness of hypnotherapy, aversive smoking therapy and acupuncture in smoking cessation could not be demonstrated (49).

Barriers to smoking cessation

Although most smokers identify tobacco use as harmful and express a desire to reduce or stop using it, only about 6% of smokers who try to quit are successful for more than a month (33). Many barriers exist to the ability to quit smoking; two-thirds (67%) of current smokers in Minnesota, US, listed physical cravings or feelings of withdrawal as a barrier – more than any other reason. Many smokers also identified social and psychological barriers, including losing a way to handle stress in their lives (55%), risk of gaining weight (32%), and concern about interference with social or work relationships (19%). Finally, some smokers expressed concern over the cost of medications or products (30%) and classes or other programs (23%) to help them quit. Many respondents identified multiple reasons – physiological, social, psychological and economic – as barriers to quitting smoking (54).

Some groups experience certain barriers more frequently. Barriers to smoking cessation that are unique to women include concerns about weight gain and negative emotional reactions following cessation (41). Indeed, a far greater percentage of women (48%) than men (17%) cited the risk of gaining weight, and a greater percentage of women (22%) than men (16%) identified the possible risk of interference with social or work relationships as a barrier to quitting (54). In this regard, behavioral treatments that focus on post-cessation weight reduction and negative mood management may be particularly beneficial for women (41). Concern about the loss of cigarettes as a way to handle stress was listed as a barrier by 65% of women and 46% of men (54). Furthermore, outcomes may be poorer for women than for men treated with nicotine replacement therapies, possibly because women experience more severe withdrawal symptoms, report poorer compliance with NRT and exhibit greater sensitivity to non-nicotine factors – such as the sight, smell, and sensations of smoking – compared with men. Recent data suggest that timing in the menstrual cycle may influence quitting success in women (41).

Patients diagnosed with schizophrenic and bipolar disorders were also more likely to report barriers to smoking cessation; stress reduction, stimulation and addiction were frequently cited as reasons for smoking, compared to a general sample of smokers. Men and participants with concurrent hazardous substance use cited fewer reasons for quitting smoking (55).

From epidemiology to tobacco control programs in Israel

As mentioned earlier in the comprehensive framework for smoking cessation, there are five main approaches for tobacco control. All types of interventions have been adopted and used in Israel. The main activities conducted in each of these areas are listed herewith.

Community interventions aimed at lowering rates of smoking

Policy interventions

(a) Raising prices on tobacco products. There has been a 70% tax on cigarettes price in Israel since 1991. This level of taxation has not been changed since then, even though the health system has demanded an increase in cigarette price taxation.

(b) Smoking restriction. In 1983, Israel enacted a law banning smoking in public places. Since 1996, smoking has been prohibited aboard Israeli airlines during international and national flights. Smoking is also prohibited in educational facilities, government buildings, health care facilities, public transportation vehicles and workplaces. In 2002, smoking in public places as malls and shopping centers was also banned. Recently, selling cigarettes to people younger than 18 years old was also banned by law (55). Additionally, smoking was forbidden in pubs, bars, restaurants and other public places in November 2007. However, law enforcement is not always adequate.

A recent survey of the Israel Cancer Association conducted in 2006 showed that 75% of the public supports the prohibition of smoking in restaurants and cafes (56). Israel was the first country to apply the World Health Organization's Framework Convention on Tobacco Control to protect a woman exposed to secondhand smoke in a restaurant. A local court awarded the plaintiff nominal compensation by the restaurant's owners, and there was no intervention by the district court. On appeal to the High Court of Justice, a judge upheld her case and raised the compensation tenfold plus costs of more than double the compensation (57).

(c) Bans on advertising and promotion of tobacco products. Media advertising strategies can not be used to advertise tobacco in accordance with national legislation. Tobacco advertising is allowed only in the print media (except for youth magazines) without using human figures – and national legislation and regulations govern its use. Free products and industry sampling practices are prohibited by law and regulations, and so is the import of chewing tobacco.

§ Educational interventions

Consumer education

State laws mandate printed health warnings on tobacco product packaging. The state determined the maximum permissible yield of nicotine per cigarette. The state also determined the maximum permissible yield of tars and other toxic constituents per cigarette (58).

Schools include education about the dangers of tobacco use in their curricula voluntarily, with assistance from government- and non-governmental organizations (NGOs). The government and NGOs, such as the Israel Cancer Association, also conduct regular public information initiatives about the dangers of tobacco use without a legislative mandate from the government (58). In fact, several large anti-smoking campaigns were conducted recently by the Ministry of Health, the Israel Cancer Association and Israel's health funds (HMOs).

§ Individual smoking-cessation interventions

Nicotine replacement and other therapies

All health funds (HMOs) now offer support groups led by smoking cessation specialists and individual treatment (NRT and individual counseling by smoking cessation specialists) programs for smoking cessation. HMOs have reached out to smokers and offered these options.

Special attention is given to specific smoker groups, such as pregnant women, patients with diabetes or chronic ischemic heart diseases and the Arab-Israeli population. The treatment is subsidized and offered at reduced prices (14). Simultaneously, documentation of the smoking status of each patient is now introduced as a quality assurance indicator in most HMOs clinics (14).

However, a recent observational study assessed the impact of primary care physician interventions on smoking cessation in Israel. The interventions included ascertainment of the smoking status of the patient; providing brief advice on smoking cessation; offering use of pharmacological therapies in addition to support and adequate follow-up. The results indicated that physician interventions to promote smoking quitting were at a low rate, that a large proportion of the physicians do not follow the recommendations to promote smoking cessation among their patients and that intervention among adolescents was particularly inadequate (59).

⚕ Conclusions

In summary, the Israeli efforts for tobacco control may be reflected in the decreasing trends of smoking prevalence in the last decades. It is still unclear, however, if further decrease should be anticipated or whether the full impact of the measures taken so far has reached its peak.

The challenge of confronting the addiction of its citizens to tobacco and smoking has been faced by the State of Israel during the last few decades. Within the last 30 years, the rates of smoking have declined by about 30%. This has been achieved by persuading smokers to quit and by successfully preventing young people from becoming new smokers. Multiple strategies have been used to tackle the tobacco addiction problem and major policies have been set in order to achieve these goals. One of the strategies used was confronting the tobacco companies and preventing them from marketing their products to new smokers. Additionally, much effort was invested into educating both smokers and nonsmokers regarding the hazards of smoking and into convincing smokers to quit. Resources were allocated to help smokers to five up their cigarettes and support them, usually through the health funds.

However, these actions are not enough; more is needed. Israel's smoking rates – especially in specific groups with relatively high smoking prevalence rates such as Arab men, Jewish men with low education level and young immigrants from the former Soviet Union –should be reduced. Targeted interventions for these specific subgroups should be developed since the general interventions are less effective for them and may not answer their specific needs.

In addition, a more vigilant action should be taken to enforce the existing laws and restrictions against smoking within the community, such as eliminating smoking places in shopping malls and restaurants. There is also room for additional tobacco control legislation.

More resources should also be allocated to the design of comprehensive campaigns aimed at adolescent smoking; the existing educational school programs have not been proven to be effective when implemented unaccompanied by other effective smoking control strategies.

In conclusion, although smoking rates in Israel are decreasing, there is much work to be done to decrease the levels of tobacco addiction within the population even further.

The authors are responsible for the views expressed in this publication and they do not necessarily reflect those of the Ministry of Health.

⚕ References

1. Wikipedia, The Free Encyclopedia. Tobacco [online]. [cited November 2008]. Available from URL: http://en.wikipedia.org/wiki/Tobacco.
2. Ernst A. On the etymology of the word tobacco. *American Anthropologist* 1889; 2: 133–142.
3. Imperial Tobacco Canada. Tobacco History [online]. [cited November 2008]. Available from URL: http://www.tobacco.org/History/Tobacco_History.html.
4. Borio G. The tobacco timeline[online]. [cited October 2008]. Available from URL: http://www.tobacco.org/History/Tobacco_History.html.
5. Mackay J, Eriksen M. *The tobacco atlas.* World Health Organization, Myriad Edition Limited UK, 2002. Available from URL: http://www.who.int/tobacco/media/en/title.pdf (cited November 2008).
6. http://info.cancerresearchuk/cancerstats (cited November 2008).
7. http://www.abs.gov.au/ausstat (cited November 2008).
8. http://www.cancercare.on.canada (cited November 2008).
9. http://www.cdc.gov (cited November 2008).
10. Shafey O, Dolwick S, Guindon GE, eds. *Tobacco control countries profile,* second edition. Atlanta, GA: The Twelfth World Conference on Tobacco or Health. The American Cancer Society, World Health Organization, and International Union against Cancer, 2003.
11. World Health Organization. Tobacco Free Initiatives. Regional Databases. Available from URL: http://www.emro.who.int/TFI/CountryProfile-Part6.htm (cited November 2008).

12. Lopez AD, Collishaw NE, Piha T. A descriptive model of the cigarette epidemic in developed countries. *Tobacco Control* 1994; 3: 242–247.

13. US Department of Health and Human Services. *The health consequences of involuntary exposure to tobacco smoke: a report of the Surgeon General*; Executive summary. US Department of Health and Human Services, Centers for Disease Control and Prevention, Coordinating Center for Health Promotion, National Center for Chronic Disease Prevention and Health Promotion, Office on Smoking and Health, 2006.

14. The Minister of Health's report on smoking in Israel 2006–2007. Israel Center for Disease Control, publication No. 308, May 2007 [Hebrew].

15. Baron-Epel O, Haviv-Messika A, Tamir D, *et al.* Multiethnic differences in smoking in Israel, pooled analysis from three national surveys. *European Journal of Public Health* 2004; 14: 384–389.

16. The Minister of Health's report on smoking in Israel 2007–2008. Israel Center for Disease Control, publication No. 313, May 2008 [Hebrew].

17. National Cancer Institute. Those who continue to smoke. In: *Smoking and Tobacco Control Monograph* No. 15, Washington, DC: US Department of Health and Human Services, 2002.

18. The Minister of Health's report on smoking in Israel 2003–2004. Israel Center for Disease Control, publication No. 236, May 2004 [Hebrew].

19. Inglis B. *The forbidden game: a social history of drugs.* New York: Charles Scribner's Sons, 1975.

20. Muller F. Tobacco misuse and lung carcinoma. University of Cologne's Pathological Institute, 1939.

21. Russek HI, Zohman BL, Dorset VJ. Effects of tobacco and whiskey on the cardiovascular system. *Journal of the American Medical Association* 1955; 157: 563–568.

22. Levin ML, Goldstein H, Gerhardt PR. Cancer and tobacco smoking, a preliminary report. *Journal of the American Medical Association* 1950; 143: 336–338.

23. Wynder EL, Graham EA. Tobacco smoking as a possible etiologic factor in bronchiogenic carcinoma; a study of 684 proved cases. *Journal of the American Medical Association* 1950; 143: 329–336.

24. Doll R, Hill AB. Smoking and carcinoma of the lung, a preliminary report. *British Medical Journal* 1950; 2: 739–748.

25. Doll SR, Peto R. The causes of cancer: quantitative estimates of avoidance risks of cancer in the United States today. *Journal of the National Cancer Institute* 1981; 66: 1191–1308.

26. US Department of Health and Human Services. *The health consequences of smoking: a report of the Surgeon General*; Executive summary. US Department of Health and Human Services, Centers for Disease Control and Prevention, Coordinating Center for Health Promotion, National Center for Chronic Disease Prevention and Health Promotion, Office on Smoking and Health, 2004.

27. Balfour D, Bates C, Benowitz N, *et al.* Tobacco smoking in Britain – an overview. In: *Nicotine Addiction in Britain.* 2000. Royal College of Physicians of London. Available from URL: http://www.rcplondon.ac.uk/pubs/books/nicotine (cited November 2008).

28. Doll R, Peto R, Boreham J, *et al.* Mortality in relation to smoking: 50 years' observations on male British doctors. *British Medical Journal* 2004; 328: 1519.

29. Centers for Disease Control and Prevention. Annual smoking-attributable mortality, years of potential life lost, and productivity losses – United States, 1997–2001. *Morbidity and Mortality Weekly Report* 2005; 54: 625–628.

30. http://www.smokingcosts.org/report.pdf (cited February 2008).

31. Kaiserman MJ. *The cost of smoking in Canada, 1991.* Public Health Agency of Canada 1991: 18 (1).

32. Balfour D, Bates C, Benowitz N, *et al.* Is nicotine a drug of addiction? In: *Nicotine addiction in Britain.* London: Royal College of Physicians of London, 2000. Available from URL: http://www.rcplondon.ac.uk/pubs/books/nicotine (cited November 2008).

33. National Institute on Drug Abuse (NIDA). Research report: tobacco addiction. NIH publication No. 06–4342, printed 1998, reprinted 2001, revised 2006. Available from URL: http://www.nida.nih.gov/researchreports/nicotine/nicotine.html (cited November 2008).

34. Pontieri FE, Tanda G, Orzi F, *et al.* Effects of nicotine on the nucleus accumbens and similarity to those of addictive drugs. *Nature* 1996; 382: 255–257.

35. Koob GF. Drugs of abuse: anatomy, pharmacology and function of reward pathways. *Trends in Pharmacological Sciences* 1992; 13: 177–184.

36. Salokangas RK, Vilkman H, Ilonen T, *et al.* High levels of dopamine activity in the basal ganglia of cigarette smokers. *American Journal of Psychiatry* 2000; 157: 632–634.

37. Besson M, Granon S, Mameli-Engvall M, *et al.* Long term effects of nicotine chronic exposure on brain nicotinic receptors. *Proceedings of the National Academy of Sciences* 2007; 104: 8155–8160.

38. Bates C, Jarvis M, Connoly G. Detailed report of the additives in cigarette tobacco (07/19-5). Excerpts from ASH (UK) Report on tobacco additives: cigarette engineering and nicotine addiction. Available from URL: http://www.ash.org.uk/papers/additives.html (cited November 2008).

39. Balfour D, Bates C, Benowitz N, *et al.* Psychological effects of nicotine and smoking in man. In: *Nicotine addiction in Britain.* London: Royal College of Physicians, 2000. Available from URL: http://www.rcplondon.ac.uk/pubs/books/nicotine (cited November 2008).

40. Dar R, Stronguin F, Marouani R, *et al.* Craving to smoke in orthodox Jewish smokers who abstain on the Sabbath: a comparison to a baseline and to a forced abstinence workday. *Psychopharmacology* 2005; 183: 294–299.

41. Schnoll RA, Patterson F, Lerman C. Treating tobacco dependence in women. *Journal of Women's Health* 2007; 16: 1211–1218.

42. DiFranza J, Savageau JA, Fletcher K, *et al.* Symptoms of tobacco dependence after brief intermittent use: the development and assessment of nicotine dependence in youth-2 Study. *Archives of Pediatrics and Adolescent Medicine* 2007; 161: 704–710.

43. Mester R, Toren P, Ben Moshe Y, *et al.* Survey of smoking habits and attitudes of patients and staff in psychiatric hospitals. *Psychopathology* 1993; 26: 69–75.

44. Kaizer I, Eytan A. Variations in smoking during hospitalization in psychiatric in-patient units and smoking prevalence in patients and health-care staff. *International Journal of Social Psychiatry* 2005; 51: 317–328.

45. Kelly C, McCreadie RG. Smoking habits, current symptoms, and premorbid characteristics of schizophrenic patients in Nithsdale, Scotland. *American Journal of Psychiatry* 1999; 156: 1751–1757.

46. Uçok A, Polat A, Bozkurt O, *et al.* Cigarette smoking among patients with schizophrenia and bipolar disorders. *Psychiatry and Clinical Neurosciences* 2004; 58: 434–437.

47. Itkin O, Nemetz B, Finat H. Smoking habits in bipolar and schizophrenic outpatients in southern Israel. *Journal of Clinical Psychiatry* 2002; 63: 368–369.

48. *Wilens TE, Fusillo S.* When ADHD and substance use disorders intersect: relationship and treatment implications. *Current Psychiatry Reports* 2007; 9: 408–414.

49. Gilbert A, Cornuz J. Which are the most effective and cost-effective interventions for tobacco control? Copenhagen: WHO Regional Office for Europe (Health Evidence Network report), 2003.http://www.euro.who.int/document/e82993.pdf (cited November 2008).

50. Schroeder SA. Tobacco control in the wake of 1998 master settlement agreement. *New England Journal of Medicine* 2004; 350: 292–301.

51. Franks P, Jerant AF, Leigh JP, et al. Cigarette prices, smoking, and the poor: implications of recent trends. *American Journal of Public Health.* 2007; 97: 1873–1877.

52. Jorenby DE. Smoking cessation strategies for the twenty-first century. *Circulation* 2001; 104: e51–e52.

53. Coleman T, West R. Newly available treatments for nicotine addiction. *British Medical Journal* 2001; 322: 1076–1077.

54. Quitting smoking. Nicotine addiction in Minnesota. July 2001; 204: 51–2e.

55. *Baker A, Richmond R, Haile M, et al.* Characteristics of smokers with a psychotic disorder and implications for smoking interventions. *Psychiatry Research* 2007; 150: 141–152.

56. Israel Cancer Association. A new survey about smoking: January 2006. Available from URL: http://www.cancer.org.il/template/default.asp?textSearch=&maincat=26&catid=214&pageid=2662 (cited November, 2008).

57. Simpson D. Israel: First FCTC court case. *Tobacco Control* 2006; 15: 421.

58. Corrao MA, Guindon GE, Sharma N, *et al.*, eds. *Tobacco control country profiles*, database 2000 Israel. Atlanta, GA: The American Cancer Society published for the eleventh World Conference on Tobacco and Health, 2000.

59. Thomas K, Yaphe J, Matalon A. Current primary care physician interventions to promote smoking cessation in Israel: an observational study. *Israel Medical Association Journal* 2007; 9: 645–648.

Chapter 11

The epidemiology of affective disorders in Israel

Itzhak Levav and Daphna Levinson

Of the group of affective disorders, major depressive disorder (MDD) has attracted special public health attention as a result of the findings of Harvard University and World Bank researchers (1). These researchers estimated that in the coming years, MDD will ranked first among the 10 leading causes of years lived with disability (YLD) in high-income countries, such as Israel. The current contribution of MDD is estimated at 11.8% of YLD – in men 7.7% and in women 11.0% (1, 2).

The general magnitude of the burden might be further compounded by psychosocial risk factors specific to Israel, such as the breakdown of social networks experienced by the waves of immigrants arriving over the years (see chapter 6). For Israel, both the general and specific factors impacting on the burden caused by MDD are particularly relevant with regard to both etiological research and program planning.

In addition, there is some research evidence that Jews, who comprise 80% of Israel's population, may be particularly vulnerable to MDD. This finding pertains in particular to Jewish men (3). Further local interest on MDD derives from clinic-based observations that found an increased risk for depression among Ashkenazi Jews as compared with Oriental Jews (4). Lastly, with regard to the Arab-Israeli minority, the specific risk for depressive disorders may result from the adverse psychological effects of the Arab-Israeli conflict that include a variety of losses (5) (see chapter 6).

This review of studies on MDD, minor depressive disorder, intermittent depressive disorder and bipolar I and II is based on the two community-based epidemiological studies that have been conducted in the Israeli adult population. (Studies covering the young and the elderly are dealt in chapters 2 and 4, respectively). While the first study (Study I) was limited to a selected cohort of Jewish Israelis (6, 7), the second one (Study II) covered both Arabs and Jews (8). A brief review of an epidemiologic study on postpartum depression (PPD) conducted in a community-based health setting was added to this chapter because of its relevance to service planning, both curative and preventive (9, 10); PPD is treated in greater detail in chapter 17. This chapter concludes with both a brief reference to an epidemiological study on the comorbidity of bipolar I disorder and cancer (11).

§ Community-based epidemiologic surveys

Study I

This study (also reviewed in chapters 6, 12 and 14) was conducted by a mixed American-Israeli research team between 1982 and 1987 (6, 7) and was based on a two-stage procedure. In the screening phase, the authors used the PERI-Psychiatric Epidemiology Research Interview and a number of anamnestic items, including previous psychiatric treatment and Israel Defense Forces (IDF) medical profile. In the diagnostic phase, the authors applied the SADS-I (Schedule of Affective Disorders and Schizophrenia, Israel version) linked to the RDC-Research Diagnostic Criteria. This survey was limited regarding the study population, as it only comprised native Israeli Jews born to immigrants from selected European and North African countries, from a 1949 and 1958 cohort.

The overall aim of this study was to explain the higher rates of selective psychiatric disorders often found in the lowest socioeconomic class. The study findings were interpreted according to a theoretical frame of reference that had been spelled out by Dohrenwend *et al.* (6).

In this study, a probability sample was extracted from the National Population Registry (NPR) and constructed using stratification procedures designed to ensure statistical power to contrast the rates of several types of disorders in advantaged and disadvantaged ethnic groups (of European and North-African origin, respectively) with social class held constant. While theory dictated the nature of the stratification, the formal probability sampling methods allowed the responses to be weighted to estimate the rates in the original cohort; the study thus serves the purpose of this chapter. The relevant sampling frame of the cohort, regardless of the place of residence, included 177,000 individuals who at the time of the initiation of the field operation were between 24 and 33 years old (in 1982). A large pre-screening phase (N = 19,000) was necessary, since information on education and ethnicity (the latter variable determined by father's country of birth) was and remains unavailable in the NPR. On the basis of pre-screening, the authors were able to estimate the final sample size – 5200 individuals.

All individuals scoring above the cut point applied to the PERI, or found "positive" in any anamnestic item (N = 2643), together with 18.3% of the 2271 individuals screened "negatives" were referred for diagnosis. Of those individuals, N = 3059, five had died and 34 migrated since the first phase. Of the remaining sample, 90.8% were successfully diagnosed by clinical psychiatrists with the SADS-I at home, jails or hospitals, N = 2741.

Prevalence rates of the affective disorders – major depressive disorder, minor depressive disorder, intermittent depressive disorder, manic disorder, hypomanic disorder and cyclothymic personality – over the preceding six months were estimated. Research Diagnostic Criteria (RDC) categories were established at the definite and probable levels, according to the number and duration of signs and symptoms.

Six-month and 12-month prevalence rates were estimated. The six-month prevalence rates for all the affective disorders at the definite level of RDC diagnoses were: major depressive disorder = 3.0%, SE = .5; minor depressive disorder = 1.5%, SE = .3; intermittent depressive disorder = 3.0%, SE = .4; manic disorder = .1%, SE = .04; hypomanic disorder = .2%, SE = .1; bipolar I – lifetime diagnosis = .5%, SE = .1; bipolar II – lifetime diagnosis = .6%, SE = .3; and cyclothymic personality – lifetime diagnosis = .3%, SE = .1.

Only the intermittent depressive disorder varied strongly with education; it was more common in the least educated. Thus from 5.3% among individuals with less than a high-school education, the rate descended to 2.4% among those who had attended high school and was even lower (1.7%) among those with a university education. The inverse relationship with education was also noted for major and minor depressive disorders, but the differences were not statistically significant. As for gender, intermittent depressive disorder showed statistical significant difference rates at the combined probable and definite level of the RDC categories: women = 4.6%, SE = .8; men = 2.5%, SE = .5, p < .01. Uncontrolled percentages for major and minor depressive disorders were higher among women than for men, 61.1% and 38.9%, and 55.1% and 44.9%, respectively. The rates for major depressive disorder and intermittent depressive disorder were statistically significantly higher among respondents of North African descent, while bipolar disorder I was higher among Israeli-born individuals of European origin.

The 12-month prevalence rates at the definite level of RDC diagnosis was almost double for major depressive disorder = 4.0%, SE = .5 than for minor depressive disorder = 2.2%, SE = .4 (7). As expected, respondents with major depressive disorder had statistically significant higher demoralization (or emotional distress) M scores = 1.6, SD = .7 than respondents with minor depressive disorders = 1.1, SD = .6. In this study, the median age at first onset of major depression, 26 years, was significantly younger than for minor depression disorder, 28 years. Respondents with major depressive disorder had a higher odds ratio (OR) of ever having attempted suicide (OR 3.1, 95% CI 1.6–5.7) than respondents with minor depressive disorder (OR 1.1, 95% CI .4–3.3). In the month preceding the interview, a higher percentage of respondents with a major depressive disorder had a more significant decline in functioning as judged by the interviewing psychiatrist (52.1%), than respondents diagnosed with a minor depressive disorder (22.8%). The uncontrolled analysis also showed that respondents with major depressive disorder had been hospitalized more often (9.1%) than those with minor depressive disorder (1.6%). This study also showed that the treatment gap in seeking help from mental health professionals was considerable, only 25.4% and 22.7% sought help for major and minor depressive disorders, respectively. A higher percentage – 36.1% and 43.6% respectively – turned to other community agents for help, including a medical doctor (Also see Study II).

Test of causation

The design of this study measured the socioeconomic and ethnic advantaged/disadvantaged statuses simultaneously in order to check whether the higher rates found among those of lower socioeconomic status reflect social selection (the social drift caused by the psychiatric disorder) and/or social causation (as the result of adversities and social pressures).

The results showed that the rate of current RDC-major depressive disorder was higher for Israeli-born women of North-African descent (p < .01). The results were interpreted as resulting from the social stress experienced by this group, thus providing support to the social causation hypothesis (6).

Study II

The Israel National Health Survey (INHS) epidemiologic study, conducted in 2003 and 2004, included the identification and diagnosis of affective disorders (8). We will review the relevant sections of the INHS with regards to the lifetime and 12-month prevalence rates of those disorders and their sociodemographic correlates.

Section A of this review deals with the general sample population. Section B addresses specific aspects of the study related to the Arab-Israeli sector. A description of the methods, procedures, analysis and characterization of the samples, also reviewed in other chapters, is presented first, since they are common to both sections.

The study sample was extracted from the NPR and comprised non-institutionalized *de jure* residents aged 21 and over. The sample was designed to reflect the distribution in the general population of selected gender/age population groups (Arab Israelis; post-1990 immigrants from the former Soviet Union; and other Jews, both Israeli born or born elsewhere). Face-to-face interviews at the respondents' homes were conducted from May 2003 to April 2004 in Arabic, Hebrew or Russian. The overall response rate was 73% (88% among Arab Israelis and 71% among Jewish Israelis), totaling almost 5,000 completed interviews (12).

Study variables

Sociodemographic: The schedule included age, gender, origin, ethnic-national group, marital and employment status, education and income (table 1).

Table 1. The Israel National Health Survey sample by sociodemographic variables (raw numbers and weighted proportions)

Variables	Total		Men		Women	
	n	%	n	%	n	%
Age group						
< 35	1585	35	796	36	789	34
35–49	1317	28	669	28	648	27
50–64	1080	21	547	21	533	22
65 and above	877	16	368	15	509	17
Population group						
Jews *	4200	87	2056	87	2144	88
Arabs	659	13	324	13	335	12
Origin						
Israeli born	2759	59	1399	61	1360	57
Immigrants	2100	41	981	39	1119	43
Marital status						
Never married	900	19	509	22	391	16
Married/cohabiting	3229	68	1664	71	1565	65
Separated/widowed/divorced	730	13	207	7	523	19
Education						
None, primary or some secondary	1068	22	517	22	551	21
Complete secondary	1728	37	850	36	878	37
Post-secondary	800	16	423	18	377	16
Complete first degree	1263	25	590	24	673	26

Table 1. The Israel National Health Survey sample by sociodemographic variables (raw numbers and weighted proportions) (cont.)

Variables	Total		Men		Women	
	n	%	n	%	n	%
Employment status						
Working	3030	60	1714	70	1316	51
Homemaker	245	6	6	0	239	11
Retired	813	15	313	13	500	18
Student	120	4	67	4	53	3
Other	651	15	280	13	371	17

*Includes Israelis not registered as Jews or Arabs

Diagnostic assessment: INHS used the Composite International Diagnostic Interview (CIDI), a structured diagnostic instrument, to assesses selected psychiatric disorders according to both the ICD-10 and the DSM-IV. The affective disorders included were: major depressive disorder, dysthymia and bipolar I and II disorders. Prevalence estimates were determined by whether the respondents' past or current symptoms met the 12-month and/or lifetime diagnostic criteria for DSM-IV disorder. For each disorder, a screening sub-questionnaire was administered to each respondent. All participants answering positively to a specific screening item were asked the questions in the respective diagnostic section of the questionnaire. Organic exclusion criteria were taken into account in determining DSM-IV diagnoses.

Age of onset: It was elicited as follows: "How old were you the first time you had the symptoms?" Different time-linked probes were used to facilitate recall.

Disability: The Sheehan Disability Scale (12) was used to measure role impairment at work, home, social life and intimate relationships due to each one of the diagnosed disorders.

Severity: Respondents who reported a DSM-IV affective disorder in the preceding 12 months were grouped according to three levels of disorder severity. Respondents with a severe level had either bipolar I disorder or had attempted suicide during the previous 12 months or reported at least two areas of role functioning with severe role impairment, as measured by the disorder-specific Sheehan Disability Scale (12). The moderate level referred to a disorder whose impairment ranked at least moderate on the Sheehan Disability Scale. All other respondents were classified as having a mild level of disorder.

Analysis

The data were weighted by making the appropriate adjustments for differential selection probabilities and response rates. The estimates of prevalence rates are presented as percentages with the respective standard errors. The Kaplan-Meier method (13) was used to generate age-at-onset curves. Logistic regression analysis (14) was used to establish the demographic correlates of prevalence, and the coefficients were transformed into odds ratios (ORs). Ninety-five percent confidence intervals (95% CIs) were estimated using the SUDAAN software package (15).

Henceforth, the results will be reviewed separately for each section.

§ Section A: General population sample

Results

Lifetime and 12-month rates were 10.2% and 6.1%, respectively. The highest rates among women for both lifetime and 12-month rates were found in the 21–34 age group, 13.3% and 7.8%, respectively. Among men, the highest rates were found in the 50–64 age group, 10.1% and 6.3%, for lifetime and 12 months, respectively. The difference between genders both in lifetime and 12-month prevalence rates was substantial, largely due to differences in the 21 to 49 age group.

Table 2. Life-time and 12-month prevalence rates (%) of major depressive disorder

Age group	n		Lifetime Total	Lifetime Women	Lifetime Men	12-Month Total	12-Month Women	12-Month Men	Gender differences Lifetime Sig.	Gender differences 12-Month Sig.
21–34	1627	n	178	109	69	105	65	40	*p*=.001	*p*=.015
		%	10.6	13.3	8.0	6.3	7.8	4.8		
		SE	(.8)	(1.2)	(.9)	(.6)	(1.0)	(.8)		
35–49	1302	n	125	80	45	74	48	26	*p*=.000	*p*=.002
		%	9.4	12.4	6.3	5.7	7.6	3.7		
		SE	(.8)	(1.3)	(.9)	(.7)	(1.1)	(.7)		
50–64	1069	n	113	61	52	62	32	30	*p*=.634	*p*=.876
		%	6.3	6.3	10.1	6.2	6.1	6.3		
		SE	(.6)	(.6)	(1.4)	(.8)	(1.1)	(1.2)		
65 and above	861	n	85	60	25	49	38	11	*p*=.096	*p*=.050
		%	10.0	11.6	8.0	6.0	7.5	4.0		
		SE	(1.1)	(1.5)	(1.6)	(.9)	(1.2)	(1.3)		
All	4859	n	501	310	191	290	183	107	*p*=.000	*p*=.000
		%	10.2	12.3	7.9	6.1	7.3	4.7		
		SE	(.5)	(.7)	(.6)	(.4)	(.6)	(.5)		

Age of onset

The age of onset for the depressive disorders decreased steadily from the oldest cohort (with a mean age of onset at 47.8) to the youngest cohort (with a mean age of onset at 20.1).

The mean number of years lived in episodes went up from the youngest cohort with 3.7 years to the oldest cohort with 7.2 years. There was no difference between genders, except in the oldest cohort.

The mean number of lifetime episodes in both genders showed a steady increase from the cohort ages 21 to 34 (with 8.6 episodes) to the cohort ages 50 to 64 (with 12.5 episodes). In the cohort 65 and older, women reported an average of 30.2 lifetime episodes, while men reported considerable less (5.0 lifetime episodes) (table 3).

Table 3. History of depressive disorders by age and gender

History	Age group	Total		Women		Men		Gender differences
		n	M (SE)	n	M (SE)	n	M (SE)	
Mean age of onset	21–34	105	20.1 (.6)	65	20.1 (.7)	40	20.1 (1.1)	p=.981
	35–49	74	30.0 (1.2)	48	29.8 (1.5)	26	30.4 (2.0)	p=.799
	50–64	62	38.6 (2.0)	32	36.3 (3.1)	30	41.1 (2.3)	p=.213
	65 and above	49	47.8 (3.5)	38	48.3 (3.7)	11	46.8 (7.8)	p=.865
	All ages	290	30.9 (1.0)	183	30.6 (1.2)	107	31.4 (1.7)	p=.689
Differences across groups		p=.000		p=.000		p=.000		–
Mean number of years in episode	21–34	105	3.7 (.4)	65	3.3 (.3)	40	4.3 (.8)	p=216
	35–49	74	5.3 (.5)	48	5.4 (.7)	26	5.1 (.9)	p=.818
	50–64	62	5.5 (.8)	32	5.5 (1.3)	30	5.5 (.9)	p=.961
	65 and above	49	7.2 (1.4)	38	8.6 (1.9)	11	3.8 (.8)	p=.019
	All ages	290	5.0 (.4)	183	5.2 (.5)	107	4.8 (.5)	p=.568
Differences across cohorts		p=.000		p=.000		p=.125		–
Mean number of life-time episodes	21–34	105	8.6 (1.9)	65	7.5 (1.4)	40	10.3 (4.3)	p=.536
	35–49	74	12.1 (1.8)	48	11.2 (2.1)	26	14.1 (3.2)	p=.449
	50–64	62	14.8 (3.0)	32	12.5 (3.4)	30	17.4 (5.0)	p=.415
	65+	49	22.7 (8.3)	38	30.2 (11.5)	11	5.0 (1.3)	p=.029
	All Ages	290	13.0 (1.7)	183	13.3 (2.3)	107	12.5 (2.3)	p=.793
Differences across groups		p=.058		p=.008		p=.591		–

Comorbidity

Table 4 shows the psychiatric comorbidity of respondents with a lifetime major depressive disorder. Of the 290 respondents with MDD, 29% met criteria for some type of anxiety disorder and 2.3%, for some type of substance abuse disorder. The likelihood of having some other psychiatric disorder during a lifetime MDD disorder (controlling for gender, education and marital status) produced significant likelihood ratios for most other disorders. Having a lifetime depressive disorder increased 25 times the likelihood of post-traumatic stress disorder (PTSD); for generalized anxiety disorder, 13.6 times; for panic disorder, 4.5 times; and, in general, it was associated with 10 times the likelihood of having any other disorder.

Table 4. Comorbidity of an episode of major depressive disorder (MDE) with other mental disorders, all ages

12 month disorders	n with MDE	n with diagnosis	% of cases with 12-month MDE that have corresponding diagnosis (SE)	Likelihood of diagnosis with 12-month MDE as predictor, controlling for gender, education, marital status OR (CI)
Generalized anxiety disorder	290	63	22.3 (2.5)	13.6 (9.4–19.8)
Agoraphobia without panic	290	6	1.9 (.8)	6.2 (2.3–16.7)
Post-traumatic stress disorder	290	14	5.7 (1.5)	25.1 (10.1–62.5)
Panic disorder	290	7	2.2 (.9)	4.5 (1.7–11.5)
Any anxiety disorder	290	80	29.1 (2.8)	13.5 (9.7–18.9)
Alcohol abuse	290	7	2.3 (.9)	2.5 (1.1–5.7)
Any substance use disorder	290	7	2.3 (.9)	2.1 (.9–4.6)
Any disorder	290	83	30.0 (2.8)	9.8 (7.2–13.4)
One disorder	290	68	25.2 (2.7)	8.1 (5.8–11.2)
Two disorders	290	13	4.3 (1.2)	23.4 (9.0–61.0)

Comorbidity with chronic physical conditions

Of the 290 respondents with MDD, 69.2% of them reported at least one chronic physical condition; 19.1%, two conditions; and 28.1%, had at least three of these conditions. The likelihood of having comorbid physical disorders during a lifetime MDD disorder (controlling for gender, education and marital status) produced significant likelihood ratios for all pain conditions but for only some of the other conditions. Thus, lifetime MDD doubled the likelihood of having some pain condition; it increased by 40% the likelihood of any cardiovascular condition; by 70% the likelihood of ulcer; and by 50% the likelihood of having a chronic lung disease.

The impact of depression

The severity level of the symptoms of depression was measured with a self-report inventory that referred to problems with sleep, level of energy, ability to concentrate, self-view, sadness and interest in daily activities. Table 5 presents the differences between severity levels of depression in terms of the number of days (weeks) in episode/s, the number of days out of role and the level of role impairment during the previous 12 months, and the percentage of individuals with two or more additional DSM-IV diagnoses.

The table shows that only 13.5% of the cases had mild depression and about 42% had severe or very severe episodes of depression. The differences between severity levels among milder and severe cases were expressed, respectively, in the mean number of weeks in episode, 13.8 vs. 25; in the mean number of days out of role during one year, 22.9 vs. 191 days; in the percentage who reported role impairment during the worst month, 8.2% vs. 79.6%; and in the percentage with comorbid disorders, 4.0% vs. 17.4%.

**Table 5. Distributions and correlates of symptom severity
("QIDS" = Quick Inventory of Depressive Symptomatology Self-Report) ***

	Mild	Moderate	Severe	Very severe	Total
QIDS (%) (se)[1]	13.5 (1.8)	42.1 (2.7)	32.0 (2.6)	10.0 (1.7)	100.0 (0.0)
Duration in weeks (m) (se)[2]	13.8 (2.3)	19.9 (1.6)	22.1 (1.9)	25.7 (3.2)	20.4 (1.0)
Days out of role (m) (se)[3]	22.9 (12.8)	41.5 (10.9)	58.4 (11.1)	191.5 (29.2)	62.7 (7.7)
Role impairment (%) (se)[4]	8.2 (4.0)	35.3 (4.0)	60.9 (4.8)	79.6 (7.0)	44.5 (2.8)
Comorbidity (%) (se)[5]	4.0 (2.8)	7.1 (2.1)	10.2 (2.7)	17.4 (6.7)	8.8 (1.5)
(n)[6]	(53)	(157)	(116)	(35)	(361)

[1] Percent of people with the symptom severity domain.

[2] Mean number of days depressed in the 365 days before the interview.

[3] Mean number of days totally unable to work or carry on usual activities.
because of depression in the 365 days prior to the interviews.

[4] Percent who reported severe or very severe impairment in at least one SDS role domain (12).

[5] Percent with two or more comorbid 12-month CIDI/DSM-IV disorders.

[6] Number of cases with valid QIDS-SR scores within each severity domain.

Inventory to characterize the MDD episode (31)

Sociodemographic correlates of major depressive disorder

Women were 60% more likely to have had a MDD in the past 12 months. Income (expressed in quartiles of the per capita income distribution of the population) and education were unrelated to a higher probability of MDD. The most significant correlate of an episode of MDD was marital status: Those who were separated or divorced or widowed were 2.2 times more likely to have MDD compared to those who were married.

Table 6. Sociodemographic correlates of 12-month episode of major depressive disorder (MDE) by age

Demographics		n in each category	n with MDE	% (se)	OR*(95% CI)
Gender	Women	2479	183	7.3 (.6)	1.6 (1.2–2.1)
	Men	2380	107	4.7 (.5)	1.0 (1.0–1.0)
	Sig.	.	.	–	p=.000
Education	Low	1068	79	7.3 (.8)	1.5 (1.0–2.2)
	Low-average	1728	109	6.4 (.6)	1.3 (.9–1.8)
	High-average	800	42	5.2 (.8)	1.0 (.7–1.6)
	High	1263	60	5.0 (.7)	1.0 (1.0–1.0)
	Sig.	.	.	–	p=.100
Marital status	Married	3229	153	5.0 (.4)	1.0 (1.0–1.0)
	Sep/wid/divorced	730	72	10.4 (1.2)	2.2 (1.6–3.0)
	Never married	900	65	6.8 (.9)	1.4 (1.0–1.9)
	Sig.	.	.	–	p=.000

Table 6. Sociodemographic correlates of 12-month episode of major depressive disorder (MDE) by age (cont.)

Demographics		n in each category	n with MDE	% (SE)	OR*(95% CI)
Income	Low	773	56	7.3 (1.0)	1.1 (.7–1.7)
	Low-average	1472	85	5.8 (.6)	.9 (.6–1.3)
	High-average	1717	92	5.4 (.6)	.8 (.6–1.1)
	High	897	57	6.6 (.9)	1.0 (1.0–1.0)
	Sig.	.	.	–	p = .295

* *Odds ratios are not shown for cases in which the number of respondents within the demographic category is less than 15 or the count of respondents with MDE is less than five.*

☙ Section B: The Arab-Israeli sample in the INHS

Psychiatric epidemiological research on the Arab-Israeli population includes studies on the young (see chapter 2) and the elderly (16), and on a number of disorders as described in several chapters of this book. However, the INHS is the most comprehensive study conducted so far on the adult Arab-Israeli population. This situation contrasts with the scarcity of epidemiological data published in English from most Arab countries, with the exception of Lebanon and Dubai (17).

As noted in chapter 5, the Arab sector constitutes a sizeable minority of the Israeli population, 19.1%. This sector includes three groups classified by their religious affiliation: Muslims (1,055,400), Christians (115,000) and Druze (109,600) (in 2003). Although different in many ways besides religion (e.g., median age: 18.5, 27.9 and 22.7 respectively; and health status: e.g., for infant mortality the respective rates for 2003 were 8.6, 3.2 and 7.1 per 1,000 live births), these three groups were aggregated in the INHS due to statistical power constraints.

Members of the Arab-Israeli minority enjoy citizenship rights and have made remarkable progress in health and life expectancy over the years. However, they still suffer from a disadvantaged social status. As for the women, their social disadvantage is compounded by their subordinate position in a patriarchal society. They share this plight with women in most Arab countries (17).

Section B of this review included a comparison between Arab Israelis (men, 324 and women, 335) and Jewish Israelis (either local born or immigrants who arrived before 1990, men, 1,662 and women, 1,670). Arab Israelis, in contrast to Jewish Israelis, were younger, more often married, and had lower incomes, lower levels of education and larger families with more individuals living in the household. In addition, they were less likely to be employed full time and that women were in the workforce.

For the analysis, the sociodemographic variables were grouped as follows: educational level (low, 0 to 9 years and high, 10 years and above); age (21 to 49 years and 50 and above); marital status (married, divorced, separated and never married); income (below and above the median national income); number of children and persons in the household (1 to 3, 4 to 6 and 7 and over); employment status (employed, unemployed in the last 12 months and not in the workforce). Twelve-month prevalence rates and standard errors were calculated.

Results

The overall 12-month prevalence rates of affective disorders were: Arab Israelis = 8.2%, 95% CI

6.2–11.0; and Jewish Israelis = 5.9%, 95% CI 5.1–6.8. The rates for men were, 6.2%, 95% CI 3.8–9.4; and 4.7%, 95% CI 3.8–5.8, respectively; and for women, 10.5%, 95% CI 7.3–14.8; and 7.1%, 95% CI 5.9–8.5, respectively. Differences between both population groups approached significance ($p = .06$).

✺ The epidemiology of postpartum depression

Several adverse consequences have been imputed to this disorder with regard to the mother, the newborn, other children of the household and the marital relationship. In Israel, practically all women of all sectors of the population are in contact with the health services both before and after pregnancy. Those contacts facilitate both screening and treatment.

Glasser *et al.* carried out a study aimed at building a case for action (9, 10). Their study, reviewed in detail in chapter 19, had the following objectives – to establish the incidence and prevalence rates and identify risk factors that would guide appropriate intervention strategies. The population sample was selected from a community-based prenatal care clinic in a town of about 20,000 residents located in the central coastal area of the country. It was comprised of 344 pregnant women, 288 of whom were successfully interviewed. At about the sixth week of their pregnancy, subjects were administered the BDI-Beck Depression Inventory (18) (a scale that measures depressive symptoms), in which different cutting points indicate level of severity. The 10-item EPDS-Edinburgh Postnatal Depression Scale (19) was used to identify postpartum depression at about six weeks after the delivery. The questionnaire used also included an inventory of factors deemed to be associated with the disorder. Some of the information was complemented from information extracted from the medical records.

Almost 15% of the pregnant women reached the combined moderate and severe level of the Beck scale. Importantly, 34% who scored depression at any level during pregnancy had high level of EPDS, while 11% of the depression-free women had high EPDS scores during pregnancy ($p <$ .001). The additional risk factors that were identified in the analysis included immigrant status ($p <$ .01); low maternal schooling ($p = .06$); and any moderate or severe postpartum problems during the hospital stay ($p = .03$). The multivariate analysis showed that the following factors had statistically significant effects: marital disharmony, odds ratio (OR) = 5.9, 95% CI 2.5–14.1; history of emotional problems, OR = 4.3, 95% CI 2.1–9.2; poor social support, OR = 4.1, 95% CI 2.0–8.8; depression in pregnancy, OR = 3.7, 95% CI 1.8–7.7; and mothers of babies with recorded health problems in the medical chart, OR = 1.1, 95% CI 1.1–12.2.

✺ Bipolar disorder and cancer

The association between bipolar disorder and cancer (11) was studied linking two national databases – the Psychiatric Case Registry, which records all admissions to and discharges from inpatient psychiatric settings, served to identify all Israeli-born Jewish patients first admitted during the years 1980 to 2005 with a diagnosis of bipolar disorder (*ICD-10* F31) and manic (non-organic) state (*ICD-10* F30) during their last or only hospitalization. Those inpatients were linked to the Cancer Registry, which records cancer morbidity and mortality information.

The cancer incidence rates in these two diagnostic groups taken together (manic and bipolar disorders *ICD-10* F30 and F31) were compared with the rates in the Jewish-Israeli population using standardized incidence ratios (SIR) and the respective 95% confidence intervals. A SIR is defined as the ratio of the observed to the expected number of cancer cases. The expected number of cases during the observation period was calculated by gender and age. Period-specific cancer incidence rates were estimated. The person-years of exposure to cancer risk were defined for the index cases as follows, from date of birth to death, diagnosis of cancer, emigration or the end of the year 2005.

A total of 2121 patients were identified according to these diagnostic categories: manic disorder 253 (men, 145; women, 108); and bipolar disorder, 1868 (men, 852; women, 1006). The person-years estimated from the samples were 9957 for men and 12056 for women. Eighty percent of all patients were last admitted after 1996, when psychiatric services were more accurate in their diagnoses. Two or more admissions were recorded for 35.6% of patients with manic disorder and 67.5% for bipolar disorder. The risk for cancer among the manic and bipolar disorder diagnostic groups combined was statistically significantly higher for both genders: men, SIR = 1.6, 95% CI 1.01–2.17; and women, SIR = 1.8, 95% CI 1.3–2.2.

✎ International comparisons

How high are the rates of affective disorders in view of the historical events that have pervaded the life of the State of Israel and that were mentioned above? A comparison of rates of RDC-definite major depressive disorder obtained in Study I, for both men and women combined, can be made with two other studies that were conducted in Christchurch, New Zealand, (5.5%) (20) and Puerto Rico (2.8%) (21), since the three studies used analogous methods and included sample populations of similar ages. The comparison showed that the Israeli rate (3.0%) was not higher. Study II, the INHS, made possible a fuller and more updated comparison with results obtained in other countries that participated in the World Mental Health Survey: Belgium, France, Germany, Italy, Netherlands, Spain, all part of the European Study of the Epidemiology of Mental Disorders (ESEMeD) (22); the Ukraine (23); Lebanon (24); and the US (25), bearing in mind that, for example, the sociodemographic composition of the countries differ, in addition to possible differences in the expression of mental health problems:

The 12-month prevalence rates of affective disorders (mood disorders, as per the published reports) were: Israel, 6.4%; US, 9.5%; Ukraine, 8.9%; and Lebanon, 6.6%. For the ESEMeD group the rates were as follows: Belgium, 8.5%; France, 3.6%; Germany, 3.8%; Italy, 6.9%; and the Netherlands and Spain, 4.9%. The estimated rate for DSM-IV major depression in Israel was 5.9%, compared with 8.4%, for the US; 8.4%, for the Ukraine; 4.9%, for Lebanon, 3.9%; and 6.7%, for the ESEMeD group of six countries. In Israel, for 45% of the respondents with any mood disorder, the level of severity was high, while 14% had a mild one. The results in the US and Lebanon were similar.

In Israel, fewer than 20% of those with a mood disorder in the 12 months that preceded the interviews had more than one diagnosis. The same pattern was found in the Ukraine, where less than 30% of men or women had more than one. In the ESEMeD group of six countries, the parallel comorbidity rate was 41.7%. In the US, where a large number of diagnoses were investigated, more than 40% of respondents with any mood disorder had more than one psychiatric disorder.

The sociodemographic correlates of the prevalence rates of mood disorder in the preceding 12 months in the sample did not replicate the patterns of other large-scale, cross-sectional surveys of common mental disorders (anxiety and depression) that had been conducted in other countries (26). Being female (27, 28), middle aged (29) or with low income (30) did not correlate with higher odds of having a mood disorder (except for intermittent depressive disorder in Study I), however among respondents who had a disorder, those variables did correlate with higher odds of having a more severe disorder.

In conclusion, the prevalence rates of mood disorders in Israel are within the range found in other countries. This is despite the collective life circumstances of its society that might constitute risk factors for mood disorders (Holocaust and migration for Jews, and armed conflict for all population groups). Probably, the bonds of support characteristic of the Israeli society protect the exposed individuals when they face major national stressful life events.

❦ From epidemiology to mental health action

As shown in Study I and, especially in Study II, affective disorders are relatively frequent in the population and take a heavy toll. Likely, the toll is even higher than shown in the INHS since institutionalized respondents were not included. Thus for program planners, these disorders constitute a serious challenge. Importantly for this purpose, Study II and also Study I have identified important correlates. Indeed, the distribution of affective disorders is not a random phenomenon; there are groups in the population, such as certain marital groups and those with physical disorders, that are at higher risk. Also Glasser *et al.* showed differential risks for women with postpartum depression (9, 10). For persons with comorbid bipolar I disorder and cancer, it is pertinent to quote the study authors: "It is incumbent upon the medical and psychiatric services to be on the alert, particularly since there is a tendency to overlook physical disorders in patients affected by severe mental disorders" (11).

Thus, outreach efforts – a central component of any community-based program due to the treatment gap and lag that characterize help-seeking for affective disorders – might particularly target those population subgroups that are more vulnerable, for both curative and preventive action.

❦ References

1. Lopez AD, Mathers CD, Ezzati M, Jamison DT, *et al.*, eds. *Global burden of disease and risk factors.* New York: The World Bank and Oxford University Press, 2006.
2. World Health Organization. *The world health report 2001 – Mental health: new understanding, new hope.* Geneva: World Health Organization, 2001.
3. Levav I, Kohn R, Golding JM, *et al.* Vulnerability of Jews to affective disorders. *American Journal of Psychiatry* 1997; 154: 941–947.
4. Kohn R, Levav I, Dorenwend BP, *et al.* Doren Wend BP, *et al.* Jews and their intraethnic vulnerability to affective disorders, fact or artifact? II. Evidence from a cohort study. *Israel Journal of Psychiatry and Related Sciences* 1997; 34: 149–156.
5. Levav I, Al-Krenawi A, Ifrah A, *et al.* Common mental disorders among Arab Israelis: findings from the Israel National Health Survey. *Israel Journal of Psychiatry and Related Sciences* 2007; 44: 104–113.
6. Dohrenwend BP, Levav I, Shrout PE, *et al.* Socioeconomic status and psychiatric disorders; the causation-selection issue. *Science* 1992; 255: 946–952.
7. Levav I, Kohn R, Dohrenwend BP, *et al.* An epidemiological study of mental disorders in a 10-year cohort of young adults in Israel. *Psychological Medicine* 1993; 23: 691–707.
8. Levinson D, Zilber N, Lerner Y, *et al.* Prevalence of mood and anxiety disorders in the community: results from the Israel National Health Survey. *Israel Journal of Psychiatry and Related Sciences* 2007; 44: 94–103.
9. Glasser S, Barell V, Shoham A, *et al.* Prospective study of postpartum depression in an Israeli cohort: prevalence, incidence and demographic risk factors. *Journal of Psychosomatic Obstetrics and Gynecology* 1998; 19: 155–164.
10. Glasser S, Barell V, Shoham A, *et al.* Postpartum depression in an Israeli cohort: demographic, psychosocial and medical risk factors. *Journal of Psychosomatic Obstetrics and Gynecology* 2000; 21: 99–108.
11. Barchana M, Levav I, Lipshitz I, *et al.* Enhanced cancer risk among patients with bipolar disorder. *Journal of Affective Disorders* 2008; 108: 43–48.
12. Sheehan D. *The anxiety disease.* New York: Bantam Books, 1983.
13. Kaplan EL, Meier P. Nonparametric estimation from incomplete observations. *Journal of the American Statistical Association* 1958; 53: 457–481.
14. Hosmer DW, Lemeshow S. *Applied logistic regression.* New York: Wiley and Sons, 1989.
15. Research Triangle Institute. *SUDAAN Version 8.0.2.* Research Triangle Park, NC: Research Triangle Institute, 2003.

16. Shemesh AA, Kohn R, Geraisy N, *et al.* A community study on emotional distress among Arab and Jewish Israelis over the age of sixty. *International Journal of Geriatric Psychiatry* 2006; 21: 64–76.

17. Okasha A, Maj M, eds. *Psychiatry in the Arab world.* Cairo: World Psychiatric Association, Scientific Book House, 2001.

18. Beck AT, Steer RA, Garbin MG. Psychometric properties of the Beck Depression Inventory: twenty-five years of evaluation. *Clinical Psychological Review* 1988; 8: 77–100.

19. Cox JL, Holden JM, Sagovsky R. Detection of postnatal depression: development of the 10-item Edinburgh Postnatal Depression Scale. *British Journal of Psychiatry* 1987; 150: 782–786.

20. Oakley-Browne MA, Joyce PR, *et al.* Christchurch epidemiology study, part II: six month and other period prevalence of specific psychiatric disorders. *Australian and New Zealand Journal of Psychiatry* 1989; 23: 327–340.

21. Canino G, Bird HR, Shrout PE, *et al.* The prevalence of specific psychiatric disorders in Puerto Rico. *Archives of General Psychiatry* 1987; 44: 727–735.

22. The ESEMeD/MHEDEA 2000 Investigators. Prevalence of mental disorders in Europe: results from the European Study of the Epidemiology of Mental Disorders (ESEMeD) project. *Acta Psychiatrica Scandinavica* 2004; 109 (Suppl 420): 21–27.

23. Bromet EJ, Gluzman SF, Paniotto VI, *et al.* Epidemiology of psychiatric and alcohol disorders in Ukraine: findings from the Ukraine World Mental Health Survey. *Social Psychiatry and Psychiatric Epidemiology* 2005; 40: 681–690.

24. Karam EG, Mneimneh ZN, Karam AN, *et al.* Prevalence and treatment of mental disorders in Lebanon: a national epidemiological survey. *The Lancet* 2006; 367: 1000–1006.

25. Kessler RC, Chiu WT, Demler O, *et al.* Prevalence, severity, and comorbidity of 12-month DSM-IV disorders in the National Comorbidity Survey Replication. *Archives of General Psychiatry* 2005; 62: 617–627.

26. Fryers T, Melzer D, Jenkins R. Social inequalities and the common mental disorders: a systematic review of the evidence. *Social Psychiatry and Psychiatric Epidemiology* 2003; 38: 229–237.

27. Gold JH. Gender differences in psychiatric illness and treatments: a critical review. *Journal of Nervous and Mental Disease* 1998; 186: 769–775.

28. Patel V, Araya R, de Lima M, *et al.* Women, poverty and common mental disorders in four restructuring societies. *Social Science and Medicine* 1999; 49: 1461–1471.

29. Paykel ES, Brughab T, Fryers T. Size and burden of depressive disorders in Europe. *European Neuropsychopharmacology* 2005; 15: 411–423.

30. Kohn R, Dohrenwend BP, Mirotznik J, Epidemiological findings on selected psychiatric disorders in the general population. In: Dohrenwend BP, ed. *Adversity, stress, and psychopathology.* Oxford: Oxford University Press, 1998.

31. Rush AJ, Carmody T, Reimitz PE. The Inventory of Depressive Symptomatology (IDS). *International Journal of Methods in Psychiatric Research* 2000; 9: 45–59.

Chapter 12

The epidemiology of anxiety disorders in Israel

Joshua D. Lipsitz, Galit Geulayov and Raz Gross

Anxiety disorders are now recognized as a leading source of suffering and disability worldwide. More people will experience an anxiety disorder at some point in their lives than any other type of psychiatric disorder (1). Epidemiologic studies in 16 countries around the world indicated that from 1/tenth to one-quarter of the population will experience an anxiety disorder (2). In the US estimates are even higher – suggesting that nearly one-third of the population will suffer from an anxiety disorder (1, 3). Because of Israel's often stressful history, one might expect the rates of some anxiety disorders to be even higher.

Problems caused by anxiety disorders are not trivial. Anxiety disorders tend to have onset fairly early in life (4); if left untreated, they tend to run a chronic or recurring course (5). Disability is often substantial, and costs in terms of healthcare utilization are staggering (6, 7). Fortunately, progress has been made in making available efficacious treatments for anxiety disorders using psychotherapy, medication or a combination of them. Although the availability of several efficacious treatment options is welcome, optimism must be tempered by evidence that a large number of those with anxiety disorders are undiagnosed (6) or do not receive adequate treatment (8, 9). Epidemiological data on anxiety disorders worldwide has helped increase awareness of the scope and characteristics of this problem, thus contributing to improved access to treatment.

Anxiety disorders include generalized anxiety disorder (GAD); panic disorder with/without agoraphobia; phobic disorders including social phobia (also called social anxiety disorder); obsessive-compulsive disorder (OCD); and post-traumatic stress disorder (PTSD). The most extensive Israeli epidemiological research to date has focused on GAD, PTSD and – to a lesser extent – on panic disorder and agoraphobia. Relatively little epidemiological research has examined the prevalence of phobic disorders and OCD.

ᖰ Generalized anxiety disorder

Generalized anxiety disorder (GAD) is characterized by persistent anxious, worried moods along with physical and behavioral symptoms of anxiety. Current diagnostic systems, such as the *Diagnostic and Statistical Manual of Mental Disorders – Fourth Edition* (DSM-IV) (10) and the

International Classification of Diseases – Tenth Edition (ICD-10) (11) require anxiety symptoms to persist for at least six months to be recognized as an anxiety disorder diagnosis. However, earlier editions such as the DSM-III (12) required symptoms for only one month in duration. As a result, GAD prevalence rates differ substantially in older vs. more recent studies as a function of the criteria applied. There are also differences between the current diagnostic systems, DSM-IV and ICD-10, on criteria for GAD. However, both definitions yield fairly comparable estimates of prevalence rates, although the identified groups are only partially overlapping (13). Lifetime prevalence rates of GAD in community studies worldwide range from 4% to 7%, while 12-month prevalence rates range from 3% to 5% (14, 15). Higher prevalence rates of GAD up to 8% and even higher have been found in medical settings (e.g., 6).

Epidemiology of generalized anxiety disorders in Israel

Three large studies have now examined GAD in the Israeli population, each using somewhat different methodologies. The study by Levav *et al.* (16) examined a 10-year birth cohort aged 24 to 33 (in 1982) using a rigorous two-stage procedure with clinically-trained interviewers. Interviews were conducted using the Psychiatric Epidemiology Research Interview (PERI) for the first-stage screening (17) and the Israeli version of the Schedule of Affective Disorders and Schizophrenia (SADS) (18) for assigning final Research Diagnostic Criteria (RDC) (largely similar to DSM-III criteria) diagnoses. In that study, the estimated rates were point prevalence, 2.3%; six-month prevalence, 3.5%; and one-year prevalence, 4.5%. These large differences based on different timeframes are most probably due to the use of a system closely linked to DSM-III criteria for which symptom duration could be as short as one month. The short duration requirement also means that rates overall are likely inflated compared with current (DSM-IV and ICD-10) criteria.

Two populations surveys conducted in 2003 and 2004 used structured interviews by non-clinicians as part of general health surveys. Both surveys assessed GAD using versions of the Composite International Diagnostic Interview (CIDI) (19) with samples aged 21 and older. The first study, known as the Israel National Health Survey (INHS), included face-to-face interviews of 4859 respondents (73% response rate), the rates were 1.8% at 12 months and 2.7% for lifetime (20). The prevalence rates in the INHS were not reported by gender.

The second study involved a telephone interview of a randomly selected sample of 9509 respondents aged 21 or older. This study was conducted in 2003 to 2004 by the Israel Center for Disease Control as a component of a World Health Organization initiative. For about 25% of the respondents, the interview included the detailed mental health components of the CIDI interview, similar to the one above that included a module for GAD. The sample included both Jewish and Arab respondents, but data have been analyzed to date for 2,082 Jewish respondents (which reflect a 54% response rate). In this sample, authors found a slightly higher 12-month prevalence rate of 2.5% (21). Interestingly, this is also similar to rates found in an Israeli sample during preliminary field testing of the study in an independent sample of 992 respondents aged 16 and over (22).

Generalized anxiety disorders in medical settings

Cwikel *et al.* (23) assessed anxiety disorders in a sample of 976 patients aged 25 to 75 in eight primary-care clinics of Israel's largest health funds (HMOs) (see chapter 17). This study also used a version of the CIDI conducted in person in Hebrew, Arabic and Russian. They estimated a 12-month prevalence rate of 11.2%. Women did not have a significantly higher rate of GAD in this sample (women, 11.9% and men, 10.9%). Higher prevalence of GAD was associated with middle age, a lower level of education, the report of insufficient income and employment status – with those working full time having lower rates than the unemployed or those working part time. Another Israeli study explored anxiety disorder in 517 patients in a general hospital emergency department (24). The researchers found a 2.7% point prevalence rate of either generalized anxiety disorder or panic disorder. Prevalence was higher (6.7%) in the subgroup of patients who reported somatic complaints in the absence of a clear physical disorder.

❧ Post-Traumatic Stress Disorder (PTSD)

PTSD is a syndrome with a specific cluster of symptoms than can develop after exposure to an event in which grave physical harm occurred or was threatened. Common events that may lead to PTSD include military combat, rape, violent assaults, disasters and road accidents. People with PTSD have persistent frightening thoughts and memories of their ordeal, feel emotionally numb and may experience other problems such as sleep difficulties or being easily startled.

Manifold events in Israel's history have made it a tragically fertile laboratory for the study of human reactions to trauma and, specifically, for PTSD. Most prominent perhaps is the impact of wars and ongoing terrorism on both military personnel and civilians. Longitudinal studies of Israeli combat veterans, for example, have revealed important information about initial reactions as being predictive of high rates of PTSD and the persistence of PTSD symptoms for 20 years (25). PTSD among military personnel is covered in detail in chapter 13. Another prominent traumatic experience, which has impacted on Israel's population, was the Holocaust. For example, Amir and Wiesel (26) found that Jews who survived the Holocaust as children continued to report higher rates of PTSD symptoms even 55 years later. Others in clinical settings (e.g., 28) showed that the psychological effects of Holocaust trauma, including vulnerability to PTSD, also may have also impacted the adult children of survivors. Chapter 7 reviews the impact of the Holocaust on mental health in Israel. In this chapter we will consider what is known about other aspects of the epidemiology of PTSD in the Israeli population.

PTSD prevalence rates in other countries range from 3.6% for 12-month and 7% to 8% for lifetime in the US National Comorbidity Studies (1, 2) to somewhat lower rates of 2% to 4% lifetime prevalence in most European and Asian countries (e.g., 28, 29). Unfortunately, Levav et al.'s (16) fairly comprehensive epidemiologic study using clinical interviews failed to assess PTSD. Recent population data come from two distinct sources. The first is a number of focused surveys conducted between 2000 and 2004 with the explicit goal of gauging the population's psychological response to the *Al-Aqsa Intifada* (insurrection, in Arabic). The second study is the INHS based on a population sample of 4859 Israelis, which was conducted in 2003 to 2004; by coincidence, the period of the *Al-Aqsa Intifada*.

Bleich et al. conducted two large telephone surveys (30, 31) using two independent, randomly selected representative samples of the population. In April 2002, 19 months after the outbreak of the second *Intifada*, they surveyed 512 respondents (69% of 742 who were reached by phone). Trained lay interviewers administered questionnaires including a modified version of the Stanford Acute Stress Reaction Questionnaire (SASRQ) (32), which asks people about a range of symptoms associated with PTSD and other reactions to stress and trauma. In this survey,

16.4% of respondents reported that they had being directly exposed to a terror attack, and 37% reported having a family member or friend exposed to it. Respondents who met diagnostic criteria for PTSD according to number of symptoms reported on the SASRQ reached 9.4% (30). In a second study, conducted in May 2004 (after 44 months of ongoing terror), 501 respondents (71% of 702 who could be reached by phone) were interviewed using a similar procedure. Curiously, a somewhat lower rate of exposure to trauma was reported: 11.2%, for direct exposure and 20.2%, for exposure among friends and relatives. The rate meeting symptom criteria for PTSD in the entire sample, 9.4%, was nearly identical to that in the first study (31). The authors emphasized that most respondents remained optimistic and had high levels of confidence in their ability to cope with terrorism. In a subsequent analysis, the authors found that for the Arab Israelis, the rate of PTSD and its symptoms increased significantly in the later study (33). Risk factors for PTSD included female gender, injury and loss of income.

High estimates of current PTSD prevalence were also reported by Hobfoll *et al.* based on a sample of 1463 adults assessed in August 2004 (34). This study used the Post-Traumatic Symptoms Scale (PTS) (35), which includes *DSM-IV* symptoms of PTSD and questions about impairment. Individuals were categorized as likely to meet criteria if they had sufficient symptoms for *DSM-IV* PTSD for one month that were (a) reported to be related to exposure to terrorism and (b) accompanied by moderate-to-severe impairment. Based on these criteria 6.6% of Jews and 18.0% of Arabs were categorized as having probable PTSD. Earlier, Shalev *et al.* used the PTS to assess PTSD diagnosis and symptoms among residents of two Israeli towns, one that had direct exposure to terrorist attacks and the other that did not (36). Using non-systematic samples, they found that 10% of 167 respondents in the town selected for study with direct exposure to terrorism and 7% of 89 respondents residing in the town without direct terrorism exposure endorsed diagnostic level of PTSD symptoms. Similarly, high rates of PTSD were also reported by Gidron *et al.* (37). In small convenience samples from five Israeli cities, they found that 10.1% reported clinically significant PTSD symptoms.

The impression gathered from all of these studies is that the rate of PTSD diagnosis and symptoms seemed to have been elevated in the Israeli population during the *Al-Aqsa Intifada*. While most individuals are showing impressive resiliency in the face of an intense ongoing threat (38), the combined results of these studies indicate that a substantial minority in the population are showing the clinical effects of ongoing terror. It is thus not surprising that the prevalence of PTSD is higher than that found in more tranquil countries. However, this picture contrasts dramatically with results of the INHS study described above (20). In this study, using CIDI with face-to-face interviews, the 12-month PTSD prevalence rate was .5% and for lifetime prevalence, 1.5%. These rates were substantially lower than rates reported in the US and European countries, which were not subject to ongoing terrorism. Coincidentally, the year immediately preceding the INHS interviews (2003–2004) was a year of particularly intense terrorist activity, so these low rates are particularly interesting, while studies on resilience ever more timely.

It is likely that differences in methods account for these discrepant findings (38). Most importantly, the surveys all used inventories of symptoms, while the INHS study used a structured diagnostic interview. The CIDI was developed for populations with a different context of traumatic events; interview probes may not be sensitive to terrorism-related trauma. It is also possible that survey studies with an explicit focus on reaction to terrorism and with extensive questionnaires about exposure may prime or bias respondents to report more symptoms, compared to general mental health surveys in which these questions are embedded in a comprehensive list of different syndromes. However, it is clear that more-thorough epidemiologic studies of PTSD using diagnostic evaluations with clinically trained interviewers are needed.

❧ Panic disorder with agoraphobia

Panic disorder is characterized by recurrent waves of intense anxiety accompanied by physical symptoms leading to significant distress and behavioral change. Panic disorder is frequently accompanied by agoraphobia, which entails avoidance of situations from which exit may be difficult or embarrassing, causing subjective distress or impairment. Agoraphobia can occur with or without the full array of panic attack symptoms and can range in severity from more circumscribed to very extensive and incapacitating avoidance. In the US and in European countries, the 12-month prevalence rates range from .7 to 2.2%; and from .7% to 2.0% for panic disorders with agoraphobia without panic attacks (40, 41), respectively. Prevalence rates of panic disorder may be significantly higher in patients identified in medical settings (6). Because of the special clinical characteristics of the core feature of panic attacks, there is some controversy regarding the validity of panic disorder diagnosis based on lay interviews such as the CIDI (42).

Panic and agoraphobia in Israel

In Levav *et al.*'s study (16), the prevalence rate for 12-month panic disorder was .2% for definite RDC diagnosis and .4%, for definite/probable RDC diagnosis (combining those with definite and a probable-only panic diagnoses). These rates are significantly lower than the 1% rate in the US and other countries based on earlier *DSM-III* diagnostic criteria (43, 44). Also, in most other countries, rates of panic disorder were higher for women than for men (40), while in the Levav *et al.* study, there was no gender difference (16). It is possible that the relatively younger age of their sample (25–35 years of age) excluded some years of peak onset of panic disorder. Also, agoraphobia without panic disorder was not assessed independently in that study, as it was included under a broad category of phobic disorders.

In the more recent INHS (20), the lifetime prevalence rate of panic disorder was .8%, and the 12-month rate was .6%. Both of these were closer to those in other countries. For diagnosis of agoraphobia without panic disorder, the respective lifetime and 12-month prevalence rates were .6% and 10.4%. Age and gender were not associated with higher rates of anxiety disorders overall in that sample, but associations for panic disorder were not reported. Thus panic disorder prevalence overall appears to be low in the Israeli population compared to many other Western countries.

Panic disorders in medical settings

In the primary care study by Cwikel *et al.* cited above (23), 12-month prevalence rate for panic disorder was 7.4%. In this study, the prevalence rate was twice higher in women than in men. This rate is similar to those for panic disorder in primary care samples in other countries (6). In the emergency department sample described above (24), the prevalence rate was 2.7% for either panic or GAD diagnoses.

❧ Phobic disorders

Social phobia (or social anxiety disorder) and specific phobias are prevalent anxiety disorders, which may cause considerable distress and disability. Although specific phobias in the absence of comorbid anxiety or other disorders is not a common cause for seeking treatment, it may still cause considerable disability and interference. Social phobia often precipitates clinical attention and it has received a great deal of clinical and research attention in the past two decades (45).

Social phobia

Social phobia is defined as a persistent fear of one or more social situations that stems from concern over scrutiny or potential embarrassment. This fear leads to avoidance or of distress in the situation and causes impairment in functioning or considerable subjective distress in the individual's life. Lifetime prevalence of social phobia worldwide ranges from 4% to 10% in most studies (46), with a rate of 13% in the US in two large epidemiological studies (1, 2). However, in Asian countries, rates are substantially lower; it is unclear whether this reflects true differences, response bias or cultural factors (47). The generalized subtype of social phobia, which involves anxiety in most social situations, is associated with more severe impairment (48). Individuals with generalized social phobia make up the large majority of treated samples. Phobic disorder generally first appears during childhood or adolescence and, if left untreated, is generally chronic (46).

Social phobia in the Israeli population

Considering the high prevalence rates of social phobia and the increased attention for this disorder worldwide, it is striking how little is known about its prevalence among Israelis. In the Levav *et al.* study (16), the prevalence rate of any phobic condition including specific and agoraphobia – but not social phobia – was 2.8%. Unfortunately, the INHS (20) excluded social phobia, particularly since other countries in World Mental Health Survey (of which the INHS was part) did assess this disorder. The other recent large health Israeli study, EUROHIS (21) did not include social phobia nor did the smaller studies in medical settings (23, 24).

A small glimpse is provided by the Iancu *et al.* study (49), which was a survey of 850 military trainees aged 18 to 25 (mean age 19) in courses for military medicine or mechanics. The researchers reported that they could not obtain approval to use a structured diagnostic interview in this population; instead, they administered the self-report version of the Liebowitz Social Anxiety Scale (LSAS) (50), a widely used clinical assessment scale to identify individuals with current social phobia. Using a fairly strict cutoff of a total LSAS score of 80 (derived from a clinical group in treatment for this disorder), 4.5% of those in the sample were considered to have current clinical-level social phobia symptoms. Interestingly, this rate approximates point prevalence rates of social phobia obtained using CIDI or similar diagnostic interview methodology in some other countries. Higher level of social phobia symptoms in that study was associated with the inability to perform military tasks, the use of medication before service, psychological treatment during service and with the type of army training program (higher in mechanics vs. medic trainees). There were no associations in this sample with immigrant status or gender.

Specific phobia

Specific phobia is defined as a persistent fear of one or more non-social situations that leads to avoidance or prominent distress in this situation and causes functional impairment or considerable subjective distress in the individual's life. Phobic situations include animals (such as dogs or insects), situational (enclosed spaces), blood-injury (fear of needles), natural environment (heights or thunderstorms), and other (fear of vomiting). Lifetime prevalence rates of specific phobia worldwide range from 2% to 16% in many studies, with higher rates, 11% to 12% in the US National Comorbidity Studies (1, 2).

The study by Levav *et al.* cited above, which included questions about a few specific phobia stimuli, obtained a fairly low overall rate of any phobic disorders (2.8%) (16). Using the same sample of conscripts described in their social phobia study above, Iancu *et al.* assessed prevalence rates of specific phobias (51). Using a self-administered questionnaire that the investigators developed themselves and called the Specific Phobia Questionnaire, they asked whether subjects feared a number of commonly feared situations as well as questions about whether these fears had caused difficulties or if they felt out of control; this was meant to ascertain rates roughly consistent with *DSM-IV* criteria. The prevalence rate of phobic symptoms was 8.7%. Contrary to most studies, women in this sample reported significantly lower rates of phobic symptoms (5.0% vs. 11.0%), fewer phobic fears and lesser symptoms than men. The authors suggested that this may be due to sampling bias, as women are less likely to participate in these military programs and those who do may participate do so because they are less fearful and representative of women in the Israeli population. Most commonly reported fears were animals (7.7%), being alone (5.8%), closed spaces (5.5%), injury (5.3%) and heights (4.4%). Because this survey was conducted within a military context, it is likely that certain situations such as injury took on different meanings and did not reflect actual phobia. In addition, no reliability or validity data were reported for the scale. Finally, clinicians were not used to clarify, among other things, the level of distress that accompanied symptoms. As a result, those findings are difficult to interpret.

Overall, the epidemiologic data available for phobia disorders in Israel is very limited, making it difficult to reach any conclusions about the population with respect to these disorders.

⸹ Obsessive-compulsive disorder

Obsessive-compulsive disorder (OCD) is an anxiety disorder that involves either obsessions (intrusive and unwanted thoughts) or compulsions (overt or mental behaviors typically aimed at reducing the anxiety associated with obsessions). OCD may be the most impairing and is the most difficult to treat of all anxiety disorders. Prevalence rates of OCD in other countries generally range from 1% to 2% for lifetime prevalence and .7% to under 2% for 12-month prevalence (52). In contrast to most other anxiety disorders, OCD is generally as common in men as in women in most samples.

OCD *in the Israeli population*

Numerous Israeli clinical studies of OCD suggest that this disorder is relatively frequent. Interesting clinical and theoretical work has examined issues regarding the diagnosis and treatment of OCD within unique subgroups of the population, such as ultra-Orthodox Jews for whom many ritualized behaviors are culturally sanctioned (53). Yet, limited epidemiologic data are currently available about OCD in the Israeli population.

Levav *et al.* (16) found a six-month OCD prevalence rate of 1.2% among adults aged 25 to 34. This rate is in line with those found in other countries (52). Neither of the two recent health surveys (INHS or EUROHIS) included assessment of OCD. In the small primary care study by

Cwikel *et al.* (23), the prevalence rate of OCD, 3.9%, was substantially higher than that reported above for their population sample (16).

Two studies examined OCD among 16- to 17-year-old Israelis using national samples of military enlistees (see chapter 2). The first examined 562 adolescents undergoing premilitary screening (54). Using a two-stage evaluation, including a self-report checklist followed by an interview with a psychiatrist, 3.6% were diagnosed with current OCD, while an additional 1.2% reported obsessions or compulsions without significant impairment or distress. In a second study by the same group, 861 adolescent enlistees were evaluated using the same two-stage procedure (55). In that sample, 2.3% were diagnosed with current OCD, and 3.9% had subclinical OCD. There were no significant gender differences. As rates are not available for adult Israelis using methods similar to those used for estimating other anxiety disorder, it is difficult to interpret these high rates.

§ The impact of anxiety disorders

The epidemiologic data currently available in Israel support the serious impact of anxiety disorders on those who experience them. The INHS evaluated the severity of the CIDI-diagnosed mental disorders, including extent of disability (20). A classification of "severe" required severe impairment in at least two areas of role functioning (such as work and home). For anxiety disorders overall, 23% of those with an anxiety disorder were classified as mildly disabled; 33%, as moderately disabled; and 44%, as severely disabled. For those with panic disorder, 53% were categorized as having severe disability; for GAD, 33% were categorized as having severe disability; for agoraphobia without panic attacks, 50% were considered to have severe disability; and for PTSD, 70% were considered to have severe disability. This compares with 41% of cases with major depression classified as severe. In the EUROHIS survey, Muhsin *et al.* found that among patients with GAD, 34% had reported spending less time at work or in other activities; 56% had accomplished less than they would like; and 48% had not performed work or other tasks as carefully due to GAD (21).

All anxiety disorders in the INHS were associated with increased suicidal behaviors. Individuals who had any anxiety disorder reported 12 times the rate of suicide attempts, seven times the rate of having a suicide plan and six times the rate of suicidal ideation compared to those who did not experience an anxiety disorder (20).

§ Correlates of Anxiety Disorders

Age

In the INHS, age of onset of anxiety and mood disorders was significantly later than in the US and some other countries (20). Median age of onset was 35, and one quarter had onset before age 25. Twelve-month prevalence rates of anxiety disorders did not differ significantly across age groups, but the rate was highest among those aged 50 to 64 (Odds Ratio=1.6, 95% CI .9–2.8) with rates in other age groups fairly equal. A similar pattern was observed in the EUROHIS study for generalized anxiety disorder (21). Twelve-month prevalence was highest in those aged 40 to 59 (3.6%); somewhat lower in those 60 and above (2.7%); and lowest among those aged 21 to 39 (1.2%). However, these differences were not significant statistically. Age differences were significant in that study for those with generalized anxiety disorder in the absence of comorbid major depression. GAD in the 40–59 age group was higher than other age groups (OR = 5.7, 95% CI 1.7–19.7).

Levav *et al.* (16) assessed only a selected sample of Israeli-born young adults, so no data are available for possible age group differences. In one small study of immigrants from the former Soviet Union, those who were older had higher rates of anxiety disorders compared to younger immigrants, possibly due to increased vulnerability to the stress of immigration (56). Overall, age does not seem to be a strong factor in anxiety risk overall or for GAD, but those in middle age seemed to have a slightly higher risk.

Gender

The INHS found no statistically significant gender differences for the category any anxiety disorder (20). In the earlier Levav *et al.* study (16), gender differences in rates were found for phobic disorder (women = 4.2%; men = 1.5%, *p* < .05) but not for GAD or panic disorder. In the recent EU-ROHIS Survey (21), the association of GAD with gender was nonsignificant, with a rate of 3.1% for women and 1.9% for men (*p* = .09). In the primary care study by Cwikel *et al.* (22), panic disorder was more prevalent in women – but other anxiety disorders showed no associations with gender.

Ethnicity

Levav *et al.* (57) considered differences between Arab Israelis and Jews in the INHS. They found no statistically significant differences between the two groups in the prevalence rates of any anxiety disorders. Arab men had slightly higher prevalence than Jewish men (3.7% and 2.8%, respectively), while Arab women had slightly lower prevalence rates than Jewish women (3.0% and 3.6%, respectively). The gender differential for Arabs is less consistent with findings in other countries. However, this lack of difference needs to be understood since Arab Israelis reported significantly higher levels of general distress, measured by the General Health Questionnaire, than Jewish Israelis (57). Earlier, Levav *et al.* compared Israeli-born subjects of Ashkenazi and North African origin. They found that second-generation North Africans were more likely to have phobic disorders, but there were no differences across ethnic groups for diagnoses of GAD, panic disorder or OCD (16).

§ Help-seeking patterns with regard to anxiety disorders

In the INHS study, Levinson *et al.* (20) found that respondents with anxiety disorders were 2.5 times more likely to report seeking mental health treatment than those without anxiety disorders – a differential comparable to that for mood disorders. Among individuals with panic disorder, 57% had mental health contact in the first year of the disorder compared to 31% for GAD. By 10 years with the disorder, 72% of those with panic disorder had mental health contact compared to 64% for GAD. Muhsin *et al.* (21) found that 24% of Israelis with GAD used prescribed medications for that disorder. Eleven percent had sought psychiatric treatment, 26% had received psychological treatment, and 19% went for a medical consultation. Many more, 77%, had shared worries with family members or friends.

§ From epidemiology to mental health action

Anxiety disorders are often untreated. In Israel, an obstacle to intervention strategies is the incomplete epidemiologic data about prevalence of anxiety disorders and associated characteristics.

This situation has improved in part with the recent publication of data from the two major public health surveys cited earlier. Currently, only GAD and, perhaps, panic disorder have a sufficient epidemiological database from which to advance reasonable populations estimates and begin to examine correlates. PTSD, an anxiety disorder of great interest in the Israeli context, has not benefited from epidemiologic studies with careful clinical assessment, and prevalence estimates based on different methodologies are widely disparate. For other prevalent and potentially serious anxiety disorders such as social phobia and OCD, scarce epidemiologic data are available. Current estimates cannot be ventured based on limited impressions from selected age groups using self-report scales rather than diagnostic interviews. For disorders such as GAD and panic disorder – for which more detailed data are available – prevalence rates seem to be comparable and perhaps slightly below rates obtained in other countries.

Another implication of the current gaps in our epidemiologic knowledge is our inability to compare prevalence of anxiety disorders in Israel with rates in other countries. Such comparisons are crucial, particularly in order to gauge the impact of conditions specific to this country such as experiences with ongoing terrorism and war. Even general estimations of prevalence of "any anxiety" would be a good start. However, these estimates depend on consistent assessment of the range of anxiety disorders. For example, the World Mental Health Survey (58) recently reported that the Israeli component of the study found a rate of 5.2% for lifetime prevalence of any anxiety disorder. This is striking, as it is one of the lowest rates found in any of the numerous participating countries – for which rates ranged from 5% to 31%. This rate is misleading however, since the interview schedule used in the Israeli study excluded social and specific phobias, which are the most prevalent of all anxiety disorders in most of these countries. Many other countries assessed these disorders and included these in estimates of overall prevalence. We await more detailed epidemiological studies, including all anxiety disorder categories using clinical diagnostic interviews.

Despite the limitations, current data have built a case for action both for research, as discussed above, and for practice. Indeed, results have shown that the number of affected individuals remains quite high thus steps need to be taken to increase screening and recognition of anxiety disorders at the population level, particularly in medical settings where these disorders are highly prevalent. This, combined with broader dissemination of evidence-based treatment approaches, such as cognitive behavior therapy, would enable a higher percentage of those affected to receive optimal treatment.

❧ References

1. Kessler RC, Berglund PA, Demler O, *et al.* Lifetime prevalence and age of onset distributions of DSM-IV disorders in the National Comorbidity Survey Replication (NCS-R). *Archives of General Psychiatry* 2005; 62: 593–602.

2. Kessler RC, Angermeyer M, Anthony JC, *et al.* Lifetime prevalence and age-of-onset distributions of mental disorders in the World Health Organization's World Mental Health Survey Initiative. *World Psychiatry* 2007; 6: 168–176.

3. Kessler RC, McGonagle KA, Zhao S, *et al.* Lifetime and 12-month prevalence of DSM-III-R psychiatric disorders in the United States: results of the National Comorbidity Survey. *Archives of General Psychiatry* 1994; 51: 8–19.

4. Magee WJ, Eaton WW, Wittchen HU, *et al.* Agoraphobia, simple phobia, and social phobia in the National Comorbidity Survey. *Archives of General Psychiatry* 1996; 53: 159–168.

5. Rumsawh HJ, Raffa SD, Edelen MO, *et al.* Anxiety in middle adulthood: effects of age and time on 14-year course of panic disorder, social phobia, and generalized anxiety disorder. [online]. [cited August 2008] *Psychological Medicine* 2008.

6. Kroenke K, Spitzer RL, Williams JBW, *et al.* Anxiety disorders in primary care: prevalence, impairment, comorbidity and detection. *Annals of Internal Medicine* 2007; 146: 317–325.

7. Stein MB, Roy-Byrne PP, Craske MG, *et al.* Functional impact and health utility of anxiety disorders in primary care outpatients. *Medical Care* 2005; 43: 1164–1170.

8. Fernandez A, Haro JM, Martinez-Alonzo K, *et al.* Treatment adequacy and depressive disorders in six European countries. *British Journal of Psychiatry* 2007; 190: 172–173.

9. Wang PS, Lane M, Olfson M, *et al.* Twelve month use of mental health services in the US: results of the National Comorbidity Survey Replication (NCS-R). *Archives of General Psychiatry* 2005; 62: 629–640.

10. American Psychiatric Association. *Diagnostic and statistical manual of mental disorders – Fourth edition (DSM-IV)*. Washington, DC: American Psychiatric Press, 1994.

11. Isaac M, Janca A, Sartorius N. *ICD-10 Symptom glossary for mental disorders*. Geneva: Division of Mental Health, World Health Organization, 1994.

12. American Psychiatric Association. *Diagnostic and statistical manual of mental disorders – Third edition (DSM-III)*. Washington, DC: American Psychiatric Press, 1980.

13. Slade T, Andrews G. *DSM-IV* and *ICD-10* generalized anxiety disorder: discrepant diagnoses and associated disability. *Social Psychiatry and Psychiatric Epidemiology* 2001; 36: 45–51.

14. Hunt C, Issakidis C, Andrews G. *DSM-IV* generalized anxiety disorder in the Australian National Health Survey of Mental Health and Well-Being. *Psychological Medicine* 2002; 32: 649–659.

15. Wittchen HU. Generalized anxiety disorder: prevalence, burden and cost to society. *Depression and Anxiety* 2002, 16: 162–171.

16. Levav I, Kohn R, Dohrenwend BP, *et al.* Epidemiological study of mental disorders in a 10-year cohort of young adults in Israel. *Psychological Medicine* 1993, 23: 691–707.

17. Dohrenwend BP, Shrout PE. Toward the development of a two-stage procedure for case-identification and classification in psychiatric epidemiology. In: Simmons RG, ed. *Research and community mental health*, vol. 2. Greenwich, CT: JAI Press, 1981.

18. Endicott J, Spitzer RL. A diagnostic interview: the schedule of affective disorders and schizophrenia. *Archives of General Psychiatry* 1978; 35: 837–844.

19. Kessler RC, Ustun TB. The World Mental Health Survey Initiative Version of the World Health Organization (WHO) Composite International Diagnostic Interview (CIDI). *International Journal of Methods in Psychiatric Research* 2004; 13: 93–121.

20. Levinson D, Levav I, Bin-Nun G, *et al.* The Israel National Health Survey: new data for planners, clinicians, researchers and the public at large. *Israel Journal of Psychiatry and Related Sciences* 2007; 44: 79–80.

21. Muhsen K, Lipsitz JD, Sandalon NG, *et al.* Correlates of generalized anxiety disorder independent of co-morbidity with depression: findings form the first Israeli National Health Interview Survey 2003–2004. *Social Psychiatry and Psychiatric Epidemiology* [online]. 2008 [cited July 2008].

22. Meltzer H. Development of a common instrument for mental health. In: Nosikov A, Gudex C, eds. EUROHIS: *Developing common instruments for health surveys*. Copenhagen: IOS Press, 2003.

23. Cwikel J, Zilber N, Feinson M, *et al.* Prevalence and risk factors of threshold and sub-threshold psychiatric disorders in primary care. *Social Psychiatry and Psychiatry Epidemiology* 2008; 43: 184–191.

24. Klein E, Linn S, Colin V, *et al.* Anxiety disorders in a general emergency service in Israel. *Psychiatric Services* 1995; 46: 488–492.

25. Benyamini Y, Solomon Z. Combat stress reactions, post traumatic stress disorder, cumulative life stress, and physical health among Israeli veterans 20 years after exposure to combat. *Social Science and Medicine* 2005; 61: 1267–1277.

26. Amir M, Weisel RL. Time does not heal all wounds: quality of life and psychological distress of people who survived the Holocaust as children 55 years later. *Journal of Traumatic Stress* 2003; 16: 295–299.

27. Yehuda R, Schmeidler J, Wainberg M, *et al.* Vulnerability to post traumatic stress disorder in adult offspring of Holocaust survivors. *American Journal of Psychiatry* 1998; 155: 1163–1171.

28. Alonso J, Angermeyer MC, Bernert S, *et al.* Twelve month comorbidity patterns in Europe: results from the European Study of the Epidemiology of Mental Disorders (ESEMED) project. *Acta Psychiatrica Scandinavica* 2004; (Suppl 420): 28–37.

29. Jeon HJ, Suh T, Lee HJ, *et al.* Partial versus full PTSD in the Korean community: prevalence, duration, correlates, and dysfunctions. *Depression and Anxiety* 2007; 24: 577–585.

30. Bleich A, Glkopf M, Solomon Z. Exposure to terrorism, stress-related mental health symptoms, and coping behaviors among a nationally representative sample in Israel. *Journal of the American Medical Association* 2003; 290: 612–620.

31. Bleich A, Gelkopf M, Melamed Y, *et al.* Mental health and resiliency following 44 months of terrorism: a survey of an Israeli national representative sample. *BMC Medicine* 2006; 4: 21.

32. Cardena E, Koopman C, Classen C, *et al.* Psychometric properties of the Stanford Acute Stress Reaction Questionnaire (SASRQ). *Journal of Traumatic Stress* 2000; 13: 719–734.

33. Gelkopf M, Solomon Z, Berger R, *et al.* The mental health impact of terrorism in Israel: a repeat cross-sectional study of Arabs and Jews. *Acta Psychiatrica Scandinavica* 2008; 117: 369–380.

34. Hobfoll SE, Canetti-Nisim D, Johnson RJ, *et al.* The association of exposure, risk, and resiliency factors with PTSD among Jews and Arabs exposed to repeated acts of terrorism in Israel. *Journal of Traumatic Stress* 2008; 21: 9–21.

35. Foa EB, Tobin DF. Comparison of the PTSD Symptom Scale-Interview Version and the clinician-administered PTSD scale. *Journal of Traumatic Stress* 2000; 13: 181–191.

36. Shalev AY, Tuval R, Frenkiel-Fishman S, *et al.* Psychological responses to continuous terror: a study of two communities in Israel. *American Journal of Psychiatry* 2006; 163: 667–673.

37. Gidron Y, Kaplan Y, Velt A, *et al.* Prevalence and moderators of terror-related post traumatic stress disorders symptoms in Israeli citizens. *Israel Medical Association Journal* 2004; 6: 387–391.

38. Bannanno GA, Galea S, Bucciarelli A, *et al.* Psychological resilience after disaster: New York City in the aftermath of the September eleventh terrorist attack. *Psychological Science* 2006; 17:181–186.

39. Lipsitz JD. Misery or resiliency during four years of terror: it depends how you ask. (Submitted for publication).

40. Goodwin RD, Faravelli C, Rosi S, *et al.* The epidemiology of panic disorder and agoraphobia in Europe. *European Neuropsychopharmacology* 2005; 15: 435–443.

41. Grant BF, Hasin DS, Stinson FS, *et al.* The epidemiology of DSM-IV panic disorder and agoraphobia in the United States: results from the Epidemiologic Survey on Alcohol and Related Disorders. *Journal of Clinical Psychiatry* 2006; 67: 363–374.

42. Means-Christensen A, Sherbourne CD, Roy-Byrne P, *et al.* The Composite International Diagnostic Interview (CIDI-Auto): problems and remedies for diagnosing panic disorder. *International Journal of Methods in Psychiatric Research* 2003; 12: 167–181.

43. Canino GJ, Bird HR, Shrout PE, *et al.* The prevalence of specific psychiatric disorders in Puerto Rico. *Archives of General Psychiatry* 1987; 44: 727–735.

44. Oakley-Browne MA, Joyce PR, Wells JE, *et al.* Christchurch psychiatric epidemiology study. Part II: Six-month and other period prevalence of specific psychiatric disorders. *Australian and New Zealand Journal of Psychiatry* 1989; 23: 327–340.

45. Stein MB, Stein DJ. Social anxiety disorder. *The Lancet* 2008; 371: 1115–1125.

46. Wittchen HU, Fehm L. Epidemiology and natural course of social fears and social phobia. *Acta Psychiatrica Scandinavica* 2003; 108 (Suppl 417): 4–18.

47. Chang SC. Social anxiety (phobia) in East Asian culture. *Depression and Anxiety* 1997; 5: 115–120.

48. Brown EJ, Heimberg RG, Juster HR, Social phobia subtype and avoidant personality disorder: Effect on severity of social phobia, impairment, and outcome of cognitive behavioral treatment. *Behavior Therapy* 1995; 26: 467–486.

49. Iancu I, Levin J, Hermesh H, *et al.* Social phobia symptoms: prevalence, sociodemographic correlates, and overlap with specific phobia symptoms. *Comprehensive Psychiatry* 2006; 47: 399–405.

50. Liebowitz MR. Social phobia. *Modern problems in pharmacopsychiatry* 1987. 22: 141–173.

51. Iancu I, Levin J, Dannon PN, *et al.* Prevalence of specific phobia symptoms in an Israeli sample of young conscripts. *Journal of Anxiety Disorders* 2007; 21: 762–769.

52. Fontanelle LF, Mendlowicz MV, Versiani M. The descriptive epidemiology of obsessive-compulsive disorder. *Progress in Neuropharmacology and Biological Psychiatry* 2006; 30: 327–337.

53. Zohar AH, Goldman E, Calamary R, *et al.* Religiosity and obsessive compulsive disorder in Israel. *Behaviour Research and Therapy* 2005; 43: 857–868.

54. Zohar AH, Pauls DL, Ratzoni G, *et al.* Obsessive compulsive disorder with and without tics in an epidemiological sample of adolescents. *American Journal of Psychiatry* 1997; 154: 274–276.

55. Apter A, Fallon TJ, King RA, *et al.* Obsessive compulsive characteristics: from symptoms to syndrome. *Journal of the American Academy of Child and Adolescent Psychiatry* 1996; 35: 907–912.

56. Zilber N, Lerner Y, Eidelman R, *et al.* Depression and anxiety among Jews from the former Soviet Union five years after their immigration to Israel. *International Journal of Geriatric Psychiatry* 2001; 16: 993–999.

57. Levav I, Al-Krenawi A, Ifrah A, *et al.* Common mental disorders among Arab-Israelis: findings from the Israel National Health Survey. *Israel Journal of Psychiatry and Related Sciences* 2007; 44: 104–113.

58. Kessler RC, Angermeyer M, Anthony JC, *et al.* Lifetime prevalence and age of onset distributions of mental disorders in the World Health Organization's World Mental Health Survey Initiative. *World Psychiatry* 2007; 6: 168–176.

Chapter 13

THE EPIDEMIOLOGY OF COMBAT-INDUCED POST-TRAUMATIC STRESS DISORDER (PTSD)

Zahava Solomon and Karni Ginzburg

Israel is considered a laboratory of human stress. It is a relatively young state made up of immigrants and children of immigrants from all corners of the world and widely different cultures. Many of those who built the country came to Israel as refugees fleeing persecution in their home countries. Its national Jewish history over 2,000 years has been beset with persecution, pogroms and deportations, culminating in the Nazi Holocaust (see chapter 7).

The State of Israel was created as a national home for the Jewish people, and its establishment embodied the promise of security. This promise was kept only partially. In its 60 years of statehood, Israel has known seven full-fledged wars and innumerable acts of terror. It is no wonder that many members of the helping professions in Israel are interested in the study and treatment of trauma survivors (1). For Israeli researchers, the study of trauma-induced reactions is not merely an academic interest but carries profound personal meaning.

Over the past 26 years, with colleagues of the Israel Defense Forces (IDF) Medical Corps and Tel Aviv University, we conducted a series of studies assessing the short- and long-term psychiatric sequelae of the Yom Kippur War (1973) and the First Lebanon War (1982). We assessed the social, psychological and somatic sequelae of war – hours, days and many years after exposure. We examined the implication of a host of psychological, social, and cultural factors in the development of and recovery from war-induced psychopathology.

In this chapter, we present some of our research attesting to the heavy toll of war on soldiers, its correlates and implications for intervention. More specifically, the following six issues will be presented and discussed:

(a) The clinical manifestations and prevalence of acute psychological reactions during or shortly after exposure to war;
(b) The long-term psychological sequelae of war stress, as assessed in two cohorts: veterans of the First Lebanon War and ex-prisoners of war (POWs) of the Yom Kippur War;
(c) Repeated exposure to war stress and reactivation of previous war stress reactions;
(d) Delayed-onset post-traumatic stress disorder;

(e) Secondary traumatization of people close to traumatized individuals: spouses of traumatized veterans and traumatized veterans who are offspring of Holocaust survivors; and

(f) Effectiveness of frontline interventions in prevention of PTSD.

ꙮ On the battlefield: The stress of combat

War is the ultimate in human aggression. In addition to the destruction of life, property and culture, it often inflicts a less-visible yet deep and enduring toll in terms of psychological damage. Combatants naturally are the ones most severely hit. In constant danger themselves, they witness the injury and death of friends and enemies and are exposed to the gruesome sights and sounds of slaughter. They struggle with loneliness and isolation along with the more tangible deprivation of food, drink and sleep. The enormous destructive power of modern weapons and uncertainties of modern guerrilla warfare add to the already massive stress of war. At the same time, soldiers are expected to inflict the same brutal death and injury on the enemy – often soldiers, but at times civilians.

These stressors of the battlefield are bound to give rise to anxiety, which is a perfectly normal response to imminent threat. When experienced in moderate levels it has a functional role, as it gives rise to much-needed vigilance within the battlefield. As observed in World War II and repeatedly confirmed later on, only a small percentage of combat troops are too paralyzed by anxiety to fire their weapons during battle. The vast majority of soldiers remain psychologically intact despite the awesome destruction of modern warfare. They continue to function as soldiers, are not a danger to themselves or to their fellow comrades and do not insist on being evacuated. For most of them, the war ends when the shooting stops.

Yet, not all combatants are as fortunate. Some, eventually, succumb to the massive pressures of war. These individuals suffer acute, chronic, reactivated and/or delayed psychiatric consequences (2, 3). Man has recognized the inevitability of psychological wounds in war since biblical times. However, war-induced psychological disorders generally gain attention at the outbreak of war and immediately afterwards, with very little in the way of sustained long-term follow-up. Hence, until recently, the knowledge in this field has been quite fragmented, and lessons learned in one war were easily forgotten in the next (4). Moreover, most of the studies on the short- and long-term sequelae of combat were conducted in the US and Europe, where veterans usually return to a stable civilian society when the war ends. The Israeli reality is quite different.

After completing three years of compulsory military service, all able-bodied men (who have not been exempted from service) are required to serve in the IDF reserves until age 45. Therefore, they continue to be directly exposed to military stimuli. Thus the post-war experiences of Israeli veterans differ from those in other countries who – after the shooting stops – have none or very little exposure to military stimuli reminiscent of their war experiences. Given that the post-war recovery environment plays a substantial role in traumatized veterans' mental health, one cannot extrapolate from findings of studies conducted in other parts of the world to the Israeli veterans. This chapter brings together some of the findings of 26 years of Israeli research aimed at casting light on the immediate and long-term psychopathological toll paid by many veterans.

ꙮ Combat stress reaction

A small, but not insignificant percentage of soldiers are overwhelmed by their anxiety. They perceive the threat as intense, prolonged and uncontrollable and feel totally vulnerable and powerless. These perceptions mark the psychological breakdown known as combat stress reaction (CSR), shell shock, combat fatigue and war neurosis, among other terms. CSR occurs when a soldier is stripped of his psychological defenses and feels so overwhelmed by the threat that he (or she) becomes powerless to counteract or distance himself (or herself) from it, and is inundated by feelings of utter helplessness and anxiety. In such a state, the soldier is a danger to self and others and is no longer able to perform military duties.

Symptoms of CSR

Polymorphic and labile symptoms characterize combat stress reaction. Psychosomatic symptoms range from loss of bladder and bowel control, trembling, stuttering and vomiting to conversion reactions such as blindness and paralysis without organic cause. Cognitive symptoms include confusion, problems with perspective, memory and judgments and disorientation. In extreme cases, soldiers may not know who or where they are. The main emotional symptoms are paralyzing anxiety and deep depression, which often alternate. The behavioral symptoms are the manifestations of these emotions – great agitation on the one hand and apathy and withdrawal on the other. Some of the symptoms are quite bizarre; some victims tear off their uniform and run amok upon seeing the enemy. Others may become frozen in their tracks, refuse to shower or cling to a piece of clothing or other object. These manifestations change as rapidly as the emotional state that underlie them, and they can be quite perplexing to the observer.

These symptoms signify the soldier's total inability to continue to perform battlefield duties. With minor variations, this clinical picture has been repeatedly observed in different cultures. Nonetheless, the great variability of this reaction makes it difficult to arrive at an agreed clinical definition. Since the two leading psychiatric classification systems, the *Diagnostic and Statistical Manual of Mental Disorders – Fourth Edition* (DSM-IV) (5) and the *International Classification of Diseases – Tenth Edition* (ICD-10) (6), only recently included their formulations of acute stress reaction and acute stress disorder, armies have used a functional definition: "Combat stress reaction consists of behavior by a soldier under the conditions of combat, invariably interpreted by those around him as signaling that the soldier – although expected to be a combatant – has ceased to function as such" (7, 8).

The multiplicity and variability of symptoms, both in a single soldier and from casualty to casualty, make it very difficult to capture the elusive nature of CSR. The prevailing definition is general and functional rather than clinical. Despite its seemingly simple functional definition and sometimes bizarre manifestations, CSR is extremely difficult to identify. In the chaotic and abnormal context of the battlefield, combatants' behavior is generally disorganized and not reflective of their everyday life. Moreover, those who would make the identification of the afflicted soldiers, commanders and fellow comrades, are themselves caught up in the stress and anxiety of the situation, and their judgment is unreliable. As a result, it is assumed that the recorded prevalence of combat stress reactions is often underestimated (8).

Prevalence

The reported prevalence rates of CSR vary considerably, both within and among wars. The reported rates in World War II ranged from 10% to 48%. In the Vietnam War, rates were significantly lower, with official figures during the war at about 1.2%. In the Yom Kippur War, the official count was 10% of those wounded in action, although in some units it was as high as 70% of the wounded. In the First Lebanon War, the official figure was 23% of those wounded in action (one of every four war casualties was a psychiatric casualty). More recently, rates of only 3% CSR casualties were reported among British veterans evacuated from the battle zone in Iraq (9).

Those figures have been challenged as underestimating the extent of the problem. The growing numbers of cases of delayed PTSD following the Vietnam War led to charges of misdiagnoses, denial and underreporting. Similar charges were made with regard to the initial figures for CSR in the Yom Kippur War, in which the rate was closer to 40% of the wounded. The variation derived from the differences in identification and counting of CSR as well as from differences in the dimension of combat stress. The reported rates clearly indicate that CSR is an inevitable and common consequence of war. Today, most armies recognize it as a major source of personal loss, which can contribute to an army's defeat.

§ The aftermath of war – PTSD and comorbidities

CSR can be a transient episode for some, but for others it marks the beginning of a process of posttraumatic decline. This process has been likened to the flooding of a piece of land: When the floodwater recedes, the land re-emerges. The pre-flood water will sometimes reappear, reinforcing the feeling that any damage can be corrected. Sometimes the flood leaves behind heavy destruction, causing feelings of helplessness and loss. Such is the expression of a traumatic event.

Sometimes, when the stress recedes, the injured recover quickly, and the emotional trauma becomes a transient life episode. At other times, the trauma is accompanied by impairment that is difficult to remedy. In still other cases, there is no obvious recognizable emotional injury subsequent to the traumatic experience, only slight impairment followed by seemingly rapid recovery. In such cases, the soldier's psychological apparatus may be more vulnerable to subsequent stresses both within and without. Again the flood metaphor is helpful.

Sometimes, for the observer, it may be impossible to see the immediate harmful consequences of the flood. Later, if the area is exposed to further internal or external stressors, the structures and foundations that have been undermined by the flood will collapse.

At the end of a war, the debilitating effects of combat stress may abate in some cases. In others, profound and prolonged psychological and somatic sequelae occur in the form of PTSD and other comorbid conditions. Following up Israeli casualties of the Yom Kippur War and the First Lebanon War, we clearly demonstrated that for many traumatized soldiers, psychological breakdown on the battlefield marks the beginning of a lifetime of stress and impairment.

§ The aftermath of the First Lebanon War

The most common psychological injury of war is PTSD. Still, very few empirical investigations have assessed posttraumatic sequelae in identified CSR casualties. The results of a 20-year follow-up of all treated Israeli CSR casualties of the First Lebanon War (8, 9) revealed that 64% of identified CSR casualties suffered from PTSD one year later. At two years, the rate of PTSD decreased to 59% and then further to 40% at three years. The most interesting and perhaps surprising finding, however, was the fact that PTSD rates increased again to 53% 20 years after the war. In other words, the war does not end for many traumatized veterans, as CSR marks the beginning of a life-long vulnerability.

Combat-induced PTSD also emerges among veterans who have not sustained CSR on the battlefield. Studies we conducted of veterans who participated in the First Lebanon War but did not experience psychological breakdown on the battlefield were diagnosed with PTSD in 14% of them during the first year after the war; 22% during the second year; 11% during the third year; and 27% 20 years after the war. These figures point toward a detrimental impact of war on soldiers who survive the immediate stress of combat without visible breakdowns.

The high PTSD rates in both groups are intriguing, and the question why they are high naturally arises. Here, of course, we can only offer our speculation that the high rates may well reflect the continuing threat of war and terror in the country. All of our participants, like other Israeli men of their age, have served in the IDF reserves and could have been recalled at any point for active duty. Like all other residents, they have been repeatedly subjected to the threat of terror and continued to be bombarded by threatening military stimuli. We believe that such exposure may well have impeded the recovery of the traumatized.

The unexpected rise in PTSD rates 20 years after the war may be attributed to two main reasons. First, 20 years after the war, most veterans were in their midlife. Midlife is a particularly high-risk period for either delayed-onset or reactivated PTSD, as it entails some reduction in activity and provides an opportunity to reminisce and review one's life. This transition may force the forgotten or suppressed traumatic memories up to the foreground again (11). The second reason is implicated in the specific time the last assessment of these veterans was carried out. The study was conducted in the midst of the second *Al-Aqsa Intifada* (Arabic for insurrection), when numerous terror attacks were carried out against the population. Possibly, the vast exposure of these veterans to harsh political violence reactivated the initial trauma which they had experienced.

We paid special attention to the traumatized veterans of the control group. It is important to note that these afflicted soldiers did not seek help. It seems that many of them were not aware that they had a disorder or believed the symptoms were a natural and inevitable outcome of their horrific experiences. Others probably did realize their plight, but were reluctant to seek help. It is all too likely that these veterans with silent PTSD are a mere fraction of a much larger number of psychiatric casualties of war whose distress is similarly unidentified and untreated. In one sample, as many as one third of Vietnams veterans who suffered from PTSD 15 years after the end of the war had never sought help.

We are aware of the fact that PTSD often goes untreated. Nevertheless, in the Israeli context, the disinclination to seek treatment was surprising. Had these PTSD casualties sought help for their war-related disturbances at any IDF mental health clinic, they would have averted the very real risk of being sent back to the front (12). In the Israeli context, traumatized veterans could have also enjoyed other secondary gains had they applied for psychological help. They could also be provided not only with help to alleviate their distress but also with monetary compensation. Nevertheless, many of them refrained from seeking professional help.

We attempted to identify reasons for veterans' reluctance to seek help. We can suggest two possible explanations. One relates to the fact that the untreated group differed from the treated group qualitatively; their PTSD was less severe and less distressing than that of the treated group. Earlier studies have shown that seeking treatment for psychiatric disorders and adopting the sick role is related to symptom severity (e.g., 13). Another possible explanation is that veterans who did not identify themselves as PTSD casualties by seeking treatment were highly motivated to continue serving in the army and not motivated in obtaining the possible secondary gains. In Israel, masculine identity is very strongly associated with military service. Identifying oneself as ill may well exert a heavy price in both self-esteem and social acceptance.

Veterans who sustained a CSR have to contend with the implications of their breakdown, with the shame and the guilt of having let down their buddies and betrayed the trust placed in them by nation and family. Considering the great importance attributed to the army in Israel, their sense of failure and injury to their manhood and self-esteem must weigh heavily and contribute to their PTSD.

Psychological and somatic comorbidity

Importantly, posttraumatic residues among Israeli veterans were not limited to PTSD. Longitudinal assessment of the Lebanon War veterans indicated that, as in other cases of PTSD (e.g., 14), PTSD is unlikely to appear as a single diagnosis (15). Fully, 74% to 80% of the veterans with PTSD also endorsed comorbid anxiety or depression, or both. More specifically, one, two, and 20 years after the war, more than one-quarter of combat veterans endorsed triple comorbidity (i.e., PTSD, anxiety and depression). These rates (27% in the first and second years post war; 30% at 20-year follow-up), were higher than rates of PTSD, either by itself (10.0% in the first year, 11.0% in the second year; and 9.0% at 20-year follow-up), or comorbid with depression (1.2%–4.5%) or anxiety (2.9%–4.5%).

Examining the chronological relations among the three comorbid disorders indicated that PTSD is the core reaction to traumatic stress. That is, although many PTSD sufferers endorse either depression or anxiety or both, PTSD is more stable over time than the other two disorders. Moreover, measuring patterns of relations between PTSD, anxiety and depression over time revealed that in cases of comorbidity, depression and anxiety are secondary to PTSD. That is, PTSD predicts subsequent depression and anxiety, while suffering either from depression or from anxiety did not change the likelihood of a PTSD diagnosis in subsequent waves of measurement. Finally, comorbidity is not only a frequent phenomenon, but it also has clinical significance. At each point of time, veterans with comorbid PTSD endorsed more severe adjustment difficulties, such as problems in occupational, social, sexual and family functioning, than those with PTSD alone.

The long-term implications of war move beyond the psychological realm and into the physical realm. In various points of assessments conducted among the same veterans over 20 years (16, 17), CSR and PTSD were both found to be associated with general self-rated ill health, chronic diseases and physical symptoms, as well as greater engagement in health-related risk behaviors, such as smoking and alcohol consumption.

Many PTSD symptoms were implicated in considerable functional impairment, including problems with concentration, memory and increased irritability. These factors severely impaired work performance. Detachment, alienation, avoidance, easily aroused anger and sexual difficulties clearly impaired the functioning of husbands and fathers.

§ The aftermath of the Yom Kippur War

As stated, we also carried out a similar, longitudinal study of veterans of the Yom Kippur War 18 years later. Here, we added a third group of veterans – decorated war heroes. In contrast to the CSR casualties who failed to function under the stress of battlefield, the decorated heroes were acknowledged by the army authorities for their exceptional conduct in the frontline. Findings indicated that 37.0% of combat stress reaction causalities, 8.0% of the war heroes, and 14.0% of the controls had PTSD some time after the Yom Kippur War. Current PTSD rates 18 years after the war were 12.0% for CSR casualties, 2.0% for war heroes and 3.0% for controls (18). More than two-thirds of the CSR causalities with PTSD in the past had recovered. One may conclude that a small but significant proportion of CSR casualties were still suffering from PTSD, almost two decades later.

In this study, we also assessed a fourth group of veterans, who, in addition to their exposure to the stress of battlefield, were subjected to one of the most extreme form of traumatic stress perpetrated by human beings – ex-prisoners of war (POWs). Usually, coming on the heels of brutal combat, this situation consists of multiple, repeated and prolonged traumatic acts (19, 20). Most POWs are held in solitary confinement, at times blindfolded and handcuffed, in small and filthy cells, and they are subjected to deliberate and systematic violence, including physical torture, deprivation of basic needs and deliberate humiliation. A considerable body of empirical research on POWs has consistently found that captivity produces deep and long-lasting psychological (e.g., 21), somatic (e.g., 22) and functional harm.

In our 18-year follow-up of the Yom Kippur veterans, we found that 23.0% of the ex-POWs had PTSD some time after the war, while at 18 years after the war, the rates among this group of veterans reached 13.0%. While two-thirds of CSR casualties demonstrated a pattern of recovery over time, only half of the POWs showed this improvement. The differential recovery rate in the two groups may have reflected differences in duration and severity of stressors and/or the impact of immediate intervention and long-term adjustment.

Our initial findings were based on a retrospective assessment following 18 years of their incarceration. Most of the studies of ex-POWs at that time were similarly flawed, as they were also based on retrospective studies. Previous studies revealed considerable variability with regard to PTSD in ex-POWs, ranging between 5.0% and 88.0%. Most studies found that substantial proportions of former POWs carry their wounds with them for a very long time. Little, however, was known about the course of PTSD over those years. The literature on the longitudinal effects of war captivity offers three alternative perspectives. One is that time is a healer; as the years pass, any adverse impact of the captivity will weaken and more ex-POWs will recover partially or in full. The second view is that PTSD is a chronic ailment, in which symptoms will intensify with the passage of time, with the natural decline in the individual's physical and mental condition over time. The third view is that other than an initial decline in psychological distress relatively soon after captivity, no clear pattern is discernible. This view stresses the labile quality of PTSD and the ability of events in the individual's outer and inner life to trigger its recurrence or intensification after periods of latency or remission (23).

At the Yom Kippur War's 30th anniversary, we revisited those ex-POWs and the matched controls who we had interviewed in the past, to assess their current mental state and changes over time. The findings show that three decades after their liberation, 23.0% of former Israeli POWs still met criteria for PTSD. This percentage attests to both the resilience of 78.0% of the former POWs who did not meet PTSD criteria, and the long-lasting psychological damage of captivity for the remaining one fifth. The PTSD rate in the POWs group was around seven times the rate among the non-POWs controls.

Why the psychological damage of captivity should be so much more enduring than that of combat, which is itself pathogenic? Three main explanations maybe offered. Perhaps the simplest is the additional hardships of captivity, such as torture, humiliation and isolation. Beyond the hardships themselves, however, is the fact that they are personal. This is the second possible explanation: The threat of combat to the life and physical integrity of the soldier is a relatively impersonal threat, in that it is directed towards whoever is in the line of fire, not at any particular soldier. Thus, there is no affront to the soldier's personhood, even if he or she is injured.

The trauma of captivity, however, occurs within the relationship between the captives and their captors. The special torments of captivity are part of a planned and concerted effort to "break" particular individuals, and intentionally inflicted on them by persons they got to know and relate to on a daily basis. The third possible explanation is the doubling of the traumatic experience with captivity: For most POWs, the trauma of captivity follows the trauma of combat. Captivity thus extends the duration of the traumatic experience; further drawing on the soldier's already-depleted coping recourses. As is well known, the longer a traumatic experience lasts, the more severe the ensuing psychopathology is likely to be.

Our findings show that PTSD followed a different course among ex-POWs and combat controls. The former were 10 times more likely to experience deterioration in their psychological condition in the 12-year interval between the two assessments. Almost 20.0% of the ex-POWs, who did not meet PTSD criteria 18 years after their release occurred, met it at the 30-year mark. The ex-POWs also showed a statistically significant increase in the endorsement of each of the PTSD symptom clusters (intrusion, avoidance and hyperarousal), as well as a statistically significant increase in their endorsement of most PTSD symptoms. Among the non-POWs controls, in contrast, there was no change in the endorsement of the three symptom clusters, along with a downward trend in their endorsement of most of the individual symptoms, which reached statistical significance with regard to recurrent and intrusive recollections. These findings clearly show that time exacerbates the detrimental effects of war captivity.

The ex-POWs' deterioration, in terms of both rate and intensity of PTSD 30 years after their release, may be related to either or both, the aging process and the unremitting threat of war and terror in Israel. At our second assessment, the men were in their late 50s through early 60s. This is a high-risk time of life for both delayed-onset and reactivation of PTSD. Midlife generally entails some reduction in activity and a shift from planning to reminiscence and from occupation with current events to the review and rethinking of one's life. The altered perspective may bring forgotten or suppressed traumatic memories to the foreground.

Aging also inevitably entails many losses and exit events, from retirement through illness. Such losses may be particularly distressing for former POWs and may remind them of their misery and helplessness in captivity.

With regard to the second explanation, the second assessment took place at the height of the second *Intifada*, when suicide bombing and drive-by-shootings created marked insecurity and fear among most Israelis. These events, regularly reported on television, may also have reawakened the dormant traumatic contents among ex-POWs, by reminding them of their misery and helplessness in captivity.

✍ The effects of repeated exposure to combat

Israel's many wars have both obliged and enabled us to study the impact of recurrent combat exposure. Since most countries are fortunate enough not to call up the same soldiers to serve in repeated wars, the available literature on combat stress has little to offer on this subject. The only basis for prediction derived from studies of psychological and somatic responses to adversity in general. The vulnerability perspective (24) considers repeated exposure to stressful events to be a risk factor, since it drains a person's coping resources and thereby makes him more vulnerable. The stress inoculation perspective (25) holds that repeated stress serves as an "immunizer" in that it fosters the development of effective coping strategies and promotes adaptation. The third view, the stress resolution hypothesis, postulates that what matters is not so much the fact that a person was exposed to a particular stress, but how he coped with it. According to Block and Zautra (26), successful coping leads to a feeling of wellbeing and an increase in coping ability, while unsuccessful coping leads to increased distress and decreased coping ability.

To assess the applicability of those theories, we presented the First Lebanon War veterans a list of seven Israeli wars and, for each, asked them to indicate whether or not they had participated in the fighting and whether or not they had sustained a combat stress reaction (27). The highest CSR rates in the First Lebanon War were among soldiers who had a prior stress reaction (66.0%). Lowest rates were found among soldiers who had fought previously without stress reaction (44.0%) and, in-between, rates among soldiers with no prior war experience (57.0%). The figures suggest that the successful resolution of previous stress indeed helps soldiers to cope with subsequent battle. But they also indicate that novice soldiers are better off than those who broke down in a previous war. Although not every soldier who sustains a combat stress reaction is doomed to a second breakdown under similar circumstances, it is clear that a combat stress reaction leaves most casualties more vulnerable the second time around (24). It should be noted that only a minority of the CSR casualties go on to fight in subsequent wars. They are a select group, having been deemed fit to return to active duty by the army and displayed the personal motivation to do so. If these veterans display increased susceptibility, the others would in all likelihood be even more vulnerable.

The detrimental impact of combat becomes all the more apparent when the number of previous wars is taken into account. Among soldiers with a prior stress reaction, CSR rates in the First Lebanon War increased linearly with the number of prior war experiences: 57% after one war; 67.0% after two; and 83.0% after three. Among soldiers who had fought without a prior stress reaction, CSR rates in the First Lebanon War were curvilinear. Veterans who actively participated in one or three previous wars showed higher CSR rates (50.0% and 44.0%, respectively) than soldiers who participated in two wars (33.0%).

Taken together, these figures again show that traumatic experiences scar the individual and weaken his resistance to future stress. They also suggest that whatever the possible benefits of successful stress resolution, repeated trauma will eventually break the hardiest souls.

The reactivation of PTSD

As stated above, Titchner and Ross (28) have likened the traumatic experiences to the flooding of a piece of land. In some cases, when the water recedes, it leaves visible and massive damage. In other cases, which we may liked to the case of reactivation, the pre-flood order soon reappears, leading to the feeling that whatever damage has occurred can be rectified, but perhaps also leaving behind invisible structural flaws that make the area more vulnerable to subsequent stresses.

Reactivation of stress reactions is a well-known phenomenon. Widows have been found to have reactivated anniversary grief reactions after being reminded of their loss (29, 30). Rape victims experience a similar reactivation of their response to the original trauma when they are reminded of it (31). Holocaust survivors and American WWII veterans have reported reactivated wartime traumas in conjunction with the losses associated with aging (32, 33). Vietnam

War veterans were found to respond with reactivated symptomatology when they attended war memorials and other public ceremonies that reminded them of their combat experience (34).

Studying our own files of the First Lebanon War veterans, we found several dozen cases of reactivated or exacerbated CSR, though more have come to our attention since, as veterans with delayed-onset PTSD sought treatment. Thirty-five of these veterans were evaluated by a team of four mental health professionals (35). Our exploratory study provides further evidence of the enduring impact of combat trauma.

The cases we studied can be placed along a spectrum ranging in severity from very mild to extreme behavioral and functional disability.

Uncomplicated reactivations or classic reactivations

Twenty-three percent of veterans in question seemed to have completely recovered from their Yom Kippur-related combat reactions. They were virtually symptom-free between the wars. The first indication that all was not well came with their combat stress reactions in the First Lebanon War, which were generally precipitated by a threatening incident directly reminiscent of their Yom Kippur experience. For example, one tank driver sustained his first CSR in the Yom Kippur War when a grenade killed the entire crew members except him. His second reaction appeared years later, during the First Lebanon War, when one of the tanks in a convoy he was in sustained a similar direct hit.

The remainders of the veterans, which constitute about three-quarters of the sample, are more aptly termed "exacerbated PTSD." Here, the Yom Kippur War stress-related reactions left more visible residuals, and the veterans continued to suffer from PTSD symptoms of a greater or lesser severity. Symptoms became intensified during reserve duty, and the call-up notice to Lebanon provoked considerable anticipatory anxiety. Moreover, these men were sufficiently vulnerable for their second reactions to have been triggered by an incident unrelated to their Yom Kippur trauma and, in many cases, one that did not pose a direct or immediate danger.

The exacerbated PTSD cases can be subdivided into three groups:

(a) Heightened vulnerability:

The first group (51%) consists of men who suffered from mild, diffuse PTSD symptoms, which did not interfere with their day-to-day functioning and from heightened sensitivity to military stimuli. During reserve duty, they tended to be tense and withdrawn and to have other stress symptoms such as nausea and depression. However, so long as their tours of duty were uneventful, they functioned adequately. Their residual or subclinical PTSD developed into a full-blown syndrome when they were exposed in the First Lebanon War to a direct military threat often similar to that which had provoked their Yom Kippur War breakdown.

(b) Moderate generalized sensitivity:

These veterans showed moderate generalized sensitivity in their civilian as well as military lives (9%). They suffered from sleep disturbances, nightmares, irritability, and uncontrollable outbursts of anger, which somewhat impaired their functioning. To cope with their distress, some resorted to drugs and alcohol, others reacted with phobic responses. There were casualties, for example, who refused to ride on public buses, where terrorists might attack, others who shied away from dark places, and yet others who did

everything in their power to avoid contact with weapons, tanks, and other military accou-
trements even while they were on reserve duty. During the First Lebanon War, the men
in this group went to the front, but soon developed CSR in response to relatively minor
military stimuli, and many were discharged before they saw actual combat.

(c)   Severe generalized sensitivity:

The most seriously ill veterans (17%) suffered from severe generalized sensitivity
throughout the entire interwar period. Their PTSD dominated their lives, and their behavior was so bizarre and phobic that their still being listed in the IDF's active roster could
only be regarded as an oversight. There were men in this group who kept guns under their
beds o walked down the street while looking for places they could hide in case of a terrorist attack. For such veterans, the mere arrival of the call-up order to Lebanon brought on
an immediate and severe stress reaction. Many of them had their second stress reaction
even without seeing combat or even reaching the front.

What should be emphasized is that all casualties who had reactivated or exacerbated
PTSD from the First Lebanon War had made great efforts to function effectively in the
nine years following the first reaction and had been generally successful. By selectively
utilizing such psychological coping mechanisms as regression, denial and avoidance,
most of them married, started families and kept their jobs – some of them even did very
well professionally. None were hospitalized. All continued to serve in the reserves, despite
the fact that their symptoms were intensified in the presence of military stimuli. Many hid
their symptoms from their friends, families and army commanders.

Their second reactions revealed the psychological damage that the first breakdowns had
created – and deepened it. In general, there were more symptoms following the second reaction than the first, and the symptoms were more intense and debilitating (36). Furthermore,
even though some soldiers participated in battle after a CSR episode without further breakdown, the detrimental effects of the earlier episode were still detectable a decade later.

Delayed-onset PTSD following combat

The manifestations of trauma sometimes are – or seem to be –delayed. Such delayed onset occurs
when an individual appears at first to respond adaptively to traumatic stress but then develops
psychopathology after an asymptomatic latency period. As pointed out earlier, the number of
psychiatric casualties stemming from the First Lebanon War tripled in the years that followed
(37). This issue raised a considerable amount of interest and become controversial over the years.
PTSD may follow several possible courses over time. These courses vary as a function of symptom chronicity and/or time of onset. According to DSM-IV-R (38), the onset of PTSD is considered delayed when symptoms first appear at least six months following the traumatic event.

Delayed-onset PTSD was described among WWII veterans (32) and Holocaust survivors
(39), and also reported among victims of other types of traumatic events, such as motor vehicle
accidents (40), natural disasters (41), incest (42) and combat (43). Yet, it first became a major
issue after the Vietnam War (44). In the years that followed, the steadily growing numbers
of Vietnam veterans with war-related stress reactions became a major public health problem.

Still, for many years, there has been substantial medico-legal debate regarding the validity of this phenomenon. Delayed-onset PTSD is often regarded with suspicion. Some have argued that seemingly new cases of PTSD are actually manifestations of malingering (45). Others

(e.g., 46), have claimed that in many cases, it is not the disorder that is delayed, but rather the seeking of mental help or the identification of posttraumatic symptoms. At the same time, the validity of this diagnosis has been questioned as some clinicians claim that malingering, factitious symptoms, drug abuse and pre-combat psychopathology were mistakenly diagnosed as delayed PTSD (47).

In examining the files of a large group of veterans who sought treatment between six months and five years after the end of the First Lebanon War, we aimed (a) to determine which of them were truly cases of delayed PTSD; (b) to examine the course of delayed PTSD; and (c) to assess the rates of delayed PTSD among those veterans.

Four IDF clinicians assessed 150 files selected at random. Assessment of the files revealed several categories of combat-related PTSD (48):

(a) Exacerbation of subclinical PTSD:

Thirty-three percent of the sample experienced exacerbation of subclinical PTSD. These were traumatized on the front in 1982 and suffered uninterruptedly from residual PTSD symptoms until accumulated tensions or exposure to subsequent adversity – either military or civilian – resulted in a full-blown PTSD syndrome. Reserve duty was the major military trigger. Other triggers included life events such as marriage or the birth of a child. The veterans in this group sought professional help when their subclinical symptoms were exacerbated.

(b) Delayed help-seeking for chronic PTSD:

Forty percent of the sample was already suffering from chronic PTSD, which DSM defines as PTSD having six month or longer duration, when they sought psychiatric help. Unlike soldiers in the previous group who had mild, subclinical symptoms throughout the so-called latency period, these subjects suffered from the full-blown syndrome right from around the time they fought in Lebanon. They sought help not when an external trigger exacerbated their symptoms, but when they could no longer bear their distress – usually during reserve duty. These soldiers invested much into containing a relatively severe and disruptive disturbance before they finally gave up trying to cope with it on their own. Not infrequently, a family member who could no longer endure the pressure that the casualty symptoms created initiated treatment.

(c) Delayed-onset PTSD:

Ten percent of our sample, consisting of soldiers who came through the First Lebanon War with no apparent psychiatric disturbance, were asymptomatic and functioned well during and for some time after the war. The latency period lasted from several weeks to several years but following exposure to stressful stimuli, their latent disturbance surfaced and they applied for treatment.

(d) Other psychiatric disorders:

Four percent of the soldiers had mild, transient pre-war psychiatric disturbances. They sought help for underlying problems, which were either triggered or colored by their war experiences, but which were not originally induced by military events.

In general, our results show that the genuinely delayed-onset PTSD was quite rare in our sample, five years after the First Lebanon War. At that time, by far the most prevalent phenomenon was delayed help-seeking for ongoing combat-induced disorders of various degrees of severity. We have offered several explanations (48): The relatively low rates of delayed PTSD could be attributed to the relatively short follow-up period. It is possible (we argued then) that a longer follow-up of our sample would have revealed a higher rate of delayed PTSD following a longer latency period and aging. We also had noted then that our findings should be considered in light of the social context in which the traumatic event took place. In Vietnam, where the highest rates of delayed PTSD were reported, the wide use of drugs and alcohol may have masked immediate CSR. In Lebanon, however, substance abuse was relatively rare among Israeli troops and did not play a significant role in masking or delaying distress (48).

Another major contextual difference has to do with the dead and consolation of the bereaved, which bring comfort and relief that help survivors to complete the mourning process. In the Holocaust, the Nazis pointedly disallowed these rites as part of their overall attempt to dehumanize their victims. In Vietnam, the rites of morning were not observed on account of the relatively long tours of duty and the fact that the soldiers were far from home. Possibly, the unresolved grief of both Holocaust survivors and Vietnam veterans contributed to their subsequent vulnerability, and exposure to reminders of their loss or other stressors would more readily trigger a reaction at a later date (49).

In Lebanon, on the other hand, as in other Israeli wars, the IDF made a concerted and well-organized effort to encourage the full mourning process. Every possible effort was made to evacuate the dead and bring them to burial in Israel. Soldiers knew that nobody would be abandoned on the battlefield, and a special rabbinical unit was in charge of seeing to the proper rites. Soldiers were routinely given leave to attend funerals and pay consolation calls. The ability to mourn and work through their grief may have made the soldiers in our sample less vulnerable to the triggering effect of subsequent stressors.

From a different point of view, Horowitz and Solomon (50) suggested that delayed onset may occur only after circumstances allow the individual to sufficiently relax his defenses. Both the long, one-year tour of duty in Vietnam and the constant, unalleviated danger of the Holocaust made it extremely unsafe for people to let down their guard during the events themselves. In Israel, on the other hand, wars are fought very close to home, allowing soldiers frequent home leaves. Conceivably, the warmth, comfort and security of the family enabled repressed traumatic contents to surface while soldiers were still serving in the army.

Furthermore, for the veterans of the First Lebanon War, homecoming at the end of the war was by and large a positive event. Although public opinion about the war was divided, the men who fought in it were welcomed back with respect and affection as brave sons who had risked their lives in defense of the country. For both, Vietnam veterans and Holocaust survivors, however, the post-war periods continued to be traumatic. Not only were Vietnam veterans denied a hero's welcome, but also they came back to a country that had disowned them and to mass anti-war demonstrations. As for the Holocaust survivors, they had no place to go back to. Most of their families and communities had been exterminated, their homes and property were appropriated, and the communities where they had once lived were hostile and rejecting. Then, when many of them finally immigrated to new communities, they had to overcome substantial adversity in rebuilding their lives. In both these groups, the accumulation of stress may have eventually led to the delayed onset of their latent disorder. When we revisited the veterans of the Lebanon War 20 years thereafter, the issue of delayed onset and/or delayed help-seeking was of great importance to us.

We set out to examine both the prevalence and correlates of this subtype of PTSD. In the most recent of these studies (51), rates of delayed-PTSD were examined among veterans from the First Lebanon War, two decades later. The rate of soldiers diagnosed with delayed-onset PTSD was approximately 16%,a relatively high rate compared to other studies (e.g., 10). In our series of studies we have also explored the correlates of delayed PTSD attempting to cast light on the underlying mechanisms responsible for the delay in symptom onset. We found that veterans with delayed-onset PTSD had more personal (i.e., locus of control) and social (i.e., social support) resources available to them compared to veterans who experienced a more acute reaction. In addition, veterans with delayed-onset PTSD presented a less severe clinical picture than those with "regular," non-delayed PTSD (e.g., 51, 52). Thus, it may be concluded from these findings that the delay in symptom onset among these Israeli veterans is a sign of relative psychological resilience.

§ Secondary traumatization: Indirect victims of war stress

The deleterious effects of trauma are not limited to those who are exposed and afflicted by it directly. Psychic trauma may be likened to a stone thrown into a pool of water; it creates ripples that reach not only the victims themselves, but also those who are close to them. The terms secondary traumatization and vicarious victimization have been used to indicate that others who come into close contact with a trauma victim may experience considerable emotional upset and may themselves become indirect victims of the trauma. Many debilitating PTSD symptoms are not only stressful for the casualty, but may also have a direct bearing on close friends and relatives.

The detrimental effects of war trauma on significant others have been observed among spouses and children of both US veterans who served in Vietnam and Israeli veterans who fought in the First Lebanon War. Especially relevant are the symptoms that interfere with the veterans' intimate relationships. These include reduced involvement, psychic numbing, diminished interest, sexual difficulties and feelings of detachment, alienation and estrangement. PTSD veterans are often withdrawn, edgy and depressed and may have unpredictable outbursts of rage and aggression. These severe symptoms may have considerable implications for the well-being of the veterans' family members.

Moreover, in a recent assessment conducted by the Ministry of Defense, traumatized veterans were asked how they perceive their role as parents and to what extent they feel they can provide the care and support their children need (53). The results were distressing: 80.0% reported moderate-to-severe verbal violence toward their children; 26.0% reported severe physical violence; and 32.0% reported severe difficulties meeting physical needs. Only 56.0% reported meeting emotional needs. These findings sketch the large circle of the infliction of war trauma.

Previous studies have reported that the wives of PTSD veterans are subjected to increased physical violence and emotional and verbal abuse. The pressure on the relationship drives many to report feeling that they are about to have a nervous breakdown. We investigated the issues of secondary traumatization in two studies. The first assessed the impact of combatants' war-induced PTSD on their spouses, and the second examined secondary traumatization among soldiers whose parents were Holocaust survivors.

Secondary traumatization among spouses of traumatized veterans
We have conducted a series of studies on secondary traumatization on spouses of CSR veterans of the First Lebanon War and ex-POWs of the Yom Kippur War. The studies on wives of veterans of the Lebanon War, conducted in the late 1980s, have shown that both CSR and PTSD were associated with increased psychiatric symptoms, impairment in self-esteem, loneliness and less satisfaction in afflicted veterans' marital and/or family relations. Marital relations appear to be particularly vulnerable to the negative consequences of traumatic combat experiences, with distress levels in wives virtually paralleling those of their husbands. Among PTSD casualties, those with antecedent CSR suffered from more intense and severe PTSD than those without a history of CSR. Spouses of PTSD and CSR veterans reported greater levels of distress and impairment than those whose husbands suffered from PTSD but had not broken down on the battlefield (54).

As part of our longitudinal study of ex-POWs we have also assessed the effects of war captivity and subsequent PTSD on their wives' mental health and marital adjustment. The first aim of this study was to compare the distress of wives of former POWs with PTSD, of former POWs without PTSD and non-PTSD combat veterans who had never been in captivity. The comparison was undertaken to determine the degree to which their distress was rooted in their husband's captivity and/or in his PTSD. The findings in all three measures of secondary traumatization that we employed show that the highest levels of distress were recognized by wives of former POWs with PTSD. They had significantly more PTSD symptoms, more general psychiatric symptomatology and poorer marital adjustment than the wives in the other two groups. We also found that wives of PTSD veterans reported more frequent physical aggression than wives of both former POWs without PTSD and non-PTSD combat controls (55).

The findings of both studies are consistent with the concept of secondary traumatization; the veterans' immersion in traumatic memories and withdrawal from everyday life can leave their spouses feeling isolated and vulnerable to various psychological and somatic conditions. In some cases, it has been reported that wives "identify so strongly with their men that they have authentically internalized their partners' stressor imagery." Thus, they begin to experience the same feelings and mimic the behavior of their traumatized husbands.

These findings clearly lent empirical support to the concept of secondary traumatization in spouses of the traumatized. They were also consistent with Galovski and Lyons (56) observation that secondary traumatization is a multifaceted phenomenon, manifested both in specific PTSD symptoms and non-trauma-specific forms of distress.

A second aim of this study was to examine potential contributors to the distress of the spouses, beyond the husband's PTSD and captivity. The findings showed that both the man's aggression and the spouse's self disclosure played a role in her level of distress. More specifically, the more frequent her husband's aggression, the more PTSD and general psychiatric symptoms the wife reported. The more frequent his verbal aggression, the lower her marital satisfaction.

Self-disclosure has a direct contribution to distress and marital adjustment and a moderating effect on wife's PTSD and distress. The salutary effect of their self-disclosure is particularly striking in view of the fact that there was no significant difference in the self-disclosure levels of the women in the study groups. It seems that women in the PTSD group who remained open and sharing seem to have been able to compensate somewhat for their husband's emotional deficiencies (57).

These and other studies indicate that the negative changes in personality and behavior experienced by combat veterans with CSR and/or PTSD often have a direct impact on the feelings and behavior of those around them, particularly their spouses. If this suffering is ignored, it will likely exacerbate the veterans' own distress. Conversely, treatment that does not focus exclusively on the individual veteran but also includes his spouse is likely to assist the veteran's own recovery.

The transgenerational impact of PTSD

The long arm of posttraumatic sequelae stretches across what one would prefer to be a natural barrier, way into the next generation. We assessed the possible implication of a trauma experienced in the Holocaust by many of the parents of the present generation of IDF soldiers (58).

In general, the clinical literature suggests that many Holocaust survivors suffer from residual PTSD seven decades after their ordeal and that many of their children suffer from a milder version of similar symptoms (e.g., 59, 60). Offspring of Holocaust survivors have been found to be highly anxious, manifest excessive narcissistic vulnerability, survival guilt and more than usual ambivalence about aggression (e.g., 60, 61). On the battlefield, these traits might exacerbate the anxiety and fear that all soldiers experience and at the same time create more than the usual qualms about killing to secure ones survival.

To examine the effects of the Holocaust on PTSD in the second generation, we asked our CSR subjects of the First Lebanon War to indicate whether either of their parents were Holocaust survivors and compared their PTSD rates following the war. The comparison confirms that trans-generational impact of trauma. Two and three years after their participation in that war, second-generation CSR casualties had significantly higher rates of PTSD than casualties without Holocaust background – 73.0% vs. 52.0% two years later, and 64.0% vs. 39.0% three years later, respectively. In other words, the PTSD of the soldiers who were second-generation survivors lasted longer.

There was also a difference in the number of PTSD symptoms. For the first two years after their psychological breakdown, the two groups had more or less the same average number of symptoms. Between the second and third years, however, that number declined among non-second generation casualties but not among those whose parents had gone through the Holocaust. In other words, while the PTSD in many veterans was abating by the third year, in second-generation Holocaust survivors it remained as severe as it had been at its onset.

The exposure to combat by the second generation seems to have unmasked a latent vulnerability that was not activated by more run-of-the-mill life events. Their PTSD is suggestive of reactivated PTSD, which is also more severe and enduring than a first episode. A CSR breakdown may entail a particular meaning for children of survivors. Almost every CSR casualty feels that he has failed, and most suffer agonies of shame and reduced self-esteem. But among the second generation, the sense of failure cuts deeper. Children of Holocaust survivors see themselves, in their uniforms and bearing their weapons, as guardians and protectors of their parents. Second-generation Israelis were meant by Holocaust survivors to "undo" the damage that the Holocaust had brought to their lives. The magnitude of this expectation probably intensifies the failure implicit in a combat breakdown. Finally, recovery might be impeded by the excess of secondary gains derived from the survivor's parents' well-documented overprotection (61). It is also possible that survivor parents may have unconsciously discouraged the recovery of their CSR sons so as to avert the very real danger of their being sent back to the front.

❦ From epidemiology to mental health action: Frontline interventions

Our studies, as well as many other studies of other populations, have consistently shown that the development of PTSD is often an evolving process. It extends over time through a series of stages ranging from relatively contained distress to severe disability. In its acute phase, combat stress reaction entails considerable distress and shame, yet its damage is limited to military functioning. In its chronic phase, PTSD may be likened to cancer; it metastasizes and is associated with higher rates of psychiatric and somatic comorbidities, substance abuse, impaired functioning and higher mortality risk (e.g., 8). As the disease evolves over time, pathological changes and debilitating comorbidity may become fixed and irreversible. Therefore, it may be useful to delay therapeutic interventions to emphasize preventive rather than curative medicine. Prevention means thwarting the development of the disorder and/or taking measures to halt or slow its progress. The acute phase of combat stress reaction is often seen as a window of opportunity. Since World War I, many armies have adopted frontline treatment as the preferred intervention for combat stress reaction.

This treatment was conceptualized first by Salmon (62) and subsequently by Artis (63) in terms of three principles:

(a) proximity – treatment is administered close to the front line;
(b) immediacy – treatment is administered close in time to the symptoms' onset; and
(c) expectancy – the expectation is that the soldier will recover rapidly and resume functioning.

Treatment focuses on replenishing depleted physiological needs by satisfying the need for sleep, food and drink for a few days in relative safety. This psychiatric first aid is time limited, lasting between 48 and 72 hours. The aim is to provide temporary relief from harsh battle stressors, enable the exhausted and distressed soldier to regain some control and decrease hyperarousal. During this period, minimal psychiatric intervention is carried out, allowing the soldier opportunities to ventilate his recent traumatic experiences. Following this brief intervention, the soldier is expected to be able to resume his military assignment. Frontline treatment is a simple intervention, believed to be potent in reducing both the loss of manpower and long-term psychiatric sequelae (64, 65). It has thus been adopted by many armies. At the same time it is a controversial intervention as some of its critics claim that military considerations of conservation of manpower outweigh mental health considerations. As a result, they argued, traumatized soldiers are unduly re-exposed and retraumatized by war.

Unfortunately, despite the extensive use of frontline treatment, empirical evidence regarding its effectiveness is quite limited. The battlefields are clearly not conducive to systematic research. Randomized clinical trials of traumatized soldiers are clearly not feasible. It is thus not surprising that the existing studies suffer from many methodological limitations that severely hinder their generalization. At the time of the First Lebanon War, the available data were derived mostly from personal impressions of the medical staff and from small-scale surveys (7). Time frames for follow-up were generally unspecified. Outcome measures focused only on rates of return to unit, apparently ignoring psychiatric symptoms (e.g., 66, 67). Since frontline treatment was the recommended treatment for combat stress reactions in the IDF in 1982, we believed that the empirical assessment of its effectiveness was imperative.

The IDF officially implemented frontline treatment for the first time, during the First

Lebanon War. As noted above, conditions of war usually do not provide a setting conducive to the systematic study of treatment effectiveness; however, the unique circumstances in Lebanon did allow for such an assessment. During this war, CSR casualties were treated either by the frontline method or in civilian facilities at the rear. The location and type of treatment were determined by logistic constraints. Because frontline and civilian services were geographically close, transfer time was negligible.

As a natural quasi-experimental design, coupled with careful documentation, these circumstances enabled us to evaluate the effectiveness of frontline treatment empirically. We assessed the contribution of each of the three frontline treatment principles – proximity, immediacy and expectancy – to two outcome measures, a return to the military unit and the presence of PTSD. Return to unit represented a concern for manpower loss; the presence of PTSD determined the existence of long-term psychiatric sequelae. The assessment of this intervention effectiveness was carried out at two points of time: The first assessment in 1983, one year after the war (68), and the second one in 2002, about 20 years after the war (69). In both assessments, frontline treatment was found to be highly effective. Both one year and 20 years after the war, traumatized soldiers who received frontline treatment had lower rates of posttraumatic and psychiatric symptoms, experienced less loneliness and reported better social functioning than similarly traumatized soldiers who did not receive frontline treatment. In addition, a cumulative effect of the application of frontline treatment principles (i.e., immediacy, expectancy and proximity) was documented: the more principles applied, the stronger the effect on psychiatric outcomes. Return to unit also had a strong association with all three treatment principles.

Combat stress reaction, often followed by a lifetime of posttraumatic decline, is the psychological toll that some soldiers pay for the proclivity of humans for war. The price is high, and it is also inevitable. There is no way men can kill and maim, see their friends killed and maimed and fear being killed or maimed themselves without at least some of them breaking down. To date, PTSD is the only psychiatric disorder that directly follows exposure to a recognized traumatic stressor. The most severe form of PTSD results from combat. The best way to prevent combat-induced psychopathology is to stop making war. As we human beings have not been able to do so, all we have left to fall back on is our ability to learn and understand. More thorough and systematic research on PTSD can increase our knowledge that could help the traumatized. Increased awareness of their flight may open our hearts to these men and chip away the denial that blinds us to their sufferings.

❧ References

1. Breznitz, S., ed. *Stress in Israel.* New York: Van Nostrand Reinhold, 1983.
2. Grinker R, Spiegel JP. *Men under stress.* New York: McGraw-Hill, 1945.
3. Figley CR. *Stress disorders among Vietnam veterans: theory, research, and treatment.* New York: Brunner/Mazel, 1978.
4. Mangelsdorff AD. Lessons learned and forgotten: the need for prevention and mental health interventions in disaster preparedness. *Journal of Community Psychology* 1985; 13: 239–257.
5. American Psychiatric Association. *Diagnostic and statistical manual of mental disorders – Fourth edition.* Washington, DC: American Psychiatric Association, 1994.
6. World Health Organization. *International classification of diseases – Tenth edition (ICD-10).* Geneva: World Health Organization, 1990.
7. Kormos HR. The nature of combat stress. In: Figley CR, ed. *Stress disorders among Vietnam veterans: theory, research and treatment.* New York: Brunner/Mazel, 1978.
8. Solomon Z. *Combat stress reaction: the enduring toll of war.* New York: Praeger, 1993.
9. Turner MA, Kiernan MD, McKechanie AG, *et al.* Acute military psychiatric casualties from the war in Iraq. *British Journal of Psychiatry* 2005; 186: 476–479.

10. Solomon Z, Mikulincer M. Trajectories of PTSD: a 20-year longitudinal study. *American Journal of Psychiatry* 2006; 163: 659–666.

11. Hertz DG. Trauma and nostalgia: new aspects on the coping of aging Holocaust survivors. *Israel Journal of Psychiatry and Related Sciences* 1990; 27: 189–198.

12. Solomon Z. The effect of combat-related post-traumatic stress disorder on the family. *Psychiatry* 1988; 5: 323–329.

13. Nadler A. Personal characteristics and help-seeking. In: Fisher JD, Nadler A, De Paulo BM, eds. *New directions in helping: help-seeking.* Vol. 2. New York: Academic Press, 1983.

14. Kulka RA, Schlenger WE, Fairbank JA, *et al. Trauma and the Vietnam War generation: report of findings from the National Vietnam Veterans Readjustment Study.* New York: Brunner/Mazel, 1990.

15. Ginzburg K, Ein-Dor T, Solomon Z. Comorbidity of posttraumatic stress disorder, anxiety and depression: a 20-year longitudinal study of war veterans. (Submitted for publication).

16. Ohry A, Solomon Z, Neria Y, *et al.* The aftermath of captivity: an 18-year follow-up of Israeli ex-POWs. *Behavioral Medicine* 1994; 20: 27–33.

17. Benyamini Y, Solomon Z. Combat stress reactions, post-traumatic stress disorder, cumulative life stress, and physical health among Israeli veterans twenty years after exposure to combat. *Social Science and Medicine* 2005; 61: 1267–127.

18. Dekel R, Solomon Z, Ginzburg K, *et al.* Combat exposure, wartime performance, and long-term adjustment among combatants. *Military Psychology* 2003; 15: 117–132.

19. Herman JL. *Trauma and recovery.* New York: Basic Books, 1992.

20. Hunter EJ. The Vietnam prisoner of war experience. In: Wilson JP, Raphael B., eds. *International handbook of traumatic stress syndromes.* New York: Plenum Press, 1993.

21. Ursano RJ, Rundell JR, Fragala RM, *et al.* The prisoner of war. In: Ursano RJ, Norwood AE, eds. *Emotional aftermath of the Persian Gulf War.* Washington, DC: American Psychiatric Press, 1966.

22. Engdahl BE, Harkness AR, Eberly RE, *et al.* Structural models of captivity trauma, resilience and trauma response among former prisoners of war 20 to 40 years after release. *Social Psychiatry and Psychiatric Epidemiology* 1993; 28: 109–115.

23. Zeiss RA, Dickman HR. PTSD 40 years later: incidence and person-situation correlates in former POWs. *Journal of Clinical Psychology* 1989; 45: 80–87.

24. Coleman JC, Butcher JN, Carson RC. *Abnormal psychology and modern life.* Glenview, IL: Scott, Foresman, 1980.

25. Epstein S. Natural healing processes of the mind: II. Graded stress inoculation as an inherent coping mechanism. In: Meichenbaum D, Jaremko M, eds. *Stress prevention and management: a cognitive behavioral approach.* New York: Plenum, 1983.

26. Block M, Zautra AJ. Satisfaction and distress in the community: a test of the effects of life events. *American Journal of Community Psychology* 1981; 9: 165–180.

27. Solomon Z, Mikulincer M, Jakob BR. Exposure to recurrent combat stress: combat stress reaction among Israeli soldiers in the 1982 Lebanon War. *Psychological Medicine* 1987; 17: 433–440.

28. Titchener JL, Ross WO. Acute or chronic stress as determinants of behavior, character and neuroses. In: Arieti S, Brody EB, eds. *Adult clinical psychiatry: American handbook of psychiatry.* New York: Basic Books, 1974.

29. Lindemann E. Symptomatology and management of acute grief. *American Journal of Psychiatry* 1944; 101: 141–148.

30. Weiner A, Gerber I, Baltin D, *et al.* The process and phenomenology of bereavement. In: Schoenberg B, Gerber I, Wiener AM, *et al.,* eds. *Bereavement: its psychological aspects.* New York: Columbia University Press, 1975.

31. Burgess AW, Holmstrom CC. Rape trauma syndrome. *American Journal of Psychiatry* 1974; 131: 981–986.

32, Archibald HC, Tuddenham RO. Persistent stress reaction after combat. *Archives of General Psychiatry* 1965; 12: 475–481.

33. Christenson RM, Walker JL, Ross DR, *et al.* Reactivation of traumatic conflicts. *American Journal of Psychiatry* 1981; 138: 984–985.

34. Faltus F, Sirota A, Parsons J, *et al.* Exacerbations of post-traumatic stress disorder symptomatology in Vietnam veterans. *Military Medicine* 1986; 151: 648–649.

35. Solomon Z, Garb R, Bleich A, *et al.* Reactivation of combat-related post traumatic stress disorder. *American Journal of Psychiatry* 1987; 144: 51–55.

36. Solomon Z, Oppenheimer B, Elizur Y, *et al.* Trauma deepens trauma: the consequences of recurrent combat stress reaction. *Israel Journal of Psychiatry and Related Disciplines* 1990; 27: 233–241.

37. Solomon Z, Zinger Y, Blumenfeld A. Clinical characteristics of delayed and immediate onset combat-induced PTSD. *Military Medicine* 1995; 160: 425–430.

38. American Psychiatric Association. *Diagnostic and statistical manual of mental disorders – Fourth edition. Text revision.* Washington, DC: American Psychiatric Association, 2000.

39. Chodoff P. Late effects of the concentration camp syndrome. *Archives of General Psychiatry* 1963; 8: 323–333.

40. Mayou R, Bryant B, Duthrie R. Psychiatric consequences of road traffic accidents. *British Medical Journal* 1993; 307: 647–651.

41. Green BL, Lindy JD, Grace MC, *et al.* Buffalo creek survivors in the second decade: stability of stress symptoms. *American Journal of Orthopsychiatry* 1990; 60: 43–54.

42. Green AH, Coupe P, Fernandez R, *et al.* Incest revisited: delayed post-traumatic stress disorder in mothers following the sexual abuse of their children. *Child Abuse & Neglect* 1995; 19: 1275–1282.

43. Nitto MM. 2001. An investigation of factors contributing to delays in the onset of PTSD among Vietnam veterans. PhD diss., University of Hartford, CT.

44. Laufer RS, Gallops MS, Frey-Wouters E. War stress and trauma: the Vietnam veteran experience. *Journal of Health and Social Behavior* 1984; 25: 65–85.

45. Smith DW, Frueh BC. Compensation seeking, comorbidity, and apparent exaggeration of PTSD symptoms among Vietnam combat veterans. *Psychological Assessment* 1996; 8: 3–6.

46. Pary R, Turns DM, Tobias CR. A case of delayed recognition of posttraumatic stress disorder. Letter to the Editor. *American Journal of Psychiatry* 1986; 143: 941.

47. Sparr L, Pankratz LS. Factitious posttraumatic stress disorder. *American Journal of Psychiatry* 1983; 140: 1016–1019.

48. Solomon Z, Kotler M, Shalev A, *et al*. Delayed onset PTSD among Israeli veterans of the 1982 Lebanon War. *Psychiatry* 1989; 52: 428–436.

49. Krystal H. *Massive psychic trauma*. New York: International Universities Press, 1968.

50. Horowitz MJ, Solomon GF. A prediction of delayed stress response syndromes in Vietnam veterans. *Journal of Social Issues* 1975; 31: 67–80.

51. Bryant RA, Harvey AG. Delayed-onset posttraumatic stress disorder: a prospective evaluation. *Australian and New Zealand Journal of Psychiatry* 2002; 36: 205–209.

52. Solomon Z, Mikulincer M, Waysman M, *et al*. Delayed and immediate onset posttraumatic stress disorder. 1. Differential clinical characteristics. *Social Psychiatry and Psychiatric Epidemiology* 1991; 26: 1–7.

53. Dekel R, Solomon Z, Bleich A. Psychosocial disability following combat-induced PTSD. In: Bleich A, and Solomon Z, eds. *Mental disability*. Tel Aviv: Ministry of Defense, 2002 (Hebrew).

54. Solomon Z, Waysman M, Belkin R, *et al*. Marital relations and combat stress reaction: the wives' perspective. *Journal of Marriage and the Family* 1992; 54: 316–326.

55. Dekel R, Solomon Z. Marital relations among former POWs: contribution of PTSD, aggression and sexual satisfaction. *Journal of Family Psychology* 2006; 20: 709–712.

56. Galovski T, Lyons JA. Psychological sequelae of combat violence: a review of the impact of PTSD on the veteran's family and possible interventions. *Aggression and Violent Behavior* 2004; 9: 477–501.

57. Dekel R, Solomon Z. Secondary traumatization among wives of Israeli POWs: the role of POWs' distress. *Social Psychiatry and Psychiatric Epidemiology* 2006; 41: 27–33.

58. Solomon Z, Kotler M, Mikulincer M. Combat related post-traumatic stress disorder among second generation Holocaust survivors: preliminary findings. *American Journal of Psychiatry* 1988; 145: 865–868.

59. Bergman M, Jucovy ME. *Generations of the Holocaust*. New York: Basic Books, 1982.

60. Danieli Y. Families of survivors of the Nazi Holocaust: some long and short term effects. In: Milgram N, ed. *Psychological stress and adjustment in time of war and peace*. Washington, DC: Hemisphere Publication Corporation, 1961.

61. Barocas H, Barocas C. Wounds of the fathers: the next generation of Holocaust victims. *International Review of Psychoanalysis* 1979; 5: 331–341.

62. Salmon TW. The war neuroses and their lessons. *New York State Journal of Medicine* 1917; 51: 993–994.

63. Artis KL. Human behavior under stress – from combat to social psychiatry. *Military Medicine* 1963; 128: 1011–1015.

64. Mullians WS, Glass AJ. *Neuropsychiatry in World War II*. Vol. 2, *Overseas theatres*. Washington, DC: Medical Department, US Army, 1973.

65. Spiegel J. Psychiatric observations in the Tunisian campaign. *American Journal of Orthopsychiatry* 1944; 14: 381–385.

66. Glass AJ. Effectiveness of forward treatment. *Bulletin of the US Army Medical Department* 1947; 7: 1034–1041.

67. Kardiner A. *War stress and neurotic illness*. New York: Hoeber, 1947.

68. Solomon Z, Benbenishty R. The role of proximity, immediacy, and expectancy in frontline treatment of combat stress reaction among Israelis in the Lebanon War. *American Journal of Psychiatry* 1986; 143: 613–617.

69. Solomon Z, Shklar R, Mikulincer M. Front line treatment of combat stress reaction: a 20-year longitudinal evaluation. *American Journal of Psychiatry* 2005; 162: 2309–2314.

Chapter 14

The epidemiology of schizophrenic disorders in Israel

Ari A. Gershon and Mark Weiser

Israeli researchers have made important contributions to our knowledge of the epidemiology of schizophrenic disorders. The combination of several factors has made those contributions possible. Some of them are unique, among them:

(a) Factors resulting from the demographic constitution of the country:

Much of the population (about 80%) consists of Jewish immigrants or their descendents from discrete ethnic backgrounds that are easily traced. The historic socioeconomic gaps among these ethnic groups, while constituting a major challenge to social equality, have also presented opportunities for epidemiologic research on the link between mental illness and socioeconomic factors (1).

(b) Factors resulting from war stressors:

The different wars in which Israel has been engaged have provided an opportunity to study the effects of major and temporally discrete stressors (2).

(c) Factors resulting from Israel's different social contexts:

Researchers have taken advantage of the different child-rearing environments (e.g., kibbutz children's house vs. urban family) to investigate the role of childhood environmental factors in mental illness (3).

(d) Factors resulting from the existence of population databases:

The availability of data from population-spanning registries maintained by both the government and the military has been a major resource for research. These databases include psychiatric, cognitive, behavioral, social, and medical measures of adolescents collected by the Israel Defense Forces' (IDF) Draft Board Registry, see e.g., (4); data on psychiatric hospitalizations kept by the national Psychiatric Case Registry (PCR) (4); other medical registries (5); and demographic data from the Population Registry. The availability of these datasets has made possible historical-prospective studies and others with long follow-up times.

✿ Scope of this review

This chapter reviews Israeli contributions in several areas of the epidemiology of schizophrenic disorders. First, we look at two prospective studies with long-term follow-up designed to study children at genetic risk for schizophrenia and other psychiatric disorders. These studies investigated the role of inborn and environmental factors as risk factors (3, 6–13). Then we review data from studies designed to examine whether the over-representation of individuals with schizophrenia among those of low socioeconomic status (SES) is a cause or a consequence of illness and/or an illness diathesis (1, 14–16). This latter effort included a study of two ethnically distinct populations using a population-based birth cohort that was directly screened for mental illness. We then review studies of another birth cohort that examined both environmental and biological risk factors for schizophrenia (17–21). Some of these studies and the ones reviewed in the following sections made extensive use of the PCR and other databases (2, 4, 5, 22–29). The cross-linking of these databases with each other or with other sources of information – often in cross-sectional designs – has shed light on a variety of aspects of schizophrenia. Lastly, we discuss a subset of these database-crossing studies, many from our own group (30–49). These studies took advantage of population-based data on adolescents from the Israeli Draft Board Registry. These data have made possible a series of historical-prospective and case-control studies that shed light, among other things, on the pre-morbid characteristics of those that would later develop schizophrenia as well as factors that increase the odds of suffering from schizophrenia (and related conditions). These studies, along with some of the long-term prospective studies, identified a variety of neurocognitive and psychosocial characteristics of the pre-morbid state.

Israel has also made important contributions to the genetic epidemiology of schizophrenia; for examples of studies see chapter 15.

✿ The Israeli High-Risk Study

The Israeli High-Risk Study is a prospective study comparing children reared in a kibbutz setting with children raised in towns; it was designed to study the influence of genetic and environmental factors on the development of schizophrenia (6). The original sample consisted of 100 subjects aged 8 to 14 years (M age 11) and included four groups: a kibbutz index group of 25 children who grew up in a kibbutz and whose parents had schizophrenia; a kibbutz control group of 25 of their classmates whose parents were healthy; a town index group of 25 children of parents with schizophrenia growing up in an urban environment, and a town control group consisting of 25 of their classmates whose parents were healthy (7). Subjects were, on average, born in 1956; they were examined at three different periods: 1968 to 1971, 1973 to 1977, and 1981 (6). At the 1981 follow-up point, 90 of the 99 surviving subjects were examined using the Schedule for Affective Disorders and Schizophrenia-Lifetime (SADS-L), the Social Adjustment Scale and the Wechsler Adult Intelligence Scale. *The Diagnostic and Statistical Manual of Mental Disorders – Third Edition (DSM-III)* diagnoses derived from the SADS-L show significantly greater psychopathology in the kibbutz index group than in each other group as assessed by chi-squared analysis (table 1). Separate statistical assessments of schizophrenia or schizophrenia spectrum diagnoses were not presented. The authors suggested that these results might represent an interaction of a diathesis and the kibbutz-rearing condition in generating illness (3).

Table 1. Psychopathology of subjects by rearing setting and parental condition

Diagnostic category	Kibbutz index	Town index	Kibbutz controls	Town controls	Total N
	23	23	23	21	90
Schizophrenia	3	2	0	0	5
Other schizophrenia spectrum	3	1	0	0	4
Major affective disorders	5	1	0	0	6
Minor affective disorders	4	0	1	0	5
Other	1	3	2	1	7
Total diagnoses	16	7	3	1	27
No diagnosis	7	16	20	20	63

(Reproduced with permission)

Results in table 1 are shown according to *DSM-III* derived from a *SADS-L* interview. Chi-squared analysis showed no significant differences in the incidences of psychiatric diagnoses between the two control and two town groups. ANOVA revealed significant effects due to rearing location ($p < .01$) and group ($p < .0001$), as well as an interaction between these two effects ($p < .04$). However, specific analyses for schizophrenia were not reported (3).

Another objective of this study was an attempt to identify differences between the index and control groups at the initial examination as these might prove predictors of illness. Two types of measures were reported. The first were objective measures including neurological "soft" signs (asymmetries, motor coordination, perception, perceptual-motor integration and auditory-visual integration); arithmetic; and scores on tests for mirror-drawing, distractibility, perceptual closure and information detection. Subjective measures included results from interviews with subjects, parents and teachers, clinical observations and sociometric scores. The authors detected a pattern of inter-correlations among clinical subjective measures of pathology, and among objective measures – with only one set of significant cross-correlations between the two types of measures. The presence of neurological "soft" signs tended to correlate with both clinically and objectively measured psychopathology. Cluster analysis revealed three groups of subjects – a small group of nine index and one control subjects who performed poorly on both clinical and objective measures; a larger cluster, of 28 index and 10 control subjects who showed clinical but not objective pathology; and a third group, including 39 controls and only 12 index subjects, who functioned relatively well on both types of measures. Index subjects tended to show more consistent psychopathology across both clinical-subjective and objective examinations than controls. The authors hypothesized that these results reflect underlying deficits in attention, motor function, and perceptual-motor integration in offspring of persons with schizophrenia (10).

Published results based on study results up to the 1981 observation point of the study have been criticized on methodological grounds (50, 51). These include the criticism that the selection of probands with schizophrenia was done according to older diagnostic criteria and thus might not meet later diagnostic criteria for schizophrenia. Also, several relevant dimensions (e.g., the course of the assumed schizophrenic process, family variables, life circumstances and psychosocial factors) were not taken into account. Furthermore, the attribution of differences between kibbutz and town children in the nature and severity of particular psychopathologies cannot be decisively ascribed to the differences in the social framework and childrearing practices in the kibbutz vs. town environments as other intra-family variables may also have been present (50). Also, it has been suggested that the psychological and cognitive differences between the kibbutz and town groups were small and unconvincing (51). In addition to taking issue with some of the specific criticisms (e.g., pointing out that the psychiatrists who diagnosed the probands at the time did not share the US tendency of that period to overdiagnose schizophrenia). One study investigator pointed out that some of the issues raised are not relevant to the goals and design of the study (52). While some of the methodological criticisms are appropriate – and even if one accepts that the probands of the study subjects might have been misdiagnosed (at least with reference to later diagnostic criteria) – two of the main findings of this study still hold interest and resonate with later data, which will be discussed below. First, the increased rates of psychopathology across diagnostic categories in the children of parents with major mental illness (even if the exact nature of the illness was misdiagnosed) remained firm. This and later work showing that non-psychotic diagnoses are risks for developing schizophrenia (37, 41) both support the notion of endo-phenotypes that cross rigid diagnostic/phenotypic boundaries (53). Second, the analysis of neurological soft signs, subjective and sociometric measures and their clustering contribute to the search for endo-phenotypes, again even if there are questions about diagnostic criteria.

A second round of reports on this sample was published in 1995 reflecting data from evaluations conducted when the subjects had reached their early 30s as well as some previously unreported earlier data (54). In one study (8), 84 of the 100 original subjects were reexamined. New information was obtained on another three. Where new data were unavailable, observations from the previous time-point (1981) were used. Index subjects were more likely than controls to suffer from non-schizophrenia spectrum disorders (Fisher's exact one tail $p = .006$). Schizophrenia was found only among index subjects, but this trend did not quite reach significance (Fisher's exact one tail $p = .059$) (table 2). In this analysis, no effect of kibbutz vs. town rearing on the development of schizophrenic illness was detected.

However, the kibbutz index group was more likely to develop major affective disorders. The authors suggested that this might represent an effect of the stresses of adolescence and individuation in the kibbutz environment, but might also represent greater comfort among kibbutz-reared individuals in acknowledging distress, a kind of reporting bias (8).

Table 2. Psychopathology of subjects on extended follow-up. Adapted from (8)

Lifetime diagnoses by 1991	Kibbutz index	Town index	Kibbutz controls	Town controls	Total N
	25	25	24	24	98
Schizophrenia	2	2	0	0	4
Major affective disorders	6	1	2	1	10
Minor affective disorders	2	5	4	4	15
Anxiety disorders	3	1	0	1	5
Personality disorders	3	5	1	1	10
Other	1	1	0	0	2
Total diagnoses	17	15	7	7	46
No diagnosis	8	10	17	17	52

(Reproduced with permission)

Lifetime diagnoses by 1991 are presented in table 2. Schizophrenia was found only among index subjects, but this was not quite significant (Fisher's exact one tail $p = .059$). Index subjects were more likely to suffer from non-schizophrenia spectrum disorders (Fisher's exact one tail $p = .006$). Kibbutz index subjects were significantly more likely than town index subjects to have a major affective disorder (Fisher's exact one tail $p = .049$).

Another study was based on 63 subjects from the Israeli High-Risk Study, as well as 31 normal controls and 17 patients with schizophrenia from the US who had been tested in the context of other protocols and chosen to closely match the Israeli cohort. It explored cognitive measures which might differentiate between patients with schizophrenia, index subjects (offspring of parents with schizophrenia) and controls. The results suggested that: (a) attention skills of the adult children of a parent with schizophrenia fall between those of schizophrenia patients and controls, and (b) that measures of sustained attention as well as the ability to focus and execute provided the best discrimination among groups. Furthermore, post-hoc analyses of data collected in childhood and adolescence revealed that low scores on a digit-cancellation test at age 11 – but not at age 17 – predicted which of the children at genetic risk would develop schizophrenia spectrum disorders at ages 26 and 32 (54). Another study looked at a subjective psychological measure thought to be related to the development of psychopathology – the belief in internal vs. external control of reinforcement (often referred to as locus of control (LOC). Subjects underwent an interview and questionnaire measuring LOC in the second phase of the study as adolescents. During phases 3 and 4, approximately eight and 15 years later, the subjects were psychiatrically assessed; 56 of them repeated the LOC questionnaire. Chi-squared analysis suggested that whereas adolescent mental health is the best predictor of general mental health, adolescent LOC is the better predictor of schizophrenia and major affective disorders ($p < .05$ for each) (7). Similarly, analysis of anxiety measures performed at age 16 showed that those subjects who would receive a schizophrenia spectrum diagnosis 10 years later had higher ratings on two anxiety scales. Non-diagnosed index subjects also had significantly higher anxiety ratings than the non-diagnosed controls (9).

§ The Jerusalem Infant Development Study (JIDS)

The JIDS was designed in response to findings of congenital neurointegrative deficits that appear in persons destined to suffer from schizophrenia (12). This led to the notion that hereditary neurointegrative deficits might represent a genetically determined vulnerability to schizophrenia. The initiators of the JIDS asked whether these deficits could be identified in infancy, whether they were specific to schizophrenia and whether they related to genetic causes or perinatal insults. They surmised that replication of similar findings from other populations would bolster support for a genetic model of the transmission of schizophrenia. In today's conceptualizations, they suspected that neuro-cognitive deficits might represent a target endophenotype for detecting a genetic schizophrenia diathesis.

To address these questions, the investigators recruited couples between the years 1973 to 1976 from the Jerusalem Municipality's pre- and perinatal care clinics. Of the 54 couples recruited, 17 had a member suffering from schizophrenia; 6 from an affective disorder; 13 from a personality disorder; and 18 had no mental illness. The no-mental-illness group was demographically similar to the all of the groups with psychopathology taken together. Diagnoses of 54 women and 44 husbands were confirmed by the Current and Past Psychopathology Scale

(55). Fifty-eight of the 67 infants born in the study period were assessed clinically and using a neonatal behavioral scale during the first two weeks of life, followed by scales of development and temperament at four-month intervals in the first year of life, and subsequently by family interviews between ages one to four. The study found a subgroup of 13 infants born to patients with schizophrenia who repeatedly performed poorly in motor and sensorimotor areas of functioning during their first year of life. No consistently poor performers were detected in the other groups. These infants were especially vulnerable to external insults, and many had low to low-normal birth weights. The authors suggested that these infants may have a genetically determined neurointegrative deficit (12).

The JIDS children were followed through school age and adolescence. In 1985, when the children were between 7.7 and 13.8 years old (*M* age, 10.3), 45 of them were recruited for a follow-up examination. Forty-four percent of the offspring of patients with schizophrenia (11 of 25 subjects) showed impaired neurobehavioral functioning in perceptual-cognitive and motor areas. Male subjects were overrepresented in this poorly functioning group. A stable subgroup (6 of 15) of the offspring of patients with schizophrenia showed impaired function during infancy and school age. None of the offspring of parents without schizophrenia showed impaired function during both age periods. While most of the poorly functioning children with parents with schizophrenia showed perceptual-cognitive and motor signs, only perceptual-cognitive signs were strongly linked to parental diagnosis and dysfunction during infancy. Motor signs, but not cognitive signs, were related to pregnancy and birth complications. These findings provide further support to the schizotaxia hypothesis that some neuro-integrative deficits may reflect vulnerability to schizophrenia and that these deficits are clearly apparent at school age, long before the onset of illness. However, these signs are not exclusive to schizophrenic illness, although they occur with a greater prevalence in this group (13).

In 1992, another follow-up study was conducted when the children had reached a mean age of 17.6. Sixty-five adolescents participated, including 40 from the original group and another 25 of their siblings observed from school age. They were administered a neurological and neuropsychiatric test battery. Adolescents with poor neurobehavioral functioning were identified from composites of motor and cognitive-attentional variables. A disproportionate number of offspring of parents with schizophrenia (42%; 10/24) – and especially male offspring of schizophrenic parents (73%; 8/11) showed poor neurobehavioral functioning relative to offspring of parents who did not suffer from schizophrenia (22%; 9/41). Adolescent offspring of parents with schizophrenia who exhibited poor neurobehavioral functioning had also been poorly functioning at earlier ages and had poor psychological adjustment as adolescents. All four offspring of parents with schizophrenia who received schizophrenia spectrum diagnoses had, by the time they reached adolescence, showed a pattern of poor neurobehavioral functioning across developmental periods. The authors argued that this supports the hypothesis that individuals at genetic risk for schizophrenia may display lifelong neurobehavioral signs that are indicators of vulnerability to schizophrenia (11).

Between 1992 and 1996, the social adjustment of an expanded JIDS sample was also measured – as poor social adjustment is a core characteristic of schizophrenic illness and may also be an indicator of genetic vulnerability to schizophrenia in young people who are at genetic risk. The sample consisted of 27 Israeli adolescents with a parent with schizophrenia, 29 adolescents with no mentally-ill parent, and 30 adolescents with a parent who suffered from other mental illness. This group included 31 families from the original JIDS sample. An additional 24 families were recruited during the adolescent follow-up of the JIDS sample to increase the power of the sample for addressing questions not requiring longitudinal study. Multiple domains of social adjustment were measured using the Social Adjustment Inventory for Children and Adolescents (56) and the Youth Self-Report (57). Teenage children of a parent with schizophrenia showed poor peer engagement, particularly in relationships with the opposite sex, and social problems characterized by immaturity and unpopularity with peers. These social adjustment difficulties in youths at risk for schizophrenia could not be attributed solely to the presence of early-onset mental disorders, although problems were greater in those with disorders in the schizophrenia spectrum. Young people whose parents had other disorders showed different patterns of social maladjustment characterized by difficult, conflict-laden relationships with peers and family. The authors concluded that adolescents at risk for schizophrenia have social deficits that extend beyond early-onset psychopathology and that these deficits might reflect vulnerability to schizophrenic disorder (58).

❦ Social function in schizophrenia and the social selection vs. causation hypotheses

A limited cross-sectional community study in Jerusalem tested the relationship between psychiatric illness, patient status, and social functioning. This study (15) sought to distinguish between two possibilities – a universal hypothesis that the presence of a psychiatric disorder is accompanied by disability independently of treatment status and a patient-specific hypothesis that the disorder is accompanied by disability only in cases who acquire the status of patients. This was tested by looking at symptom and social functioning scales of the Psychiatric Epidemiology Research Interview (PERI) (59) in a sample of 205 adults from the general population and 204 psychiatric patients. There were 62 patients with schizophrenia in the patient sample. The group with schizophrenia had the highest level of correlation between different social function scores when compared with the patient sample as a whole and the community sample. However, owing to the lack of a group of individuals with schizophrenia in the community sample, it was not possible to test whether this correlation was due to patient status or illness (15).

One of the most stable observations in epidemiological psychiatry is the relationship between psychiatric illness and low socioeconomic status (SES). Two types of explanation have been posited for this observation: One is social causation, that low SES has a causal relationship with mental illness. A second explanation is one of social selection or downward drift. This posits downward social mobility among the ill and/or the genetically predisposed.

Several, increasingly sophisticated attempts have been made to address this question in Israel. These studies took advantage of a socioeconomic division in Israel: Jews of European or American origin traditionally tended to be socioeconomically advantaged as compared to those of North African or Asian origin. This allowed investigators to use ethnicity as a surrogate marker for SES. They also used level of education as a proxy for actual SES. In the first study, the PCR was probed for all first hospitalizations during a 13-month period beginning in July 1971. Patients older than 14 who were members of one of the Jewish ethnic groups included in the study and who were diagnosed with a schizophrenia spectrum disorder were considered. In addition, a subset of males aged 15–24 diagnosed with schizophrenia was separately considered. The sample included 205 patients of European or American ancestry and 170 of North

African or Asian origin. They found that the crude rate of schizophrenia spectrum disorders was higher in the disadvantaged ethnic group, though not among the less educated males – which they interpreted as supporting social causation. Among males age 15 to 24 with more narrowly defined schizophrenia, however, the rates were higher in the advantaged ethnic group. The authors argued that this supports a social selection model (16). However, a statistical analysis of the differences between the different groups and their significances was not presented.

This question was next addressed by a study of all 509 first admissions of Jewish Israelis to a Jerusalem mental hospital between 1970 and 1974. Selected patients were aged 15 and over and had been hospitalized with a diagnosis of schizophrenia spectrum disorders. In this study, diagnoses were confirmed by chart review, and then the patients were categorized by whether they belonged to an advantaged or disadvantaged ethnic group and by level of education, a proxy for SES. The investigators found that age-adjusted rates of schizophrenia-spectrum disorders were higher among the less educated within each ethnic category, that the ratio of lower to higher education was greater for the ethnically advantaged groups, and that the incidence of schizophrenia spectrum disorders was higher among the less educated segment of the ethnically advantaged groups than of the disadvantaged groups. These results pointed toward social selection rather than causation (14).

Several years later, a population-based approach to this same question using a birth cohort sample and a quasi-experimental design provided more robust evidence (1). In 1982 and 1983, a sample was selected from among all Israeli-born Jews between 1949 and 1958 (N = 350,689.) Those with Central or Eastern European (a traditionally advantaged group in Israel) or North African (a traditionally disadvantaged group) parents (estimated N = 177,000) were considered. This was done as ethnic status cannot be the effect of a disorder because it is present at birth, whereas socioeconomic status depends on educational and occupational attainment. In the experimental portion of the study, a sample of 19,000 individuals was drawn from this population and pre-screened. From among these, 4914 persons were examined using a two-stage procedure: PERI (59) for screening and SADS-I, for Israel (an expanded SADS-L psychiatric interview) (60) to diagnose psychiatric illness. This second phase of the study included intensive follow-up of all those who were screened positive for psychiatric disorders, as well as a control group of 18.0% who were screened negative (N = 2741.) Because SES and ethnic status are confounded in the population, the highly educated members of the disadvantaged, North African group and less educated members of the advantaged European group were oversampled. This study found a significantly higher rate of schizophrenia among the Israeli-born individuals of European ancestry after controlling for SES (logistic regression results: b = 1.34, SE = .55, z = 2.42, p < .05; adjusted odds ratio = 3.8) (table 3). In the same sample, they reported no statistically significant ethnic difference in the base rates of schizophrenia in the two ethnic groups. The authors interpreted this result to mean that the significantly higher European rates of schizophrenia with SES controlled are not due to a stronger genetic predisposition to schizophrenia in this ethnic group, but rather to how persons predisposed to or affected by schizophrenia are sorted into different SES groups. (Additionally, a significant gender difference was noted, possibly due to the relative youthfulness of the sample.) These results suggest that social selection is more important than social causation for the etiology of schizophrenia. This result contrasted with results suggesting that social causation was more important for depression in women and for antisocial personality and substance use disorders in men.

Table 3. Diagnostic results for schizophrenia in second-stage clinical interviews; current prevalence of schizophrenia is listed by education, gender and ethnic background (1)

Education	Israeli born of European origin (N = 1197)		Israeli born of North African origin (N = 1544)	
	Men (n = 602)	Women (n = 595)	Men (n = 852)	Women (n = 692)
Not high school graduate	4.18%	.84%	1.91%	.00%
High school graduate	.29%	.39%	.17%	.00%
College graduate	.00%	.39%	.00%	.00%

(Reproduced with permission)

Another paper based on the same birth cohort sample reported that the six month prevalence of schizophrenia (at the definite level of diagnosis) was .69% (60).

§ The Jerusalem Perinatal Study (JPS)

The JPS is a population-based study of all births in the greater Jerusalem area between 1964 and 1976. The cohort consisted of 89,722 infants who survived the first year of life (18). It includes demographic information from birth certificates, obstetric and pediatric data, as well as interviews with some mothers (20). Since that time, members of the cohort have reached the typical age range for the onset of schizophrenia. Several studies have cross-linked JPS data with later data from the nation-wide Psychiatric Case Register (PCR) (17, 18, 21). This research strategy has provided several interesting findings.

One finding confirmed that advanced paternal age carries increased risk for schizophrenia in the offspring. The authors noted that while this finding had been made, previous reports suffered from methodological problems and did not all agree. In this Israeli study, data on 87,907 individuals born in Jerusalem were cross-linked to the PCR. Of the 1337 cohort members admitted to psychiatric units before 1998, 658 were diagnosed as having schizophrenia and related non-affective psychoses. Compared with offspring of fathers younger than 25 years, the relative risk (RR) of schizophrenia increased in each 5-year age group, reaching 2.0 (95% CI 1.2–3.5) and 3.0 (95% CI 1.6–5.5) in offspring of men aged 45 to 49 and 50 years or more, respectively (figure 1).

Figure 1. Estimated cumulative incidence and percentage of offspring estimated to have onset of schizophrenia by age 34 years displayed by categories of paternal age. The numbers above the bars show the proportion of offspring who were estimated to have onset of schizophrenia by age 34 (18).

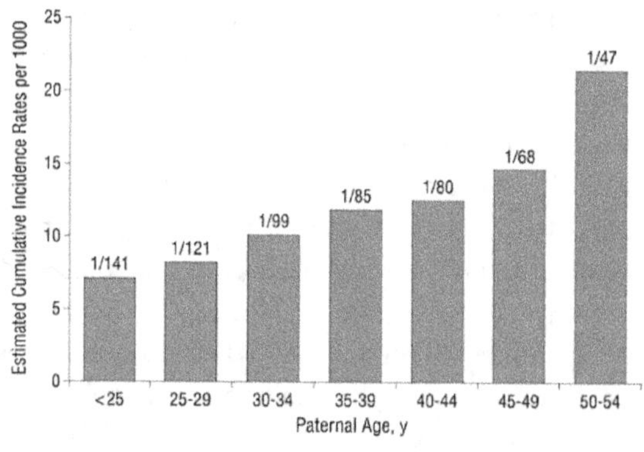

(Reproduced with permission)

The same was not true of other psychiatric disorders. The mother's age showed no significant effect after adjusting for paternal age (18). This large population-based sample using prospectively acquired data represents a significant methodological advance over previous work in the field, since it enabled teasing apart various potential risk factors from each other even when they confer relatively low relative risks. For example, one study investigated a sub-cohort of 11,015 individuals, including 104 with schizophrenia, from this sample. The authors asked whether household crowding was associated with the risk of schizophrenia. Offspring of mothers who during pregnancy resided in a household with five or more individuals had a RR of 1.5 (95% CI .99–2.2), $p = .05$) to develop schizophrenia, compared to those whose mother resided with four or fewer individuals. However, when adjusted for paternal age, the RR was reduced to 1.2 (95% CI .8–1.8), $p = .46$. Thus, household crowding during pregnancy did not significantly impact the risk of developing schizophrenia (17).

Similarly, the JPS sample was used to address the relationship between socioeconomic status (SES) and schizophrenia. This was done both on the individual and community level. In this study, a part of the original JPS sample that excluded those with missing SES data or who had died before age 14 was used. The sample included 68,794 persons. After linking this sample to the PCR in order to identify whoever was later hospitalized with a diagnosis of schizophrenia, several factors that increased the odds of becoming affected by schizophrenia were identified. They found that children of parents with 13 years or more education were less likely to suffer from schizophrenia than children of parents with 0 to 8 years of education. This was true whether the father's education level (OR $= 1.2$, $p < .0001$) or the mother's (OR $= 1.1$, $p < .001$) was considered. Lower occupational status of fathers was similarly identified as a risk (OR $= 1.3$, $p < .05$). In addition to factors related to subjects' families, there was also an effect of a community factor. Living in a residential area with poorer SES (OR $= 1.3$, $p = .01$) also increased the odds of later schizophrenia (21). In addition, the JPS sample has been used to address phenomena thought to be related to schizophrenia. For example, it has been suggested that schizophrenia and low IQ might share risk factors. It has even been suggested that shared risk factors might represent some mechanistic relationship. Work with the JPS cohort that took advantage of information obtained from the draft board database has shown independent effects of maternal and paternal age on the IQ scores of offspring, even when controlled for multiple possible confounding factors such as the other parent's age, parental education, social class, gender and birth order, birth weight and birth complications (19). The PCR database has also been used to assess more biological environmental risks. For example, one study examined the risk of schizophrenia in the children of dry cleaners as one of the solvents used in dry cleaning –tetrachloroethylene – is neurotoxic and thus suspected of playing a role in schizophrenia. Out of 144 offspring whose parents were dry cleaners, four developed schizophrenia. This reflects a significantly increased incidence of schizophrenia in this population (RR $= 3.4$, 95% CI 1.3–9.2, $p = .01$) (20).

Modifiers of risk

The PCR has been used to study several potential modifiers of risk factors for schizophrenia. For example, previous studies had suggested that there are differences in incidence and prevalence rates of schizophrenia between immigrants and nonimmigrants, and that there are differences in age of onset of the disorder that may be related to the country of origin. The reasons for these differences are unclear. With Israel's high proportion of immigrants, the PCR presented an opportunity to address these issues. A study of 10,902 first psychiatric hospital admissions over the age of 14 showed that immigrants were older at time of first hospitalization than the native born, with considerable variations by countries of origin. However, Israeli-born children of immigrants and patients with native-born parents were of similar age upon first hospitalization. Males were younger at first hospitalization than females. The results suggest that immigration may have a delaying effect on age of first admission and support previous findings regarding gender differences in age of onset (25).

A similar 14-year sample from the PCR that included 9081 nonforensic patients with schizophrenia examined the impact of involuntary first psychiatric hospitalization on subsequent admissions. (In Israel, involuntary admissions require impairment in judgment, which almost invariably means psychosis, as well as a threat to the patient or others as a result of this impairment). While an involuntary first admission, 12.9% of the sample, increased the odds of a subsequent involuntary admission by 4.1 times in females and 3.4 times in males, it was not related to the total number of psychiatric admissions over a mean follow-up time of 9.6 ± 4.1 years (22).

The course of schizophrenia

A more recent study revisited a question originally raised by Kraepelin: What is the course of schizophrenia? The investigators followed a group of 6,865 patients that represented all first admissions for schizophrenia in Israel over a 9-year period. They followed re-admission rates for this sample over 10 years, using the number of days spent hospitalized as a marker of the course of illness.

Cluster analysis identified three groups: The first group was smallest and consisted of 324 (5.4%) patients regarded as having a deteriorating course as they consistently spent more days in hospital, with the exception of the final year. The second group of 764 (12.8%) patients improved, spending fewer days in hospital over the follow-up period. The third and largest group was characterized by an initial improvement followed by a period of relative stability (n = 4,902, 81.8%). The investigators concluded that most patients with schizophrenia followed an improving course after their first admission (29).

Another classic observation revisited by this research team was whether earlier age of onset and being male confer a poorer course of schizophrenia. All first admissions for schizophrenia in the PCR from 1978 to 1992 were followed through 1996 (N = 12,071). Cutoff ages for different groups of patients were determined empirically. Of patients younger than 17 at first admission, 82.5% were admitted more than once. This decreased for subsequent age groups to 73.5% (18–28); 69.4% (29–31); 62.9% (32–45); and 50.8% (over 45). Men had an earlier first admission than women. Irrespective of gender, the relationship between age at first admission and later hospitalization was linear (26).

Stability of diagnosis

Another study examined the stability of psychiatric diagnoses among all 2998 patients who were admitted to a psychiatric hospital for the first time in 1989. Diagnoses on admission and discharge were compared across a variety of disorders. A diagnosis of schizophrenia or other non-organic psychosis was made in 26.3% of patients and was stable on first discharge 74.2% of the time (23). A longer-term study using PCR hospitalization data from 1983 to 1990 covering 4,570 hospitalizations of 2,220 patients showed similar results. A schizophrenia diagnosis on first admission was stable to the last discharge 73.0% of the time (29).

Rehospitalization rates by type of antipsychotics

Another use of the PCR has been to study the intersection of clinical and epidemiological data. One study addressed a clinical question with significant public health implications. The study compared the re-hospitalization rates of all patients with schizophrenia discharged from psychiatric wards in 1998 while being treated with risperidone, olanzapine, or conventional antipsychotics. Survival analysis over a 24-month follow-up period showed that 67% of the 268 risperidone-treated patients and 69% of the 313 olanzapine-treated patients remained in the community, as compared to 52% of the 458 patients treated with conventional antipsychotics.

Importantly, patients were treated under naturalistic conditions and followed up by the investigators only with respect to readmission. This confirmed previous studies' results that the overall effectiveness of risperidone and olanzapine were not very different, and offered evidence that these drugs were more effective in preventing re-hospitalization than conventional antipsychotic drugs (28). The same group also examined data from the PCR and a national survey of psychiatrists to examine national prescribing habits for risperidone and olanzapine. The estimated the mean daily dose of risperidone was about one-third that of olanzapine, irrespective of patient subtype. This represented an average daily retail price of US $6.85 for risperidone and US $13.60 for olanzapine at the time the check was conducted (27).

Schizophrenia and cancer

Israel maintains other health registries in addition to the PCR. One of these is a national cancer registry to which reporting has been mandatory since 1982. This has allowed for a population-based examination of an observation made in the past: Patients with schizophrenia seem to have reduced risk of cancer. One study took advantage of the PCR in order to verify this observation. Data from the PCR were used to identify patients first admitted to any psychiatric ward and discharged with a diagnosis of schizophrenia over 39 years. This was then correlated with data from the cancer registry for persons aged 15 to 45 to identify the patients with schizophrenia that were also diagnosed with cancer. The investigators further stratified the Jewish-Israeli patients with schizophrenia based on their place of birth – as cancer rates vary by ethnicity. Of the 33,372 persons with schizophrenia evaluated between the years 1962 and 2001, 1504 developed cancer. The incidence of cancer in patients diagnosed with schizophrenia was compared with the general Jewish population, adjusting for relevant variables The results showed that the cancer standardized incidence ratios (SIRs) for all sites were significantly lower among men and women with schizophrenia = .9 (95% CI .8–.9) and .9 (95% CI .85–.97), respectively. This reduced overall risk was clearest for those born in Europe/America in both men SIR = .9 (95% CI .74–.97) and women SIR = .9 (95% CI .8–.9). Among women diagnosed with schizophrenia, the SIRs were statistically higher for breast cancer among those born in Asia/Africa = 1.4 (95% CI 1.1–1.6) and uterine cancer among the Israeli born = 2.8 (95% CI 1.7–3.8) than among their counterparts in the general population. Lung cancer was significant statistically higher in men born in Asia/Africa diagnosed with schizophrenia than in the respective comparison population group SIR = 1.6 (95% CI 1.1–2.2) (5). The same research group noted, however, that other results in this field had been mixed (61). Subsequently, the group extended their focus to first-degree relatives of patients with schizophrenia. This was achieved via linkage analysis of national population, psychiatric and cancer databases. The hypothesis behind their inquiry was that genetic factors might play a role in the relationship between schizophrenia and cancer risk. The results showed a reduced cancer risk among biological parents of patients with schizophrenia (mothers, SIR = .9, 95% CI .8–.9; fathers, SIR = .8, 95% CI .8–.9). A trend towards reduced cancer rates was found among their healthy siblings (24).

Stress as a risk factor

The PCR has also been used to examine maternal stress during pregnancy as a possible risk factor for schizophrenia in offspring (2). This was achieved by looking at births occurring in the nine months after two major wars, in 1967 and 1973. Both wars began suddenly (though the authors noted that military-political tension existed before the 1967 war) and were brief. Risk for schizophrenia was assessed by comparing this cohort to unexposed cohorts born in the two previous and subsequent years. The results show no impact of prenatal exposure to stress, even when separate analyses were conducted for each trimester for males and females.

§ Historical-prospective studies and the Israel Draft Board Registry

Databases maintained by the IDF offer unique opportunities for the study of the epidemiology of schizophrenia and other psychiatric illness. This is because Israel has a universal draft law that requires all adolescents aged 16 and 17 to undergo pre-induction assessment to determine their intellectual, medical and psychiatric eligibility for military service. This assessment is compulsory and administered to the entire unselected population of Israeli adolescents. (Some groups, such as Orthodox and ultra-Orthodox Jewish women, ultra-Orthodox men, and Arab Israelis other than male Druze and volunteer male Bedouins are exempted). It includes individuals who are eligible for military service, as well as those who will be excused from service on the basis of medical, psychiatric or social reasons. The IDF Draft Board assessment consists of (a) a physical examination, a review of systems and a psychiatric history – all conducted by a physician; (b) a cognitive test battery; and (c) an interview assessing personality and behavioral traits (62). Thus the Israeli Draft Board Registry contains a wealth of population-based data including relevant pre-morbid data on conscripts who will go on to develop schizophrenia or other psychiatric illnesses. Our own research group and others have taken advantage of this resource to expand the knowledge base on the epidemiology of schizophrenia. Two methodological approaches have typically been used. The first one is population-based historical-prospective studies that rely on large sample sizes. The second research strategy consists of case-control studies with cases and matched controls being drawn from the draftee database. Both types of study are described below.

In one study, 90 soldiers, 67 males and 23 females, who were hospitalized for a first psychotic episode were investigated. Of these, 55 were diagnosed with schizophrenia or schizophreniform disorder and 13 as suffering from affective psychoses. They were compared with 90 soldiers hospitalized in psychiatric units during the same year who received a diagnosis other than psychosis. The investigators reported no gender difference in the occurrence of psychoses; within-average mean ratings on the pre-induction psychometric intelligence test; no history of substance abuse; and a remarkable occurrence of psychiatric hospitalizations, including first psychotic episodes during the stressful beginning of military service. The results support the hypothesis that psychotic symptoms are more likely to occur in a stressful situation among vulnerable individuals (31).

The full potential of the Draft Board Registry to provide population-based, pre-morbid data was revealed in studies linking this to other national databases, such as the PCR. This has allowed for historical-prospective studies examining the relationship between the psychological and cognitive measures assessed by the Draft Board and the later development of schizophrenia. For example, one study investigated the link between Draft Board measures between 1985 and 1991 and schizophrenia. Patients (N = 509), as diagnosed in the PCR until 1995, were compared to non-patients, i.e., adolescents not appearing in the PCR (N = 9,215), matched to patients by age, gender, and school attended at the time of evaluation. This allowed a follow-up time of four to 10 years. Healthy male adolescents who were later hospitalized for schizophrenia had significantly lower test scores on all measures than adolescents not reported to the PCR. The strongest predictors for schizophrenia were deficits in social functioning (odds ratio (OR) = 4.4, 95% CI 3.4–5.8), organizational ability (OR = 2.0, 95% CI 1.7–2.5) and intellectual functioning (OR = 1.6, 95% CI 1.4–1.7) (62) (figure 2).

**Figure 2. Comparison of future patients with schizophrenia and controls
on Draft Board measures of social functioning (37, 62)**

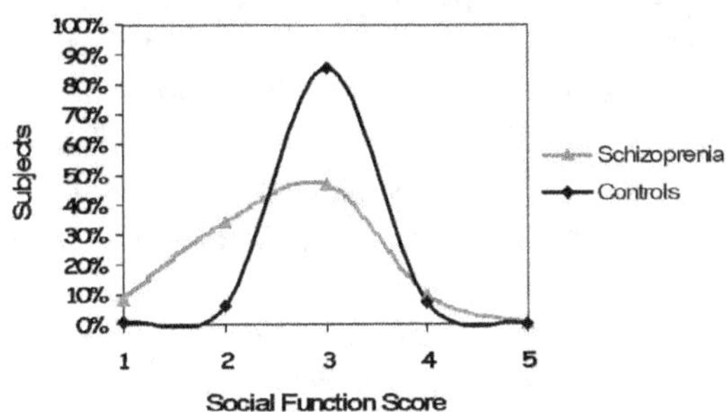

Note: Higher score indicates better function.
(*Reproduced with permission*)

Another study drawn from the Draft Board sample studied 692 men who had been admitted for schizophrenia and compared them to similarly matched control. This study measured the time that had elapsed between testing and first admission to hospital to allow the detection of psychocognitive measures that might change as illness approaches. Cases performed worse than non-cases on all measures. On the tests of Social Functioning and the Raven's Progressive Matrices-R (a test of nonverbal abstract reasoning and visual-spatial problem solving), differences between cases and non-cases were progressively greater for cases admitted closer to the time of evaluation. The differences were greatest for adolescents tested after they had already experienced their first psychiatric hospitalization. The authors concluded: first, that this result further confirms the existence of pre-morbid deficits in individuals who in the future will develop schizophrenia, and second, that some measures point to a progressive decline in cognitive function in patients approaching the onset of illness (32).

Twin study

Another study used the draftee database to identify abnormalities in twins which might be associated with illness. It did so by identifying sets of twins in which one member of the pair had a psychotic disorder. The investigators sought abnormalities common to both members of such a pair of twins but that distinguish them from pairs of twins with no psychotic illness. The ability to collect data from before the onset of illness resolved a problem of earlier twin studies conducted after the affected twin had already been diagnosed. In such type of studies, it is possible that at least some of the differences between the co-twins were not constitutional but were caused by active manifestations of psychotic illness. In this study, pairs of male twins who were healthy at the time of testing but discordant for psychoses later on were compared with one another and with pairs of healthy male twins. Affected twins performed significantly worse than healthy twins on measures of individual autonomy, social functioning and physical activity and worse, but not to a statistically significant extent, on measures of abstract reasoning. There were no significant differences in cognitive or behavioral scores between the co-twins who did or did not develop psychotic disorders (33).

Pre-morbid functioning

The studies described thus far established convincingly the existence of pre-morbid cognitive and social deficits in adolescents who would ultimately suffer from schizophrenia. However, this begs the question of specificity – how specific are these deficits for schizophrenia? This question was addressed in a case-control study: The IDF Draft Board database was used to identify adolescents with no evidence of illness at their pre-induction assessment but who were later hospitalized for non-psychotic bipolar disorder (n=68), schizoaffective disorder (n=31) or schizophrenia (n=536) as assessed by diagnoses listed in the PCR. The pre-morbid functioning of subjects who developed schizophrenia was compared to that of the other groups, and the pre-morbid function of each diagnostic group was compared with a group of non-hospitalized individuals matched for age, gender and school attended at the time of pre-induction assessment. Relative to the comparison subjects, subjects with schizophrenia showed significant pre-morbid deficits on all intellectual and behavioral measures and on measures of reading and reading comprehension. Subjects with schizophrenia performed significantly worse on these measures than those with bipolar disorder without psychotic features who did not differ significantly from the comparison subjects on any measure. Subjects with schizoaffective disorder performed significantly worse than the comparison subjects only on the measure of non-verbal abstract reasoning and visual-spatial problem solving, and performed significantly worse than subjects with bipolar disorder without psychotic features on three of the four intellectual measures and on the reading and reading comprehension tests. The authors concluded that the results support a nosologic distinction between non-psychotic bipolar disease and schizophrenia in hospitalized patients (35). A later study asked a related question: What is the relationship of different psychiatric diagnoses at the time of Draft Board assessment to cognitive performance? IDF draftee data on 19,075 male adolescents who were assigned any psychiatric diagnoses at the time of assessment, and 243,507 male adolescents without psychiatric diagnoses showed that the mean cognitive test scores of cases were significantly poorer than controls, for all diagnostic groups except for eating disorders. Effect sizes ranged from .3 to 1.6. The authors concluded that, as a group, adolescent males with psychiatric disorders showed at least subtle impairments in cognitive functioning (45). These studies suggest that while many diagnoses carry with them effects on cognitive performance, pre-morbid effects on cognition might be specific for schizophrenia or schizophrenia spectrum disorders.

Low IQ as a risk indicator

Evidence indicates that some, but not most, patients with schizophrenia have below-average intelligence years before they manifest psychosis. However, it is not clear whether this below-average, pre-morbid intelligence is stable or progressive. In order to examine whether increased risk for schizophrenia is associated with declining intellectual performance from childhood through adolescence, data from the Draft Board cognitive tests and estimated IQ during childhood were compared. Estimates of childhood IQ were based on tests of reading and spelling as these abilities usually acquired between ages 6 and 8. Draft Board data on four intelligence subtests as well as on reading and spelling abilities and behavioral and psychosocial variables were examined in a population-based cohort of 555,326 Israeli-born adolescents. Of these, 1856 were hospitalized for schizophrenia during an eight- to 17-year follow-up period. For 75.0% of patients with schizophrenia with low IQ (< 85) at age 17 years and for 23.0% of patients with IQ within the normal range (≥ 85), IQ was 10 or more points lower than estimated childhood IQ as reflected by reading and spelling abilities. Lower-than-expected IQ was not associated with bipolar disorder, depression or anxiety disorder. The authors concluded that intellectual deterioration from childhood through adolescence is associated with increased risk for schizophrenia (36). Within the same sample, individuals of normal-range IQ with the highest variability between tests were 3.8 times (95% CI 2.32–6.08, $p < .0001$) more likely to have schizophrenia compared with individuals with the lowest variability. The authors suggest that, despite normal intelligence, this might represent brain abnormalities (37). A possibly related finding comes from a population-based cohort of 174,994 male adolescents screened by the Draft Board with average or above-average intellectual abilities but with low scores (eighth and tenth lowest percentile respectively) on reading or arithmetic tests. These were thought to represent discrete impairments in reading comprehension or arithmetic abilities. They were compared with adolescents who scored in the tenth percentile and above on these tests (comparison group). Adolescents with impaired reading comprehension were also at increased risk for later hospitalization for schizophrenia (hazard ratios=1.8, 95% CI 1.3–2.6) (46).

Low pre-morbid IQ had been found to be at risk for schizophrenia spectrum disorders (SSD), a broader category which includes schizophrenia, schizoaffective disorder other non-affective psychoses, schizotypal personality disorder, and paranoid personality disorder. A population-based cohort of nearly 54,000 17-year-old conscripts from two consecutive years was investigated using draftee data. Diagnoses were drawn from the PCR over a follow-up period of 10 to 11 years. Risk for SSD increased with decreasing IQ score. The adjusted odds ratio associated with each standard deviation decrease in IQ was 1.4 (95% CI 1.2–1.5) (34).

In addition to social and cognitive measures, non-psychotic psychiatric symptoms may herald the later development of schizophrenia. The cross-linking of Draft Board mental health assessments of 124,244 male adolescents with PCR data through a four- to eight-year follow-up period allowed examination of this relationship. A total of 9365 adolescents were assigned a non-psychotic, non-major affective diagnosis by the Draft Board. Those adolescents (1.0%) assigned a non-psychotic, non-major affective psychiatric diagnosis, compared with only .2%

of the adolescents without any psychiatric diagnoses were later hospitalized for schizophrenia. Of patients with schizophrenia, 26.8% – compared with only 7.4% in the general population – had been assigned a non-psychotic, non-major affective psychiatric diagnosis in adolescence (overall OR = 4.5, 95% CI 3.6–5.6), ranging from OR = 21.5, 95% CI 12.6–36.6 for schizophrenia spectrum personality disorders to OR = 3.6, 95% CI 2.1–6.2 for neurosis. Conversely, ~99% of adolescents assigned a non-psychotic, non-major affective psychiatric diagnosis did not go on to develop schizophrenia (43) (figure 3). These results were later expanded with a similar finding about drug abuse. The prevalence of self-reported drug abuse in adolescents later hospitalized for schizophrenia was 12.4%, compared with 5.9% prevalence of drug abuse in adolescents not later hospitalized, relative risk (RR) = 2.0, 95% CI 1.3–3.1 (42).

Figure 3. Association between non-psychotic psychiatric diagnosis and later hospitalization for schizophrenia in a population of 17-year-old male adolescents. Odds ratios of each diagnostic category for later hospitalization for schizophrenia are shown (39, 43)

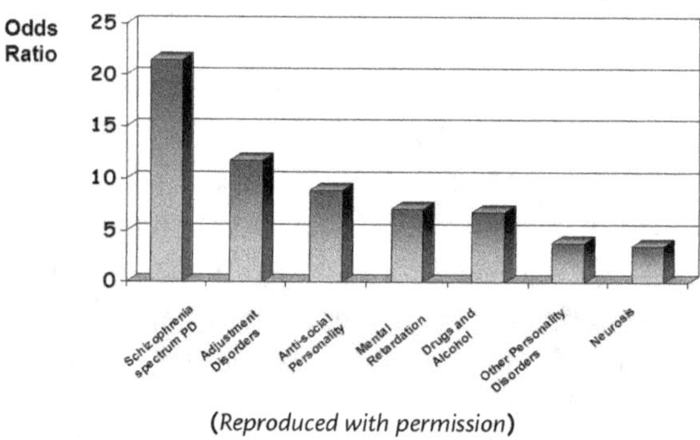

(Reproduced with permission)

Gender differences in cognitive performance in individuals suffering from schizophrenia have previously been insufficiently studied. In order to examine this issue, draftee scores on pre-morbid cognitive performance in schizophrenia were examined in 90 female-male case pairs matched for school attended as a proxy for socioeconomic status. The mean age of first hospitalization was 20.1±1.8 years and 19.6±1.8 years for males and females, respectively. Repeated-measures with ANCOVA with age of first hospitalization and years of formal education as covariates and controlling for gender differences in cognitive performance in healthy adolescents revealed a significant difference in pre-morbid cognitive performance between males and females on all four cognitive measures ($F(1,87) = 8.07$, $p = .006$) with females scoring worse than males (44).

The same database has been used to study cognitive deficits in schizotypal personality disorder (SPD). SPD patients have been reported to suffer both from specific cognitive impairments and from a generalized cognitive dysfunction similar to those found in schizophrenia. Of 341,511 males assessed, the cognitive test scores of adolescents diagnosed at the time of Draft Board assessment as suffering from SPD (N = 326) were retrieved. The Draft Board used criteria based on *DSM-III-R* to make this diagnosis during the relevant period. The cognitive scores of those diagnosed with SPD were compared to the scores of adolescents diagnosed as suffering from schizophrenia (N = 901), and adolescents with no neurological or psychiatric diagnosis (controls, N = 293,820). Male adolescents with SPD or with schizophrenia scored lower on all measures compared to healthy individuals (effect sizes ranging from .6–.89; all $p < .001$). The SPD patients scored significantly higher than the schizophrenia patients on the sub-tests of similarities and Ravens Progressive Matrices – tests that reflect abstract reasoning. On the concentration-dependent sub-tests of arithmetic and instruction comprehension SPD and schizophrenia patients' scores did not differ significantly from each other. The authors suggested that the generalized cognitive impairment, in the presence of schizotypal personality traits and in the absence of psychosis, might be conceptualized as being the core of a schizotaxia syndrome. The greater impairment in abstract reasoning in the schizophrenia patients might be correlated with the psychotic symptoms that differentiate schizophrenia from SPD (40).

Environmental risk factors in schizophrenia

The Draft Board and the PCR databases have also been used to examine environmental risks for schizophrenia. For example, previous work suggested that the association between urbanicity and schizophrenia may be greatest in those with pre-existing vulnerability. To check this, draft board data on social and cognitive functioning for 371,603 adolescent males, data on later hospitalization for schizophrenia and population density of place of residence were examined. There was an interaction between population density (divided into five levels) and poor premorbid social and cognitive functioning (interaction $\chi2 = 4.6$, $p = .03$). The adjusted increase in cumulative incidence associated with one unit change in population density was .10% in the vulnerable group (95% CI .02–.18, $p = .02$), nine times larger than that in the non-vulnerable group (.01%, 95% CI .002–.020, $p = .02$) (48).

Smoking and schizophrenia

The Draft Board database and the PCR have also been used to address general health issues related to schizophrenia. One such issue is the relationship of smoking and schizophrenia. The prevalence of cigarette smoking among patients with schizophrenia is significantly higher than in the general population and might be related to abnormalities in nicotinic transmission in patients and their relatives. The IDF routinely administers a smoking questionnaire to a random sample of male recruits who have been screened and found not to be suffering from major psychopathology. Of these adolescents, 14,248 were followed to determine later psychiatric hospitalization as assessed by PCR records. Of these, 4,052 (28.4%) reported smoking at least one cigarette a day. Over a four- to 16-year follow-up, the prevalence of schizophrenia in the entire cohort was .3% (N = 44). Smokers were at greater risk for later hospitalization with schizophrenia (adjusted RR = 1.9, 95% CI 1.1–3.6). The number of cigarettes smoked was significantly associated with such a risk (41).

Overweight as predictor

Similarly, compared with the general population, individuals suffering from schizophrenia are more likely to be overweight. It has been suggested that increased weight, like other metabolic dysfunctions, might precede active illness. Data on height and weight of 203,257 male adolescents assessed by the Israeli Draft Board, and followed for two to six years for later hospitalization for schizophrenia using the PCR, were analyzed; 204 recruits who would later receive a hospital diagnosis of schizophrenia were available for analysis. Compared with the rest of the cohort, future patients had lower body mass indexes (21.24 ± 3.3 kg/m2 vs. 21.77 ± 3.5 kg/m2;

$F = 4.682$, df = 1, $p = .03$) and weighed slightly but significantly less (64.2 ± 11.6 kg vs. 66.3 ± 12.0 kg; $F = 6.615$, df = 1, $p = .01$). Since before the onset of illness, patients were not heavier than their peers the authors concluded that the increased weight of patients with schizophrenia is related to illness or medication effects (38).

Schizophrenia among immigrants

The same databases have been used to elaborate on reports of increased incidence of schizophrenia and non-affective psychotic disorders among immigrant populations. During the late 1980s and 1990s, 885,000 persons immigrated to Israel from the former Soviet Union and 43,000 from Ethiopia. The authors suspected that a difference would be found between the two groups because, unlike the immigrants from the former Soviet Union, Ethiopian immigrants came from a very different culture compared to the rest of the population and have a distinct appearance. Of 661,792 adolescents consecutively screened by the Israeli Draft Board, 557,154 were born in Israel and 104,638 were immigrants. The risk of hospitalization for schizophrenia, after controlling for SES, was increased among both first-generation (Hazard Ratio = 1.6, 95% CI 1.2–2.2) and second-generation immigrants (HR = 1.4, 95% CI 1.01–1.95 [one immigrant parent] and HR = 1.5, 95% CI 1.1–2.0 [two immigrant parents])!. When the risk for schizophrenia was calculated for each immigrant group separately, immigrants from Ethiopia were at highest risk of later schizophrenia (HR = 3.0, 95% CI 1.9–4.7). The authors suggested that immigrants, who differ in culture and appearance from the host population, are at increased risk for schizophrenia (49)

Family functioning and schizophrenia

Previous studies indicate that a poor family environment might affect the vulnerability to later manifestation of psychotic illness. Subjects were 42, 948 17-year-old males with behavioral disturbances who were asked about the functioning of their family as part of their induction examinations by the Draft Board. Poorer self-reported family functioning was associated with greater risk for later hospitalization for psychosis (adjusted HR = 1.2, 95% CI 1.1–1.3), with a trend in the same direction for schizophrenia (adjusted HR = 1.1, 95% CI .98–1.24). The authors cautioned that the result cannot be interpreted as representing causality and thus it does not necessarily show that perceived familial dysfunction increases vulnerability for psychosis (47).

§ Conclusions

The studies reviewed here demonstrate amply the broad nature of the contribution made by Israeli researchers to the epidemiological study of schizophrenia and the diverse uses to which Israel's informational resources have been put in order to broaden our knowledge. Yet, if we look at all the contribution that Israeli epidemiological studies of schizophrenia have made, two major areas stand out.

The first is the issue of social selection vs. causation. Arguments about the reasons that psychiatric illness is related to low SES echo similar arguments over the relative importance of environmental vs. genetic factors in the etiology of mental illness. That means that the question of whether unfavorable environmental conditions are responsible for increased rates of mental illness or whether some people arrive at these conditions by virtue of illness or traits related to a biological vulnerability to illness is not only scientifically interesting but has been also socially charged. This is especially true when one takes into account the dominance of psychodynamic understandings of schizophrenia at the time that some of the earlier studies described here were conceived. Some of the studies described here, and especially that of Dohrenwend *et al.* (1), convincingly argued that in schizophrenia, factors related to social selection are more important than social causation. Studies that supported a stress-diathesis model of schizophrenia, such as those arising from the Israeli High-Risk Study (3), are much more readily interpretable when the psychosocial implications of a diathesis are established.

The second major set of findings is the extensive description of the pre-morbid differences in neurocognition, social function and mental health between those destined to suffer from schizophrenia and controls. The work described here convincingly describes the existence and the possibility to detect at adolescence broad pre-morbid deficits. Furthermore, work from the Jerusalem Infant Development Study suggests that deficits might be detectable in some children of patients with schizophrenia as early as infancy (12). This work is consistent with the notion that schizophrenia is a developmental disease and carries implications both for etiological research as well as for secondary prevention (64).

The availability in Israel of several databases, its demographic and ethnic characteristics, and the opportunity to use these databases to do long-term follow-up will continue to provide opportunities to understand more about the course, comorbidities, characteristics, social implications and pre-morbid state of and risks for schizophrenia for the foreseeable future.

⚘ References

1. Dohrenwend BP, Levav I, Shrout PE, *et al.* Socioeconomic status and psychiatric disorders: the causation-selection issue. *Science* 1992; 255: 946–952.

2. Selten JP, Cantor-Graae E, Nahon D, *et al.* No relationship between risk of schizophrenia and prenatal exposure to stress during the Six Day War or Yom Kippur War in Israel. *Schizophrenia Research* 2003; 63: 131–135.

3. Mirsky AF, Silberman EK, Latz A, *et al.* Adult outcomes of high-risk children: differential effects of town and kibbutz rearing. *Schizophrenia Bulletin* 1985; 11: 150–154.

4. Rabinowitz J, Levine SZ, Haim R, *et al.* The course of schizophrenia: progressive deterioration, amelioration or both? *Schizophrenia Research* 2007; 91: 254–258.

5. Grinshpoon A, Barchana M, Ponizovsky A, *et al.* Cancer in schizophrenia: is the risk higher or lower? *Schizophrenia Research* 2005; 73: 333–341.

6. Nagler S, Mirsky AF. Introduction: the Israeli high-risk study. *Schizophrenia Bulletin* 1985; 11: 19–29.

7. Frenkel E, Kugelmass S, Nathan M, *et al.* Locus of control and mental health in adolescence and adulthood. *Schizophrenia Bulletin* 1995; 21: 219–226.

8. Ingraham LJ, Kugelmass S, Frenkel E, *et al.* Twenty-five-year follow-up of the Israeli High-Risk Study: current and lifetime psychopathology. *Schizophrenia Bulletin* 1995; 21: 183–192.

9. Kugelmass S, Faber N, Ingraham LJ, *et al.* Reanalysis of SCOR and anxiety measures in the Israeli High-Risk Study. *Schizophrenia Bulletin* 1995; 21: 205–217.

10. Silberman EK, Tassone EP. The Israeli high-risk study: statistical overview and discussion. *Schizophrenia Bulletin* 1985; 11: 138–145.

11. Hans SL, Marcus J, Nuechterlein KH, *et al.* Neurobehavioral deficits at adolescence in children at risk for schizophrenia: the Jerusalem Infant Development Study. *Archives of General Psychiatry* 1999; 56: 741–748.

12. Marcus J, Auerbach J, Wilkinson L, *et al.* Infants at risk for schizophrenia. The Jerusalem Infant Development Study. *Archives of General Psychiatry* 1981; 38: 703–713.

13. Marcus J, Hans SL, Auerbach JG, *et al.* Children at risk for schizophrenia: the Jerusalem Infant Development Study. II. Neurobehavioral deficits at school age. *Archives of General Psychiatry* 1993; 50: 797–809.

14. Levav I, Zilber N, Danielovich E, *et al.* The etiology of schizophrenia: a replication test of the social selection vs. the social causation hypotheses. *Acta Psychiatrica Scandinavica* 1987; 75: 183–189.

15. Dohrenwend BS, Dohrenwend BP, Link B, *et al.* Social functioning of psychiatric patients in contrast with community cases in the general population. *Archives of General Psychiatry* 1983; 40: 1174–1182.

16. Eaton WW, Levav I. Schizophrenia, social class and ethnic disadvantage. A study of first hospitalization among Israeli-born Jews. *Israel Journal of Psychiatry and Related Sciences* 1982; 19: 289–302.

17. Kimhy D, Harlap S, Fennig S, *et al.* Maternal household crowding during pregnancy and the offspring's risk of schizophrenia. *Schizophrenia Research* 2006; 86: 23–29.

18. Malaspina D, Harlap S, Fennig S, *et al.* Advancing paternal age and the risk of schizophrenia. *Archives of General Psychiatry* 2001; 58: 361–367.

19. Malaspina D, Reichenberg A, Weiser M, *et al.* Paternal age and intelligence: Implications for age-related genomic changes in male germ cells. *Psychiatric Genetics* 2005; 15: 117–125.

20. Perrin MC, Opler MG, Harlap S, *et al.* Tetrachloroethylene exposure and risk of schizophrenia: offspring of dry cleaners in a population birth cohort, preliminary findings. *Schizophrenia Research* 2007; 90: 251–254.

21. Werner S, Malaspina D, Rabinowitz J. Socioeconomic status at birth is associated with risk of schizophrenia: population-based multilevel study. *Schizophrenia Bulletin* 2007; 33: 1373–1378.

22. Fennig S, Rabinowitz J, Fennig S. Involuntary first admission of patients with schizophrenia as a predictor of future admissions. *Psychiatric Services* 1999; 50: 1049–1052.

23. Ginath Y, Rabinowitz J, Popper M, *et al.* Patterns of use and changes in diagnosis during first admission. National Case Register Study. *Psychopathology* 1996; 29: 39–45.

24. Levav I, Lipshitz I, Novikov I, *et al.* Cancer risk among parents and siblings of patients with schizophrenia. *British Journal of Psychiatry* 2007; 190: 156–161.

25. Rabinowitz J, Fennig S. Differences in age of first hospitalization for schizophrenia among immigrants and nonimmigrants in a national case registry. *Schizophrenia Bulletin* 2002; 28: 491–499.

26. Rabinowitz J, Levine SZ, Hafner H. A population based elaboration of the role of age of onset on the course of schizophrenia. *Schizophrenia Research* 2006; 88: 96–101.

27. Rabinowitz J, Lichtenberg P, Kaplan Z. Comparison of cost, dosage and clinical preference for risperidone and olanzapine. *Schizophrenia Research* 2000; 46: 91–96.

28. Rabinowitz J, Lichtenberg P, Kaplan Z, *et al.* Rehospitalization rates of chronically ill schizophrenic patients discharged on a regimen of risperidone, olanzapine, or conventional antipsychotics. *American Journal of Psychiatry* 2001; 158: 266–269.

29. Rabinowitz J, Slyuzberg M, Ritsner M, *et al.* Changes in diagnosis in a nine-year national longitudinal sample. *Comprehensive Psychiatry* 1994; 35: 361–365.

30. Davidson M. Risk of cardiovascular disease and sudden death in schizophrenia. *Journal of Clinical Psychiatry* 2002; 63 (Suppl 9): 5–11.

31. Knobler HY. First psychotic episodes among Israeli youth during military service. *Military Medicine* 2000; 165: 169–172.

32. Rabinowitz J, Reichenberg A, Weiser M, *et al.* Cognitive and behavioural functioning in men with schizophrenia both before and shortly after first admission to hospital. Cross-sectional analysis. *British Journal of Psychiatry* 2000; 177: 26–32.

33. Reichenberg A, Rabinowitz J, Weiser M, *et al.* Premorbid functioning in a national population of male twins discordant for psychoses. *American Journal of Psychiatry* 2000; 157: 1514–1516.

34. Reichenberg A, Weiser M, Caspi A, *et al.* Premorbid intellectual functioning and risk of schizophrenia and spectrum disorders. *Journal of Clinical and Experimental Neuropsychology* 2006; 28: 193–207.

35. Reichenberg A, Weiser M, Rabinowitz J, *et al.* A population-based cohort study of pre-morbid intellectual, language, and behavioral functioning in patients with schizophrenia, schizoaffective disorder, and nonpsychotic bipolar disorder. *American Journal of Psychiatry* 2002; 159: 2027–2035.

36. Reichenberg A, Weiser M, Rapp MA, *et al.* Elaboration on premorbid intellectual performance in schizophrenia: pre-morbid intellectual decline and risk for schizophrenia. *Archives of General Psychiatry* 2005; 62: 1297–1304.

37. Reichenberg A, Weiser M, Rapp MA, *et al.* Premorbid intra-individual variability in intellectual performance and risk for schizophrenia: a population-based study. *Schizophrenia Research* 2006; 85: 49–57.

38. Weiser M, Knobler H, Lubin G, *et al.* Body mass index and future schizophrenia in Israeli male adolescents. *Journal of Clinical Psychiatry* 2004; 65: 1546–1549.

39. Weiser M, Knobler HY, Noy S, *et al.* Clinical characteristics of adolescents later hospitalized for schizophrenia. *American Journal of Medical Genetics* 2002; 114: 949–955.

40. Weiser M, Noy S, Kaplan Z, *et al.* Generalized cognitive impairment in male adolescents with schizotypal personality disorder. *American Journal of Medical Genetics B Neuropsychiatry Genetics* 2003; 116: 36–40.

41. Weiser M, Reichenberg A, Grotto I, *et al.* Higher rates of cigarette smoking in male adolescents before the onset of schizophrenia: a historical-prospective cohort study. *American Journal of Psychiatry* 2004; 161: 1219–1223.

42. Weiser M, Reichenberg A, Rabinowitz J, *et al.* Self-reported drug abuse in male adolescents with behavioral disturbances, and follow-up for future schizophrenia. *Biological Psychiatry* 2003; 54: 655–660.

43. Weiser M, Reichenberg A, Rabinowitz J, *et al.* Association between nonpsychotic psychiatric diagnoses in adolescent males and subsequent onset of schizophrenia. *Archives of General Psychiatry* 2001; 58: 959–964.

44. Weiser M, Reichenberg A, Rabinowitz J, *et al.* Gender differences in premorbid cognitive performance in a national cohort of schizophrenic patients. *Schizophrenia Research* 2000; 45: 185–190.

45. Weiser M, Reichenberg A, Rabinowitz J, *et al.* Cognitive performance of male adolescents is lower than controls across psychiatric disorders: a population-based study. *Acta Psychiatrica Scandinavica* 2004; 110: 471–475.

46. Weiser M, Reichenberg A, Rabinowitz J, *et al.* Impaired reading comprehension and mathematical abilities in male adolescents with average or above general intellectual abilities are associated with comorbid and future psychopathology. *Journal of Nervous and Mental Disease* 2007; 195: 883–890.

47. Weiser M, Reichenberg A, Werbeloff N, *et al.* Self-report of family functioning and risk for psychotic disorders in male adolescents with behavioural disturbances. *Acta Psychiatrica Scandinavica* 2008; 117: 225–231.

48. Weiser M, van Os J, Reichenberg A, *et al.* Social and cognitive functioning, urbanicity and risk for schizophrenia. *British Journal of Psychiatry* 2007; 191: 320–324.

49. Weiser M, Werbeloff N, Vishne T, *et al.* Elaboration on immigration and risk for schizophrenia. *Psychological Medicine* 2008; 38:113–119.

50. Kaffman M. The Israeli High-Risk Study: Some critical remarks. *Schizophrenia Bulletin* 1986; 12: 151–157.

51. Rabin AI. The schizophrenic diathesis and the kibbutz. *Journal of Personality Assessment* 1986; 50: 448–454.

52. Mirsky AF. The Israeli High-Risk Study: reply to Kaffman. *Schizophrenia Bulletin* 1986; 12: 158–161.

53. Weiser M, van Os J, Davidson M. Time for a shift in focus in schizophrenia: from narrow phenotypes to broad endophenotypes. *British Journal of Psychiatry* 2005; 187: 203–205.

54. Mirsky AF, Ingraham LJ, Kugelmass S. Neuropsychological assessment of attention and its pathology in the Israeli cohort. *Schizophrenia Bulletin* 1995; 21: 193–204.

55. Endicott J, Spitzer RL. Current and past psychopathology scales (CAPPS). Rationale, reliability, and validity. *Archives of General Psychiatry* 1972; 27: 678–687.

56. John K, Gammon GD, Prusoff BA, *et al*. The Social Adjustment Inventory for Children and Adolescents (SAICA): testing of a new semistructured interview. *Journal of the American Academy Child and Adolescent Psychiatry* 1987; 26: 898–911.

57. Achenbach TM. *Manual for the youth self-report and 1991 profile*. Burlington, Vermont: University of Vermont Department of Psychiatry, 1991.

58. Hans SL, Auerbach JG, Asarnow JR, *et al*. Social adjustment of adolescents at risk for schizophrenia: the Jerusalem Infant Development Study. *Journal of the American Academy of Child and Adolescent Psychiatry* 2000; 39: 1406–1414.

59. Dohrenwend BP, Shrout PE, Egri G, *et al*. Nonspecific psychological distress and other dimensions of psychopathology. Measures for use in the general population. *Archives of General Psychiatry* 1980; 37: 1229–1236.

60. Levav I, Kohn R, Dohrenwend BP, *et al*. An epidemiology study of a 10-year cohort of young adults in Israel. *Psychological Medicine* 1993; 23: 691–707.

61. Levav I, Ponizovsky A, Grinshpoon A. Cancer and schizophrenia. *British Journal of Psychiatry* 2006; 188: 191.

62. Davidson M, Reichenberg A, Rabinowitz J, *et al*. Behavioral and intellectual markers for schizophrenia in apparently healthy male adolescents. *American Journal of Psychiatry* 1999; 156: 1328–1335.

Chapter 15

Genetic epidemiology of schizophrenia in Arab communities in Israel

Joseph Levine, Richard Ebstein, Ilana Kremer and R.H. Belmaker

While the field of psychiatric epidemiology studies the relationship of risk factors, especially of environmental risks, in the incidence and prevalence of disease in the population – genetic epidemiology uses modern molecular techniques to look at the interaction of genetic markers and polymorphisms with other disease-causing factors in a population. As an example of genetic epidemiology research conducted in Israel, the following chapter will review our studies on schizophrenia in Arab-Israeli communities.

The Arabs in general are considered to be genetically diverse due to migrations of Semitic tribes from the Arabian Peninsula, the Islamic expansion in the seventh century of the Common Era, the Crusade wars and the recent migration dynamics resulting in admixture of the original Arabs with other populations extending from eastern and southern Asia to Europe and Africa (1). The first serious initiative to compile data about genetic traits in Arab populations was that of Teebi and Farag, which was published only a decade ago in a book titled Genetic Disorders among Arab Populations (2). It is thus important to contribute further to the existing knowledge about the genetics of mental disorders in Arab populations.

Arabs in Israel are part of the Palestinian-Arab people and characterized by large sibships and extended family structure. They have been often studied for Mendelian genetic disorders, especially those involving a predominance of autosomal recessive disorders (2). Bedouin Arabs, originally nomadic, are of diverse origin – but they share with almost all Arabs in the rest of the Middle East the language, the Muslim religion and very high rates of cousin marriages, known as consanguinity or inbreeding (3–7). The reasons for the persistence of cousin marriages have been discussed elsewhere (4, 8), and include the fact that they serve to maintain the property within the family and ensure some protection for women's rights in a patriarchal society, since the wife has relatives among the husband's family.

❧ Study 1

The rate of consanguineous marriages among parents of patients with schizophrenia in the Arab Bedouin population in Southern Israel – based on the study by Dobrusin et al. (9)

254

Schizophrenia is usually considered a polygenic illness, although mathematical models of family studies could not completely rule out a mixed model of a single major gene effect on a polygenic background (10). Classically, consanguinity increases the rate of appearance of illness caused by recessive genes in Mendelian systems. This is clinically noticeable in a high rate of rare illnesses in inbred communities (8), including some Arab communities in Israel (6).

Ahmed *et al.* (11) studied the rate of consanguinity among the parents of individuals with schizophrenia in an isolated Sudanese community. Over 40% of marriages were between first cousins – with no difference between parents of offspring with schizophrenia and controls. Chaleby and Tuma (12) studied consanguinity in parents of 143 individuals with schizophrenia and 143 controls matched for age, sex and socioeconomic class in a Saudi Arabian Bedouin population. Sixteen percent of the marriages involving individuals with schizophrenia were between first cousins compared with 12% among the controls; this was a non-significant statistical difference.

These data did not support the recessive, single-gene model of schizophrenia. However, a recent editorial in *Nature Genetics* (13) revived the debate about the still-common opinion that inbreeding and cousin marriages have deleterious effects on the rate of schizophrenia (14). Indeed, Bener *et al.* (15) reported that among 876 Arabs in Qatar, the rate of consanguinity in the present generation was 51% – significantly higher than the maternal rate of 40%.

The records of the Beersheba Mental Health Center, located in the city of Beersheba, were systematically searched for all patients admitted between 1980 and 2000 with a diagnosis of schizophrenia, schizophreniform disorder or schizoaffective disorder and having an identifying Bedouin name. Over 80% were located and agreed to participate in the study. Only patients with both parents living were included.

The study was approved by the Ben-Gurion University Helsinki Committee (Institutional Review Board, or IRB), and all participants provided written informed consent in Arabic. Diagnostic assessments were carried out during the screening visit and sometimes repeatedly by a senior psychiatrist and trained Arabic-speaking social worker. Complete demographic data were taken, a pedigree tree for each family was drawn and the degree of consanguinity was divided into marriage of first cousins, second cousins or more distant relatives.

The control group was studied separately by Weitzman *et al.* (16). Data were obtained from follow-up records in a prenatal clinic that consisted of demographic data on parents of an infant cohort born between September 1994 and February 1995. The survey was conducted originally to study rates of utilization of prenatal services by Bedouin women and was based on all singleton births at University Medical Center in Beersheba (where about 99% of Bedouin women give birth) to women living in four of the seven Bedouin towns in the region. Almost all Bedouin women – 89% of them – were registered in the Mother and Child Health (MCH) clinics, which are the main provider of prenatal care for the study population. During this period, a total of 1104 Bedouin singleton births took place at these four index Bedouin towns. Of these 936 births, there were complete data about the relatedness of the baby's parents in 85%. The data source was the MCH clinic follow-up card, which contains identifying information (e.g., address and birth dates of the woman and her husband) and intake information obtained by the MCH nurse, including the relatedness of the women to her husband.

When the offspring of not-related, first cousins, second cousins and distant relationship marriages were compared, the results showed a small but significant increase in parental consanguinity among patients with schizophrenia compared with controls (51% vs. 40%; χ2 = 13.55, df = 3, p < .01). However, if only first-cousin marriages were counted, this difference was not significant.

While we found a small but significant increase in consanguinity among parents of Bedouin Arabs with schizophrenia compared to the control group, the effect was small. The control population was born later (1994 to 1995) than the population with schizophrenia (sampled as adults between 1997 and 2000). Interestingly, in agreement with Bener *et al.* (15), there was evidence that cousin marriages are increasing in this population. This could suggest that the real effect of consanguinity in this population is somewhat larger. However, the study and the control groups were ascertained differently. It is possible that psychiatrists performing a genetic study obtain a more thorough family history than nurses at the child care clinics, although the nurses are also instructed to search for genetic risk factors. Indeed, large rates of second-cousin marriages as well as first-cousin marriages were reported, 15% in parents of patients with schizophrenia vs. 11% in control parents.

The baseline rates of consanguinity reported here are similar to those reported throughout the Arab world (3–8) and, specifically, from Sudan (12), but higher than those reported in Saudi Arabia (12). It is possible that these high rates represent a ceiling effect and that any additional increase in the parents of patients with schizophrenia could not be identified. However, the rate of first-cousin consanguinity in the Saudi Arabia sample (12) was 12% among controls, and only non-significantly elevated among the parents of patients with schizophrenia. Moreover, there was some evidence that in a population that has had cousin inbreeding over several generations, homozygosity was very high for the tribe as a whole. Thus, in such a population, consanguinity of parents might not increase the risk of schizophrenia because marrying someone who is not a relative in the same tribe would be like marrying a cousin (4). It is also possible that schizophrenia, like many complex genetic disorders, may be caused by different combinations of genes in different populations and that among the Bedouin of southern Israel, a gene with recessive qualities may explain a fraction of the cases.

℘ Study II

No association between the dopamine D3 receptor Bal I polymorphism and schizophrenia in a family-based study of Israeli Palestinian-Arab and Palestinian West Bank populations – based on the study by Kremer et al. (17)

The D3 receptor gene contains a *Bal* I polymorphism resulting in a serine-glycine substitution in the N terminus of the receptor. There is some evidence that this coding region polymorphism is functionally significant. Lundstrom and Turpin (18) noted significantly higher dopamine-binding affinity for the Ser9Gly homozygote when recombinant DNA was expressed in CHO cells.

A total of 129 Palestinian patients with schizophrenia attending the psychiatric ward in the general hospital of Afula, and the psychiatric hospitals in Beersheba and Bethlehem, and their parents were included in the study after written informed consent was obtained. All probands were interviewed by experienced psychiatrists using the Structured Clinical Interview for DSM Diagnoses (SCID) (19). The DRD3 *Bal* I polymorphism was characterized as previously described (20).

The results showed no difference in either genotype (ser/ser gly/ser gly/gly) or allele frequency (serine, glycine) between patients with schizophrenia compared to the haplotype relative risk control group. Nor was there increased homozygosity in the group with schizophrenia. No significant difference in genotype or allele frequency was observed when either male or female probands were separately analyzed. Again, no difference was observed between schizophrenic and HRR control subjects, nor there was any difference observed in genotype frequency between patients with schizophrenia from the three geographical locations.

❧ Study III

No evidence for linkage of microsatellite marker D22S278 and schizophrenia in a Palestinian-Arab population – based on the study by Dobrusin et al. (21)

Pulver *et al.* (22) first reported evidence of linkage of schizophrenia to 22q at the IL2RB locus near D22S278. Subsequently, this region has been implicated in several other linkage studies, and the marker D22S278 in several linkage disequilibrium studies (23–25). A group of 223 Palestinian-Arab patients with schizophrenic triads was examined (21). All patients were interviewed by an experienced psychiatrist using the SCID interview. Diagnosis of schizophrenia was made on the basis of the interview and medical records according to the *Diagnostic and Statistical Manual of Mental Disorders – Fourth Edition,* (DSM-IV) criteria (19). Genomic DNA was extracted from peripheral blood or transformed lymphocytes using phenol-chloroform or commercial kits. The allele-wise TDT (TDT extension for multiallelic markers) was performed using the program ETDT (26). The standard biallelic TDT (27) was also performed considering in turn each allele of the multiallelic marker against the others in order to measure allelic relative risks (RR). No preferential transmission of any allele was detected. The study thus failed to detect a linkage of microsatellite marker D22S278 and schizophrenia in these populations.

❧ Study IV

A family-based study of the CYS23SER 5HT2C serotonin receptor polymorphism in schizophrenia – based on the study by Murad et al. (28)

The 5HT2C receptor has a high affinity for clozapine, a non-typical neuroleptic, and has therefore been postulated to play a role in mediating negative symptoms and neuroleptic response in schizophrenia. In the current study (28), the CYS23SER 5HT2C serotonin receptor polymorphism was examined for linkage to schizophrenia by genotyping 207 nuclear families consisting of both parents and offspring with schizophrenia and using the transmission disequilibrium test to examine possible preferential transmission of these alleles from 68 heterozygous mothers to their ill child.

The CYS23SER 5HT2C serotonin-receptor polymorphism was characterized as previously described (20). No evidence was obtained for preferential transmission of the CYS23SER 5HT2C alleles in schizophrenia.

❧ Study V

No evidence for association between NOTCH4 and schizophrenia in a large family-based and case-control association analysis of Palestinian Arabs – based on the study by Ivo et al. (29).

NOTCH4 belongs to an evolutionarily highly conserved family of transmembrane receptors that play an important role in the differentiation of glial cells and the organization of neuronal processes.

NOTCH4 markers were studied in a sample of Palestinian-Arab patients with schizophrenia.

The study population included parent-offspring trio samples. A total of 10 single nucleotide polymorphisms were studied within the NOTCH4 locus and the adjacent loci, spanning a region of approximately 100 kb. Written informed consent was obtained from all individuals participating in this study. All patients were interviewed by an experienced psychiatrist using the Schedule for Affective Disorders and Schizophrenia-Lifetime Version (30). Best-estimate diagnoses were assigned on the basis of the interview in addition to the review of all available clinical records according to criteria of the *Diagnostic and Statistical Manual of Mental Disorders – Third Edition Revised (DSM-III-R)*. The Arab study population consisted of 208 parent-offspring trios, including father, mother and offspring with schizophrenia.

Neither single-marker nor haplotype analyses showed association with schizophrenia. These results suggest that NOTCH4 is unlikely to play a major role in the genetic predisposition to schizophrenia in the Palestinian-Arab population.

⸙ Study VI

Family-based and case-control study of catechol-o-methyltransferase in schizophrenia among Palestinian Arabs – based on the study by Kremer et al. (31)

COMT is a ubiquitous enzyme crucial to catechol metabolism. The molecular basis of COMT thermolability, which leads to three- to four-fold differences in enzyme activity, is due to a substitution of valine with methionine in the Val158/108Met polymorphism. Of special interest is the role of this gene in major psychoses – especially since a microdeletion (22q11) containing the COMT gene (velo-cardio-facial syndrome) also carries with it several types of behavioral disorders, including an increased prevalence of schizophrenia. The following study (31) examined Palestinian-Arab schizophrenic triads (N = 276) using both a case–control and family-based study.

All patients were interviewed by an experienced psychiatrist using the SCID. Diagnosis of schizophrenia was assigned on the basis of the interview and medical records according to DSM-IV criteria. The sample included 248 nuclear families (276 probands) from three different centers: 136 families from Bethlehem; 62 families from Afula; and 50 families from Beersheba. Twenty-four families had more than one affected child. The mean age of the probands with schizophrenia was 35 ± 14 years, of these 31% were men and the rest women. The average age of illness onset was 21 ± 5 years. The control sample consisted of Palestinian Arabs recruited from northern Israel. Their average age was 39.5 ± 15.5 years, and 31% of them were men. The control group was randomly recruited from subjects visiting a family medicine (not psychiatric) national health fund clinic (HMO) for minor medical ailments. The protocol for recruiting both control and schizophrenic families was approved by the local IRB committees and all subjects or their legal representative gave informed consent. Genotyping Genomic DNA containing the COMT polymorphism was amplified as previously described (32). No preferential transmission of either COMT allele was observed in this sample (TDT statistic, NS; 131 COMT valine alleles were transmitted and 125 alleles not transmitted). However, using a case-control design, a significant increase (likelihood ratio = 3.9, p = .047) in the valine allele was observed in the group of patients with schizophrenia (N = 276), compared to an ethnically matched control group (N = 77). The association was stronger in female patients (p = .012) similar to other studies showing that some COMT behavioral effects are gender sensitive.

In summary, by case-control design but not by a family based study, there is a weak effect in female patients of the high activity COMT allele in conferring risk for schizophrenia.

§ Study VII

Transmission disequilibrium and haplotype analyses of the G72/G30 – based on the study by Korostishevsky et al. (33)

Linkage evidence suggests that chromosome 13 (13q32–33) contains susceptibility genes for schizophrenia. Recently, genes called "G72" and "G30" were identified, and polymorphisms of these overlapping genes were reported to be associated with schizophrenia in French Canadian, Russian and Ashkenazi populations using case-controlled studies. In the present study (33), a total of 223 Arab families that included an affected offspring and parents were genotyped with 11 SNPS encompassing the G72/G30 genes. The families were recruited from three regions: 56 from northern Israel (Afula), 136 from the central hill region (Bethlehem, Palestinian Authority), and 31 from the south (Beersheba).

All patients were diagnosed based on the SCID interview according to DSM-IV criteria for schizophrenia. The protocol for recruiting schizophrenic families was approved by the local committees. Eleven SNPs were genotyped: rs3916965 (M12), rs3916966 (M13), rs3916967 (M14), rs2391191 (M15), rs3918341 (M16), rs947267 (M18), rs778294 (M19), rs3916970 (M20), rs3916971 (M21), rs778293 (M22), and rs3918342 (M23). The designations of the SNPs in parentheses are according to Chumakov *et al.* (34). Primer sequences and PCR conditions are described in Korostishevsky *et al.* (35). Re-genotyping was performed for M20, M22 in BL group and for M22, M23 in BS group, where a deviation from Hardy-Weinberg equilibrium (HWE) was observed. Individual SNP analyses disclosed a risk allele in SNP rs3916970 by both haplotype relative risk (HRR: $\chi2 = 5.59$, $p = .018$) and transmission disequilibrium test (TDT: $\chi2 = 6.03$, $p = .014$) in the Afula families. The results strengthen previous reports on the role of this locus in the etiology of schizophrenia.

§ Study VIII

Mitochondrial DNA HV lineage increases the susceptibility to schizophrenia among Arab Israelis – based on the study by Amar et al. (36)

An emerging body of data suggests that impaired energy metabolism due to mitochondrial dysfunction plays a role in the pathophysiology of schizophrenia (37).

It has been shown that linked sets of mitochondrial DNA (mtDNA) genetic variants (haplogroups) alter human tendency to develop neuropsychiatric disorders including Parkinson's and Alzheimer's diseases (38). Several attempts have been made to assess association of certain mtDNA genetic variants with schizophrenia (39, 40). However, those attempts focused on specific variants rather than on a hypothesis-free approach.

In the current study (36), evidence is presented for association of mutations in the mitochondrial genome defining the HV lineage cluster with the propensity to develop schizophrenia in an Arab-Israeli population.

A total of 202 DNA samples from unrelated schizophrenia patients in addition to their parents – all of Arab-Israeli origin – were collected in two independent locations (Beersheba Mental Health Center, Beersheba, and Emek Medical Center, Afula) after informed consent.

The original protocol was approved by the Helsinki Committees in both institutions. Since mtDNA is maternally transmitted, samples of the patients' psychiatrically healthy fathers were used as normal controls.

DNA was extracted from peripheral lymphocytes using standard techniques (phenol-chloroform). Genotyping was conducted using PCR amplification and restriction enzyme analysis (restriction fragment length polymorphisms or RFLPs) for the relevant polymorphic sites, in a hierarchical approach starting from the most prevalent lineages in the Arab-Israeli population, the HV lineages, followed by haplogroups H, L, U, K, J, T, N1, W, X, I, R, N non-R. The rest of the less prevalent haplogroups in this population were aggregated as "others" (41).

In addition to the PCR RFLP analysis to assign the samples into haplogroups the hypervariable region 1 (HVR1) of the mtDNA control region were sequenced in all the samples as previously described (42–44). The HVR1 sequence is highly polymorphic and harbors multiple haplogroup-defining mutations – hence it assists in assigning samples to certain mtDNA haplogroups.

A 518-bp fragment encompassing the HVR1 region, located between mtDNA positions 15883 and 16401 was amplified with primers designed using the Oligos software (Molecular Biology Insight, Cascade, CO) and the PCR conditions described above. PCR products were purified with the ExoSAP-IT PCR clean-up kit (GE Healthcare Bio-Sciences Corp) and were sequenced by Danyel Biotech (Rehovot).

Analysis of the distribution of mitochondrial haplogroups in schizophrenia patients compared to their healthy fathers (202 pairs) resulted in an over-representation of the mtDNA lineage cluster, HV, in the patients ($p = .01$), with a relative risk of 1.8. Since mitochondrial DNA is small relative to nuclear DNA, a total mitochondrial genome analysis was possible in a hypothesis-free manner. However, mitochondrial DNA haplogroups are highly variable in human population and it will be necessary to replicate these results in other human ethnic groups.

⸹ Conclusions

Interest in the Arab population was stimulated by a series of studies identifying rare genetic diseases in specific Arab villages in Israel (6, 45, 46). More generally, genetic disorders among Arab populations have recently received increased attention (1, 7). While some researchers have emphasized the genetic diversity among Arabs (1), other researchers have emphasized the value for genetic research of the widespread custom of consanguinity in the Arab world (8).

We ascertained well-diagnosed Arab patients with schizophrenia from several clinics in Israel and were able to collect samples from their parents as well for studies based on transmission disequilibrium. We found no powerful genetic effects for schizophrenia of any of the genes in this population, consistent with recent findings in many other populations that schizophrenia is affected by such a large number of genes that no single gene has emerged as contributing a clinically significant component of the variance (47). However, a unique new study of mitochondrial DNA did find an overrepresentation of one lineage cluster with a relative risk score of 1.8 (36). Moreover, a unique study of the rate of consanguineous marriages in the parents of schizophrenic patients vs. a control group found that there was an increase of cousin marriages among the parents of patients with schizophrenia compared to controls. While consanguinity is usually not considered to be a risk factor for polygenetic diseases, this study suggests that in some populations, recessive genes might contribute to the etiology of schizophrenia.

Table 1. Summary of genetic epidemiology studies among Palestinian-Arab communities in Israel and the Palestinian Authority

Year	Authors	Parameter studied	Population studied	Design	Findings
2000	Kremer *et al.* (17)	Dopamine D3 receptor Bal I polymorphism	Palestinian Arab population	Family-based study	No association between the dopamine D3 receptor *Bal* I polymorphism and schizophrenia
2001	Dobrusin *et al.* (21)	Microsatellite marker D22S278	Palestinian Arabs from three different centers in Israel and Palestinian Authority	A family-based study of nuclear families consisting of both parents and child with schizophrenia	No evidence for linkage by transmission disequilibrium test analysis of microsatellite marker D22S278 and schizophrenia
2001	Murad *et al.* (28)	CYS23SER 5HT2C serotonin receptor polymorphism	German and Palestinian Arabs	A family-based study of nuclear families	No evidence for preferential transmission of the CYS23SER 5HT2C alleles in schizophrenia
2003	Kremer *et al.* (31)	Catechol-O-methyltransferase	Palestinian Arabs	Family-based and case-control study	By case-control design but not by a family-based study, there is a weak effect in female patients of the high-activity COMT allele in conferring risk for schizophrenia
2006	Ivo *et al.* (29)	NOTCH4 locus	Palestinian Arab origin	A large family-based and case-control association analysis	No evidence for association between NOTCH4 locus and schizophrenia
2006	Korostishevsky *et al.* (33)	Transmission disequilibrium and haplotype analyses of the G72/G30 locus	Palestinian Arabs from three different centers in Israel and Palestinian Authority	Palestinian Arab families that included an affected offspring and parents	Individual SNP analyses disclosed a risk allele for schizophrenia in SNP rs3916970 by both haplotype relative risk and transmission disequilibrium in the Afula families
2007	Amar *et al.* (36)	Analysis of the distribution of mitochondrial haplogroups		Mitochondrial haplogroups in patients with schizophrenia compared to their healthy fathers	Over-representation of the mtDNA lineage cluster, HV, in patients
2008	Dobrusin *et al.* (9)	Rate of consanguineous marriages	Bedouin population in southern Israel	Comparison study between parents of patients with schizophrenia vs. parents of control newborns	Increase in consanguinity among parents of Bedouin Arabs with schizophrenia

❧ References

1. Teebi AS, Teebi SA. Genetic diversity among the Arabs. *Community Genetics* 2005; 8: 21–26.

2. Teebi AS, Farag TI. *Genetic disorders among Arab populations.* New York: Oxford University Press, 1996.

3. Bener A, Abdulrazzaq YM, al-Gazali LI, *et al.* Consanguinity and associated socio-demographic factors in the United Arab Emirates. *Human Heredity* 1996; 46: 256–264.

4. Bittles A. Consanguinity and its relevance to clinical genetics. *Clinical Genetics* 2001; 60: 89–98.

5. Jaber L, Shohat M, Halpern GJ. Demographic characteristics of the Israeli Arab community in connection with consanguinity. *Israel Journal of Medical Sciences* 1996; 32: 1286–1289.

6. Jaber L, Shohat T, Rotter JI, *et al.* Consanguinity and common adult diseases in Israeli Arab communities. *American Journal of Medical Genetics* 1997; 70: 346–348.

7. Teebi AS, El-Shanti HI. Consanguinity: implications for practice, research, and policy. *The Lancet* 2006; 367: 970–971.

8. Bittles AH. Endogamy, consanguinity and community disease profiles. *Community Genetics* 2005; 8: 17–20.

9. Dobrusin M, Weitzman D, Levine J, *et al.* The rate of consanguineous marriages among the parents of schizophrenic patients in the Arab Bedouin population in southern Israel. *World Journal of Biological Psychiatry* published online: February 11, 2008; 1–3.

10. Vogler GP, Gottesman II, McGue MK, *et al.* Mixed-model segregation analysis of schizophrenia in the Lindelius Swedish pedigrees. *Behavioral Genetics* 1990; 20: 461–472.

11. Ahmed AH. Consanguinity and schizophrenia in Sudan. *British Journal of Psychiatry* 1979; 134: 635–636.

12. Chaleby K, Tuma TA. Cousin marriages and schizophrenia in Saudi Arabia. *British Journal of Psychiatry* 1987; 150: 547–549.

13. Axton 2006. The germinating seed of Arab genomics. *Nature Genetics* 2006; 38: 851.

14. Grady D. Few risks seen to the children of first cousins. *The New York Times*, 2002.

15. Bener A, Hussain R, Teebi AS. Consanguineous marriages and their effects on common adult diseases: studies from an endogamous population. *Medical Principles and Practice* 2007; 16: 262–267.

16. Weitzman D. Shoham-Vardi I, Elbedour K, *et al.* 2003. Consanguinity and utilization of prenatal tests to detect fetal malformations and hereditary diseases among the settled Bedouins of the Negev: evaluation of community interventions among pregnant women. PhD diss., Ben-Gurion University of the Negev.

17. Kremer I, Rietschel M, Dobrusin M, *et al.* No association between the dopamine D3 receptor Bal I polymorphism and schizophrenia in a family-based study of a Palestinian Arab population. *American Journal of Medical Genetics* 2000; 96: 778–780.

18. Lundstrom K, Turpin MP. Proposed schizophrenia-related gene polymorphism: expression of the Ser9Gly mutant human dopamine D3 receptor with Semliki Forest virus system. *Biochemical and Biophysical Research Communications* 1996; 225: 1068–1072.

19. Spitzer RL, Williams JBW, Gibbon M, *et al. Structured clinical interview for DSM-III-R. patient edition (SCID-P).* Washington, DC: American Psychiatric Press, 1996.

20. Ebstein RP, Segman R, Benjamin J, *et al.* 5-HT2C (HTR2C) serotonin receptor gene polymorphism associated with the human personality trait of reward dependence: interaction with dopamine D4 receptor (D4DR) and dopamine D3 receptor (D3DR) polymorphisms. *American Journal of Medical Genetics* 1997; 74: 65–72.

21. Dobrusin M, Corbex M, Kremer I, *et al.* No evidence for linkage by transmission disequilibrium test analysis of microsatellite marker D22S278 and schizophrenia in a Palestinian Arab and in a German population. *American Journal of Medical Genetics* 2001; 105: 328–331.

22. Pulver AE, Karayiorgou M, Wolyniec PS, *et al.* Sequential strategy to identify a susceptibility gene for schizophrenia: report of potential linkage on chromosome 22q12–q13.1: Part 1. *American Journal of Medical Genetics* 1994; 54: 36–43.

23. Coon H, Jensen S, Holik J, *et al.* Genomic scan for genes predisposing to schizophrenia. *American Journal of Medical Genetics* 1994; 54: 59–71.

24. Moises HW, Yang L, Li T, *et al.* Potential linkage disequilibrium between schizophrenia and locus D22S278 on the long arm of chromosome 22. *American Journal of Medical Genetics* 1995; 60: 465–467.

25. Vallada H, Curtis D, Sham PC, *et al.* Chromosome 22 markers demonstrate transmission disequilibrium with schizophrenia. *Psychiatric Genetics* 1995; 5: 127–130.

26. Sham PC, Curtis D. An extended transmission/disequilibrium test (TDT) for multi-allele marker loci. *Annals of Human Genetics* 1995; 59: 323–336.

27. Spielman RS, McGinnis RE, Ewens WJ. Transmission test for linkage disequilibrium: the insulin gene region and insulin-dependent diabetes mellitus (IDDM). *American Journal of Medical Genetics* 1993; 52: 506–516.

28. Murad I, Kremer I, Dobrusin M, *et al.* A family-based study of the Cys23Ser 5HT2C serotonin receptor polymorphism in schizophrenia. *American Journal of Medical Genetics* 2001; 105: 236–238.

29. Ivo R, Schulze TG, Schumacher J, *et al.* No evidence for association between NOTCH4 and schizophrenia in a large family-based and case-control association analysis. *Psychiatric Genetics* 2006; 16: 197–203.

30. Endicott J, Spitzer R. A diagnostic interview: the schedule for affective disorders and schizophrenia. *Archives of General Psychiatry* 1978; 35: 837–844.

31. Kremer I, Pinto M, Murad I, *et al.* Family-based and case-control study of catechol-O-methyltransferase in schizophrenia among Palestinian Arabs. *American Journal of Medical Genetics Part B Neuropsychiatric Genetics* 2003; 119: 35–39.

32. Eisenberg J, Mei-Tal G, Steinberg A, *et al.* Haplotype relative risk study of catechol-O-methyltransferase (COMT) and attention deficit hyperactivity disorder (ADHD): association of the high-enzyme activity Val allele with ADHD impulsive-hyperactive phenotype. *American Journal of Medical Genetics* 1999; 88: 497–502.

33. Korostishevsky M, Kremer I, Kaganovich M, *et al.* Transmission disequilibrium and haplotype analyses of the G72/G30 locus: suggestive linkage to schizophrenia in Palestinian Arabs living in the north of Israel. *American Journal of Medical Genetics Part B Neuropsychiatric Genetics* 2006; 141: 91–95.

34. Chumakov I, Blumenfeld M, Guerassimenko O, *et al.* Genetic and physiological data implicating the new human gene G72 and the gene for D-amino acid oxidase in schizophrenia. *Proceedings of the [US] National Academy of Sciences* 2002; 99: 13675–13680.

35. Korostishevsky M, Kaganovich M, Cholostoy A, *et al.* Is the G72/G30 locus associated with schizophrenia? Single nucleotide polymorphisms, haplotypes, and gene expression analysis. *Biological Psychiatry* 2004; 56: 169–176.

36. Amar S, Shamir A, Ovadia O, *et al.* Mitochondrial DNA HV lineage increases the susceptibility to schizophrenia among Israeli Arabs. *Schizophrenia Research* 2007; 94: 354–358.

37. Ben-Shachar D. Mitochondrial dysfuntion in schizophrenia: a possible linkage to dopamine. *Journal of Neurochemistry* 2002; 83: 1241–1251.

38. Wallace DC. A mitochondrial paradigm of metabolic and degenerative diseases, aging, and cancer: a dawn for evolutionary medicine. *Annual Review of Genetics* 2005; 39: 359–407.

39. Marchbanks RM, Ryan M, Day IN, *et al.* A mitochondrial DNA sequence variant associated with schizophrenia and oxidative stress. *Schizophrenia Research* 2003; 65: 33–38.

40. Bandelt HJ, Yao YG, Kivisild T. Mitochondrial genes and schizophrenia. *Schizophrenia Research* 2005; 72: 267–269.

41. Owen MJ, Williams NM, O'Donovan MC. The molecular genetics of schizophrenia: new findings promise new insights. *Molecular Psychiatry* 2004; 9: 14–27.

42. Macaulay v, Richards M, Hickey E, *et al.* The emerging tree of West Eurasian mtDNAs: a synthesis of control-region sequences and RFLPs. *American Journal of Human Genetics* 1999; 64: 232–249.

43. Mishmar D, Ruiz-Pesini E, Golik P, *et al.* Natural selection shaped regional mtDNA variation in humans. *Proceedings of the [US] National Academy of Sciences* 2003; 100: 171–176.

44. Ruiz-Pesini E, Mishmar D, Brandon M, *et al.* Effects of purifying and adaptive selection on regional variation in human mtDNA. *Science* 2004; 303: 223–226.

45. Rachmilewitz EA, Tamari H, Liff F, *et al.* The interaction of hemoglobin O Arab with Hb S and beta+ thalassemia among Israeli Arabs. *Human Genetics* 1985; 70: 119–125.

46. Nevo S. A rare adenosine deaminase allele (ADA6) in an Arab Muslim village in Israel. *Human Genetics* 1977; 38: 235–238.

47. Crow TJ. How and why genetic linkage has not solved the problem of psychosis: review and hypothesis. *American Journal of Psychiatry* 2007; 164: 13–21.

❧ Glossary*

5HT2C: A subtype of serotonin receptor

Allele: One version of a gene at a given location (locus) along a chromosome

Autosomal recessive: A trait or disorder requiring the presence of two copies of a gene mutation at a particular locus in order to express observable phenotype

Base pair (bp): Two nitrogenous bases paired together in double-stranded DNA by weak bonds; specific pairing of these bases [adenine (A) with thymine (T) and guanine (G) with cytosine (C)] facilitates accurate DNA replication; when quantified (e.g., 8 bp), refers to the physical length of a sequence of nucleotides

CHO cells: A cell line derived from Chinese Hamster Ovary cells

Chromosome: An organized structure of DNA and protein that is found in cells containing many genes, regulatory elements and other nucleotide sequences along with DNA-bound proteins, which serve to package the DNA and control its functions

Coding region: All exons of a gene that contribute to the protein product(s) of the gene

Complex genetic disorders: Genetic disorders which are complex, multifactorial or polygenic, are associated with the effects of multiple genes in combination with lifestyle and environmental factors

Complex trait: Trait that has a genetic component that does not follow strict Mendelian inheritance. May involve the interaction of two or more genes or gene-environment interactions

COMT: Catechol-O-Methyl Transferase an enzymes that degrads catecholamines such as dopamine, epinephrine, and norepinephrine

Consanguinity: Genetic relatedness between individuals descended from at least one common ancestor

Cysteine (cys): One of the 20 naturally occurring proteinogenic amino acids

D22S278: A microsatellite marker on chromosome 22

D3 receptor: A subtype of dopamine receptor

Dopamine: A brain neurotransmitter possibly involved in the pathogenesis of schizophrenia

Deletion: Absence of a segment of DNA; may be as small as a single base or as large as one or more genes

DNA (deoxyribonucleic acid): The molecule that encodes the genes responsible for the structure and function of an organism

Gene: The basic unit of heredity, consisting of a segment of DNA arranged in a linear manner along a chromosome

Gene amplification: Any process by which specific DNA sequences are replicated disproportionately greater than their representation in the parent molecules

Genetic association studies: Studies that aim to test whether single-locus alleles or genotype frequencies (or more generally, multilocus *haplotype* frequencies) are different between two groups (usually diseased subjects and healthy controls)

Genetic markers: A gene or other identifiable portion of DNA whose inheritance can be followed

Genetic variation: A phenotypic variance of a trait in a population attributed to genetic heterogeneity

Genome: All the DNA content of an individual, which includes all 46 chromosomes and the mitochondrial DNA

Genotype: Genetic constitution of an organism

Genotyping: Testing that reveals the specific alleles inherited by an individual

Glial cells: Non-neuronal cells that provide support and nutrition, maintain homeostasis, form myelin and participate in signal transmission in the nervous system

Glycine: One of the 20 naturally occurring proteinogenic amino acids

Haplogroup: A group of similar haplotypes that share a common ancestor with a single nucleotide polymorphism (SNP) mutation

Haplotype: A combination of alleles at multiple loci on the same chromosome that are transmitted together

Haplotype analysis: Molecular genetic testing used to identify a set of closely linked segments of DNA

Hardy-Weinberg equilibrium: A principle stating that both allele and genotype frequencies in a population remain constant or are in equilibrium from generation to generation unless specific disturbing influences are introduced

Heterozygote: An individual who has two different alleles at a particular locus, one on each chromosome of a pair; one allele is usually normal and the other abnormal

Homozygote: An individual who has two identical alleles at a particular locus, one on each chromosome of a pair

HV: Mitochondrial DNA haplogroup HV

IL2RB: Interleukin 2 receptor, beta

Kb: Kilo-base pair, a unit of measurement of DNA or RNA length used in genetics, equal to 1,000 nucleotides

Linkage: A phenomenon of co-segregating loci, not alleles, within families. Linkage studies are used for coarse mapping as they have a limited genetic resolution

Linkage disequilibrium: The co-occurrence in a population of a specific DNA marker and a disease at a higher frequency than would be predicted by random chance

Locus: The physical site or location of a specific gene on a chromosome

Locus name: An informally assigned abbreviation used in the process of mapping to designate a putative gene prior to gene identification

Mendelian genetics: A set of primary tenets relating to the transmission of hereditary characteristics from parent organisms to their children

Methionine: One of the 20 naturally occurring proteinogenic amino acids

Microdeletion: The loss of a very small piece of a chromosome, its absence is not apparent on ordinary examination

Microsatellite: Repetitive segments of DNA two to five nucleotides in length scattered throughout the genome in non-coding regions between genes or within genes (introns), often used as markers for linkage analysis

Mitochondrial inheritance: Mitochondria, cytoplasmic organelles contain their own distinct genome; mutations in mitochondrial genes always maternally inherited

Mixed model: A model of a single major locus with a polygenic background

Molecular genetics: The study of macromolecules of importance in biological inheritance

Monogenic disorder: A disorder caused by mutation of a single gene

Mutation: Changes to the nucleotide sequence of the genetic material of an organism

N terminus: The end of a protein or polypeptide terminated by an amino acid with a free amine group (-NH2)

NOTCH4: This gene encodes a member of the NOTCH family. NOTCH family members play a role in a variety of developmental processes

Nucleobases (nucleotide bases): Parts of DNA and RNA that may be involved in pairing (see also base pairs). The main ones are cytosine, guanine, adenine (DNA and RNA), thymine (DNA) and uracil (RNA), abbreviated as C, G, A, T, and U, respectively. They are usually simply called bases in genetics. Because A, G, C, and T appear in the DNA, these molecules are called DNA-bases; A, G, C, and U are called RNA-bases

Polygenic disorder: A genetic disorder resulting from the combined action of alleles of more than one gene, thus the hereditary patterns usually are more complex than those of single-gene disorders

Polymerase chain reaction (PCR): A method for amplifying a DNA base sequence using a heat-stable polymerase (an enzyme) and two 20-base primers

Polymorphism: Difference in DNA sequence among individuals that may underlie differences in health. Genetic variations occurring in more than one percent of a population would be considered useful polymorphisms for genetic linkage analysis

Primer: A strand of nucleic acid that serves as a starting point for DNA replication

Receptor: A protein molecule, embedded in either the plasma membrane or cytoplasm of a cell, to which a mobile signaling molecule may attach such as a neurotransmitter, a hormone, a pharmaceutical drug, or a toxin

Recessive gene: A gene that is phenotypically manifest in the homozygous state but is masked in the presence of a dominant allele

Recessive allele: A gene that is expressed only when its counterpart allele on the matching chromosome is also recessive (not dominant).

Recombinant DNA molecules: A combination of DNA molecules of different origin that are joined using recombinant DNA technologies

Restriction enzyme (restriction endonuclease): An enzyme that cuts double-stranded DNA at specific recognition nucleotide sequences known as restriction sites

Restriction fragment length polymorphism (RFLP): Variation between individuals in DNA fragment sizes cut by specific restriction enzymes; polymorphic sequences that result in RFLPS are used as markers on both physical maps and genetic linkage maps

SCID: Structured clinical interview for DSM disorders

Sequencing: Determination of the order of nucleotides (base sequences) in a DNA or RNA molecule or the order of amino acids in a protein.

Serine (Ser): One of the 20 naturally occurring proteinogenic amino acids

Serotonin hydroxytryptamine (5-HT): A monoamine neurotransmitter synthesized in serotonergic neurons in the central nervous system (CNS)

Single nucleotide polymorphism (SNP): DNA sequence variations that occur when a single nucleotide (A, T, C, or G) in the genome sequence is altered

Single-gene disorder: Hereditary disorder caused by a mutant allele of a single gene

Singleton: An offspring born alone

Transmission Disequilibrium/Distortion Test: A widely applied family-based association test in which trios of parents and proband are used

Valine (Val): One of the 20 naturally occurring proteinogenic amino acids

Velo-cardiofacial syndrome: An inherited disorder characterized by cleft palate, heart defects, characteristic facial appearance, minor learning problems and speech and feeding problems

Some of the terms of this glossary were modified from either Wikipedia or other online genetic dictionaries.

Chapter 16

THE EPIDEMIOLOGY OF SUICIDAL BEHAVIOR IN THE ISRAELI POPULATION

Cendrine Bursztein and Alan Apter

The spectrum of suicidal behavior ranges in severity from ideation (thoughts about the worthlessness of life and death wishes) to threats, mild attempts, serious attempts and completion (1).

Suicide is defined by Webster's New Collegiate Dictionary (2) as "the act of taking one's own life voluntarily and intentionally." Shneidman defined suicide more broadly as "the conscious act of self-induced annihilation, best understood as a multi-dimensional malaise in a needful individual who defines an issue for which the act is perceived as the best solution" (3).

Attempted suicide is defined as "the deliberate initiation of a non-habitual behavior that, without intervention from others, would cause self harm or deliberate ingestion of a substance in excess of the prescribed or generally recognized therapeutic dosage in order to realize changes that the person desires via the actual or expected physical consequences" (4).

Both completed and attempted suicide acts are important public health problems that require intervention. They are often – though not always – the most severe indicators of poor mental health and suffering. About 15% of those who attempt suicide are at high risk for succeeding (5). Therefore, even when life is not lost, addressing suicidal behaviors as well as completed suicide warrants in-depth investigation (6).

Suicide is associated with many risk factors. One way of characterizing them is to differentiate between distal and proximal exposures, which combined may lead to suicide (7). Distal risk factors – such as psychopathology, personal characteristics, substance abuse and familial factors – define the background against which suicidal behavior may develop. Their relation to suicide is indirect; they serve as thresholds that increase an individual's vulnerability to specific proximal risk factors (8). Proximal risk factors are the direct precipitators of suicide and occur within a short time before the tragic event. They include stressful life events such as sudden major illness or bereavement. Certain subpopulations may be particularly vulnerable to the influence of proximal factors. For instance, adolescents may be especially susceptible to stresses arising from life events (9), such as a breakdown in social or family structure (8). This issue is later discussed in this chapter. In addition, one of the strongest proximal risk factors for committing suicide is the availability of a method. Keeping firearms at home increases the risk for both genders and across all age groups. The effect of this factor is independent of others, such as drug abuse, living alone or taking prescribed psychotropic medications (10).

❦ Data sources on suicidal behavior

Israel's Central Bureau of Statistics (CBS) is responsible for collecting all data on deaths, including those by suicide. It receives regular updates from several external sources such as the police and the Ministry of Health (11). The Ministry, in turn, obtains information on suicides mostly from the L. Greenberg Institute of Forensic Medicine at Abu Kabir (near Tel Aviv). Although the cause of death in the CBS database corresponds to the one written on the death certificate (*ICD-10* coding), suicide may still be underestimated due to under reporting. In some situations, suicide is not recognized as such, and death is attributed to accidental or natural causes. This applies in particular to road accidents, drowning or domestic deaths of an ambiguous nature. Additionally, family and friends may try to conceal the cause of death for social, religious, legal or economic reasons. This is not uncommon in population groups in which suicide casts stigma on the survivors (12), such as among Arab Israelis and Orthodox Jews. In these cases, the official cause of death registered by the CBS may be an external event, accident or undetermined, especially if no information has been provided by the forensic institute.

Suicide rates may also be distorted by the practice of officially recording deaths by their "underlying cause" in accordance with World Health Organization (WHO) guidelines (11). For example, when a person with cancer commits suicide, the cause of death is registered as cancer, not as suicide.

Finally, in Israel, like in other countries, the process of issuing death certificates may vary among coroners, doctors and hospitals (13). To minimize errors, these officials must give special attention to deaths considered to be due to external undetermined causes (*ICD-10* codes Y10–Y34 "event of undetermined intent"); medication overdose (codes X40–X49); accidental poisoning by and exposure to noxious substances (14); suffocation; fall from a height; drowning; or shooting.

As for suicide attempts, information on the general Israeli population has until now been derived only from the National Emergency Departments Database (15, 16), which is linked to the Ministry of Health. This system is similarly prone to underestimations because some persons who attempted suicide are treated either in the community or not at all and do not seek care at emergency rooms.

Recently, the Israel National Health Survey (INHS), reviewed in other chapters, collected data on the prevalence rates and associated factors of three components of suicidal behaviors: ideation, planning and attempt in a community sample. INHS provided some additional data to what is known about suicide attempters brought to hospitals (17). However, except from epidemiological studies that examine the scope of the problem, research on risk factors of suicidal behavior in Israel is still lacking. Such studies are crucial for the development of effective and targeted preventive measures.

❦ Suicidality over the last 20 years

To bridge the current gap in knowledge, suicidality needs to be examined as a function of the ethnic and religious diversity that contributes to the mosaic of Israeli society. In addition, it is necessary to take into account high-risk subpopulations that are particularly salient in the society, such as army recruits and new immigrants (of the latter, many arrived within the last 20 years). Finally, there are the specific high-risk age and gender subgroups across religious and ethnic divides, which can be found in many societies. Only by assessing all these societal cross sections can a comprehensive picture of suicidality in Israel be drawn.

Longitudinal observations have shown that suicide rates rose in the 1980s among individuals aged 15 years and over. They stabilized in the 1990s, although updated data show a small rise since the end of the 1990s in suicide rates of people aged 45–64 and a decline in the rates of people aged 75 and older (table 1 and figure 1) (11).

Table 1: Suicide by gender. Age-standardized rates per 100,000 population 15 years of age and older. Years 1981–2004 (11)

Years	Men	Women	Total
1981	10.4	5.9	8.1
1982	9.9	6.0	7.9
1983	12.9	5.9	9.2
1984	11.4	5.2	8.2
1985	11.8	5.2	8.4
1986	13.2	6.5	9.7
1987	15.3	5.5	10.3
1988	14.8	5.8	10.2
1989	17.0	6.6	11.6
1990	14.3	5.2	9.6
1991	16.0	5.5	10.6
1992	16.2	5.6	10.7
1993	15.6	5.1	10.1
1994	16.7	5.6	10.9
1995	13.8	4.9	9.2
1996	12.0	3.5	7.5
1997	15.2	3.5	9.1
1998	11.7	3.4	7.4
1999	13.8	3.0	8.2
2000	14.2	3.7	8.7
2001	14.6	2.9	8.5
2002	12.8	3.5	8.0
2003	14.7	2.8	8.5
2004	13.5	3.4	8.3

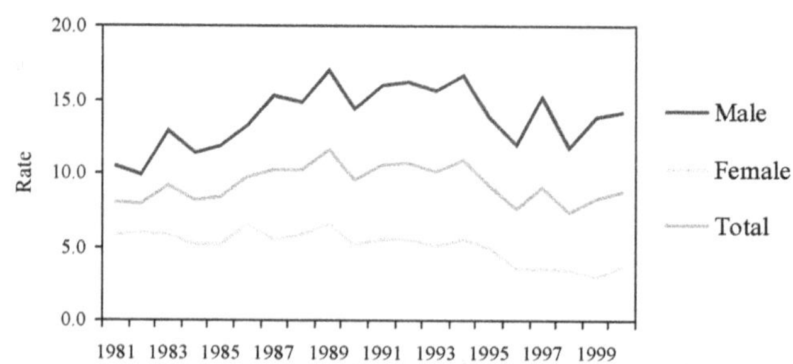

Figure 1. Age-standardized suicide rates per 100,000 of the population 15 years and older by age. Years 1981–2000. Three year-average.

In 2004, the official suicide rate in the group aged 15 years and older was 8.3 per 100,000 population. By gender, it was four times higher in men (13.5 per 100,000) than in women (3.4 per 100,000) (11). These figures represent more than 400 suicides a year. To complete the number of individuals involved (excluding the immediate survivors), one should add the attempts, which constitute about 10 times this figure according to hospital admissions records; these are probably even higher, given the many attempts that take place each year of which there are no official records.

In agreement with the literature on marital status and suicide (18), divorced men aged 25 to 44 are 6.2 times more likely to commit suicide than married men and 1.8 times more than single men (11) (table 2).

Table 2. Suicide rates per 100,000 population by marital status for the age group 25–64. Years 2000 to 2004 (11)

Age group Marital status	Total	Men	Women	Male/female rate ratio
25–44				
Single	15.1	21.9	5.2	4.2
Married	3.8	6.4	1.3	4.9
Divorced	19.9	39.5	8.8	4.5
Widowed	(19.9)	(14.4)	..	
Total	7.4	12.2	2.6	4.7
45–64				
Single	23.9	46.3	9.0	5.1
Married	6.8	10.8	2.4	4.5
Divorced	20.9	40.2	9.9	4.0
Widowed	11.2	(50.2)	(4.5)	
Total	9.3	15.1	3.9	3.9

( ) Based on less than 20 cases

Breakdown by ethnic origin showed that in the 1980s, adult Jews of European or American descent had higher rates of suicide than their counterparts born in Israel, Asia or Africa. Thereafter, suicide rates among North African-born Jewish Israelis rose in the early 1990s, reaching values close to those of European and American-born Jews. By the mid-1990s, rates for Israeli-born

Jews dropped below those of all the other Jewish ethnic groups (11). Since 2000, the highest suicide rate can be found in African-born Israelis, as will be further described in this chapter (11).

Regarding suicide attempts, the rate in the population aged 10 years or older was rather stable since the end of the 1990s in men, with rates that ranged between 59 to 67 per 100,000 population. During those years, rates in women rose to a range of 76 to 94 per 100,000. Between the years 1999–2002 the average number of emergency department visits for suicide attempts was 3600 annually: 1500, in men and 2100, in women. During the year 2003 there was a rise in the number of registered suicide attempts while between the years 2004–2007 the number stabilized at about 4300 cases per year (11). In 2007, more than one-third of all registered suicide attempts were committed by youth aged 15 to 24 (11). This issue is discussed further in the section on suicidality among the young.

More information on the lifetime prevalence rates of suicide ideation, intention, and attempts in the non-institutionalized Israeli population aged 21 years and older was provided by the INHS (17) (N = 4859). The study sample was designed to reflect the Israeli population distribution by gender, age and population groups (i.e., Arab Israelis, immigrants from the former Soviet Union (FSU) since 1990, Jewish Israelis and others not included in the first two groups). The results showed that 5.5% of Israeli adults reported having thought about suicide during their lifetime, while 1.4% had attempted suicide. About 60% of those who had ever thought about suicide actually planned or attempted one for the first time before age 35. In the first year after onset of ideation, the odds of having a suicide plan were 99 times higher than after 10 years; the odds of attempting suicide without a plan were 107 times higher; and of attempting suicide with a plan, 24,540 times higher than a decade later. In the subsequent five or 10 years, the odds of attempting suicide were highest among those who had a specific plan (17). The youngest age group in the Israeli sample – 21 to 34 years old – were found to have high odds of suicide ideation, plans and attempts (10.8 per 100,000 population) (17). The odds dropped to 4.0 per 100,000 in the 35 to 49 age group and to 2.1 per 100,000 in the 50 to 64 age group. The corresponding odds for planning suicide were 8.3, 3.6 and 2.6; and for attempts, 16.0, 6.8 and 4.0 per 100,000. The 21- to 34-year-old group also had the highest odds of impulsive suicide attempts – that is, of attempting suicide consequent to ideation with no preceding plan (16.9 compared to 7.7 per 100,000 for age 34 to 49, and 1.0 per 100,000 for age 50 to 64) (17).

In agreement with the literature on risk factors for suicidal behavior (19), the risk of attempting suicide was highest among individuals with mental health disorders. These people were more vulnerable to suicidal ideation, and their transition from suicide ideation to suicide attempt was more likely to be planned (17).

Suicidal behavior in the young

In Israel, suicide is uncommon in childhood and early adolescence. Within the group aged 10 to 14, most suicides occur between ages 12 and 14 (20). The incidence increases markedly in the late teens and continues to rise until the early 20s (21).

The rarity of completed suicide before puberty is a universal finding (22). A study by the US Centers for Disease Control and Prevention (CDC) and 25 other industrialized countries for 1990 to 1995 yielded no suicides among children aged less than five years old. For children aged five to 14, the age-specific rate was .84 per 100,000 population in the US and lower (.40 per 100,000) in other countries (23).

By contrast to completed suicide, suicide attempts are considered a behavior more common among adolescents and young adults (16). The highest rates in Israeli youths were found in those less than 20 years of age, after which the rates drop. The highest rates were found among females aged 15–20, especially in the age group 16 and 19 (249 and 247 per 100,000 females, respectively, in the years 2003–2007). Among males, the highest rates were found in those aged 19 and 20 (187 per 100,000 males) (11).

Over time, as in many other countries, Israel has seen an increase in youth suicide rates followed by stabilization. Suicides accounted for 6% of total deaths in youths in the early 1980s; the figure doubled to 13.0% in the 1990s. Today, suicide is the second leading cause of death in males aged 15 to 24 (after accidents), with a rate of 11.8 per 100,000 population; it is the third leading cause of death in females, with a rate of 1.8 per 100,000 (11).

Many gender analyses of suicide worldwide have reported a "gender paradox," with completed suicide being more common among males and suicide attempts more common among females (24, 25). In Israel, Levinson *et al.* (16) noted that women did not attempt suicide more often than men, except for the 13- to-26- year-old age group.

In adolescents, in addition to demographic variables, suicidal behavior is strongly associated with external factors such as acute and chronic life problems, and with psychiatric disorders such as depression, anxiety and behavioral disorders (26). Studies in the US and New Zealand suggested that up to 90% of youngsters who completed or attempted suicide had at least one diagnosable mental disorder at the time of their attempt (27–29). Other risk factors of deliberate self-harm in adolescents are increased stress (30); maladaptive coping (31); hopelessness (32); cognitive rigidity (33); deficits in problem solving skills (34); impulsivity (35); and certain negative personality traits (36).

In a study of 163 adolescents in Israel admitted to a psychiatric inpatient unit, Apter *et al.* (37) found that aggression (wish to die) and poor impulse control (wish not to be here for a time) were risk factors of suicidality. The wish to die was characteristic of psychiatric disorders with prominent depression such as major depression and anorexia nervosa, while the wish not to be here for a time was characteristic of conduct disorder. Hence, besides depressive symptomatology, violent behavior also correlates significantly with suicidal behavior (37).

The role of behavioral disorders in the risk of suicidality in adolescents was supported by Kerfoot *et al.*'s study in England (38), wherein 35% of adolescent suicide attempters by overdose had a diagnosis of oppositional disorder and 22% of conduct disorder. Others have noted that a small proportion of adolescents who harm themselves suffer from post-traumatic stress symptoms or eating disorders and, occasionally, schizophrenia (39).

Accordingly, the two most prominent risk factors for completed suicide in adolescents are a past suicide attempt and a diagnosis of a depressive episode. Approximately 40% of suicide completers have made a prior suicide attempt (28–37, 40–42) and 40% to 80% of adolescent attempters meeting the diagnostic criteria for depression at the time of the attempt (29, 42–46).

As shown in the records of the Ministry of Health (11), as well as in the study by Levinson *et al.* (14), the rate of suicide attempts peaked in females towards the late high school years (ages 16 and 17) and in males during compulsory army service. This three-year delay in males may reflect both their fear of exhibiting "unmanly" behavior in high school (47) and their need for escape methods during the stressful period of army service (16). (Military service and suicide is discussed in depth in the next section and in chapter 2.) Others have found that suicide attempts occurred most frequently in depressed females during the high school years – usually in the context of family dysfunction (47). As mentioned earlier, updated data from the Ministry of Health show a new peak for suicide attempts among 19-year-old women (11), a finding that requires clarification.

The use of weapons as a suicide method has also grown since the 1980s in the 15- to 24-year-old group (see table 3 below), while the use of other methods has decreased. Until the mid 1990s, there was also a rise in hanging and suffocation by young men to commit suicide, but no parallel changes were noted in females (11).

Epidemiological studies of self-injury in Israeli adolescents reported that self-poisoning was the preferred method in about 90% of cases (47–50). Iancu *et al.* (49) evaluated the characteristics of 404 adolescent suicide attempters (83.7% female) admitted to a large Israeli hospital between 1984 and 1994. Drug overdose was used in 92.8% of the cases. Younger adolescents had a higher probability of performing a violent suicide attempt.

Suicidality in the army

In some Western countries such as those in Scandinavia, suicide rates among soldiers are significantly lower than among civilians (52, 53). Researchers attribute this finding to the comprehensive medical and psychological examinations performed at recruitment (53), which filter out individuals with psychiatric disorders associated with suicide risk (54–56).

By contrast, in Israel during peacetime, suicide is the leading cause of death in the Israel Defense Forces (IDF). Recall here that military service in Israel is compulsory for 18-year-old Jewish and Druze men (except for those who receive an exemption for a variety of reasons). Recruitment and service can cause considerable stress to young men who struggle for independence and self-determination precisely at that developmental stage (57). Suddenly, in the army, they face strict demands for obedience and submission within a hierarchical system, cut off from the usual sources of social support, status and self-esteem (8). This potential crisis setting combined with the sudden availability of firearms places this population at particular risk of suicide (12, 58). Indeed, in Israel, the male suicide rate is higher in the 18- to 24-year-olds than in the 15- to 17-year-olds (11) and highest in the 18- to 21-year-olds (15.7 per 100,000 population) (11). During the past years, an average of 35 IDF soldiers committed suicide annually, an average of about one soldier every two weeks (59). In 2006, 26 soldiers committed suicide, representing a 20% decrease (60). It has yet to be clarified whether this drop resulted from the new suicide-prevention program launched by the IDF.

IDF service is compulsory for women as well, but the number who actually serve is considerably lower than for men, and they are usually assigned noncombatant jobs with less exposure to firearms (8).

Bodner *et al.* (61) reported that the underlying causes of suicide in the military may differ between combat and noncombatant soldiers. The reason they suggested was that combat soldiers may be stronger psychologically than noncombatant soldiers but serve under more stressful situations. Thus, suicide in this group is more situationally based. These are the "good soldiers" who tend to avoid seeking help for emotional distress (62). Apter *et al.* (62) showed that one of the prominent stressors precipitating suicide in combat soldiers was a perceived failure to live up to expectations. They also manifested excessive motivation, as indicated by fewer requests for unit changes, and a greater sense of duty. These findings may reflect their tendency for perfectionism and striving for excellence, leading to greater difficulty in coping with stress and failure. By contrast, individuals found at recruitment to have psychological deficiencies or a history of poor social adjustment or a low sense of duty are allocated to "friendlier" noncombatant jobs and are more likely than combat soldiers to be referred for psychological evaluation. Therefore, suicide in these individuals is more likely due to preexisting psychological problems rather than to external pressures or accessibility to weapons.

Suicide in the elderly

Despite cultural differences across nations, suicide rates are universally higher among the elderly. Suicide is most prevalent in people aged 75 and older, especially men and particularly those in Western countries (63). According to the data published by the Ministry of Health covering 2000 to 2004, the suicide rates among men aged 75 and older were about 2.5 times higher than the rate in 15- to 24-year-olds (26.1 per 100,000 vs. 11.8 per 100,000 in 2000–2004). Suicide rates in elderly women were also higher than in younger age groups, though lower than the rates for elderly men. In Israel, the highest rates in women were noted in those aged 75 years and older (11.8 per 100,000) and the lowest in the 15- to 24-year-olds (1.8 per 100,000). In both elderly men and women a large decrease in suicide rates can be seen in recent years (men, 36 per 100,000 and women, 11.8 in 1996–2000 vs. men, 26.1 per 100,000 and women, 8.1 in 2000–2004) (11).

The elderly have to face a number of stressful events that often take place during this period of life, such as loss of physical and functional abilities, cognitive function, social life and autonomy, status and independence (64). Those events can lead to a sense of hopelessness, disengagement and depression, as well as to evoke feelings of emptiness or suicidal wishes (65, 66). Ron (67) stressed health problems, such as the early stages of Alzheimer's disease, as risk factors for depression and suicidality in older individuals.

Hopelessness and depression in older people may also stem from the awareness that their chances of finding a new life partner decrease with time. A US report confirmed the importance of family support for the well-being of the elderly (68), and one Israeli study emphasized the importance of the presence of a spouse (69). As mentioned earlier, studies from England and Israel reported that singles (widowed, divorced or unmarried) are at greater risk for depression and suicidality than those with partners (11, 69, 70).

The elderly population of Israel is unique in that a sizeable proportion of them are survivors of the Holocaust. Aging is known to be associated with the reactivation of traumatic syndromes and the presence of physical disorders and psychological distress. All these factors may increase the risk of suicide (71). Barak *et al.* (72) analyzed the data on a large sample of elderly patients admitted to psychiatric hospitals over a five-year period. A total of 135 patients (14.6%) had attempted suicide before admission. These included 90 of the 374 Holocaust survivors in the sample (24.0%) compared to 45 of 502 patients (8.2%) with no World War II experience.

The rate of suicide is often underestimated in the elderly. One reason is that death in this group is often self-inflicted by indirect methods – such as refusal to eat or to take life-sustaining medications – and may not be identified as suicide. In other cases, a long time elapses from self-inflicted injury to death, leading to misattribution of the death to other pathophysiological causes (63).

Interestingly, the elderly (even women) not infrequently use violent methods of suicide, indicating high suicidal intent (68). The most updated reported methods of suicide used by

Israelis aged 75 years and older during 2000–2004 were strangulation (7.4 per 100,000 for men, and 1.6 per 100,000 for women), and jumping from a height (5.5 per 100,000 for men, and 1.8 per 100,000 for women). In younger age groups, rates of both these methods were lower in both genders (11). From the mid 1980s to the end of the 1990s, there was a rise in the use of weapons among men aged 75 years and above from 2.7 per 100,000 to 4.8 per 100,000, which is similar to the findings for men aged 15 to 24 years. After that, rates in elderly males decreased (3.4 per 100,000) while those in young males rose (5.2 per 100,000). In men aged 65 to 74, rates fluctuated between 2.8 per 100,000 in the beginning of the 1980s and 5.0 at the end of the 1980s. Gradually, the rates decreased; between the years 2000–2004 they were 3.4 per 100,000 (11). Weapons are not a usual means of suicide in women, regardless of age (table 3).

Table 3. Suicide rates per 100,000 by methods in the population 15 years and older. Years 1981–2004 (11)

Method/Years	Age group				
	15–24	25–44	45–64	65–74	75+
			Men		
1981–1990					
Poisoning	(.3)	.6	1.1	(1.4)	(2.4)
Hanging, suffocation	2.4	4.1	4.3	8.8	13.0
Firearms	2.1	2.5	3.7	3.9	(1.5)
Jumping from height	(.5)	1.1	1.6	4.8	9.6
Other	.9	2.4	4.1	5.7	11.5
Total	6.1	10.7	14.8	24.7	38.0
1991–2000					
Poisoning	..	.5	.6	1.4	2.3
Hanging, suffocation	3.5	5.7	6.3	7.9	14.8
Firearms	5.6	2.8	3.4	3.6	4.4
Jumping from height	.8	1.0	1.5	2.9	7.9
Other	1.0	1.9	2.5	4.2	8.4
Total	11.0	12.0	14.3	20.1	37.9
2001–2004					
Poisoning	(.4)	.6	(.7)	(1.3)	(1.1)
Hanging, suffocation	3.8	5.7	6.5	4.7	7.4
Firearms	5.2	2.6	2.9	3.4	(3.4)
Jumping from height	(.7)	1.6	1.7	(2.3)	5.5
Other	1.8	1.8	3.4	4.2	8.9
Total	11.9	12.3	15.2	15.9	26.3
			Women		
1981–1990					
Poisoning	(.4)	.4	1.0	(1.4)	3.0
Hanging, suffocation	.6	.7	1.6	2.6	2.6
Firearms	(.5)	.5	..	..	
Jumping from height	.6	1.4	1.5	3.4	4.9
Other	.7	1.2	2.1	4.6	6.6
Total	2.8	4.2	6.4	12.4	17.1
1991–2000					

Table 3. Suicide rates per 100,000 by methods in the population 15 years and older. Years 1981–2004 (11) (cont.)

Method/Years	Age group				
	15–24	25–44	45–64	65–74	75+
Poisoning	..	.3	.5	(1.0)	2.6
Hanging, suffocation	.6	.9	1.5	2.7	3.7
Firearms	.7	.4	.3	..	..
Jumping from height	.5	.6	1.0	1.8	4.1
Other	(.3)	.8	1.3	2.9	4.4
Total	2.1	3.0	4.6	8.4	15.0
2001–2004					
Poisoning	..	(.3)	(.2)	(.9)	(1.3)
Hanging, suffocation	(.6)	1.0	1.4	(.6)	(1.6)
Firearms	(.2)	(.2)	..	..	..
Jumping from height	(.4)	.6	1.1	(1.0)	(1.8)
Other	(.5)	.6	1.1	(1.3)	3.0
Total	1.7	2.7	3.8	3.8	7.7

..Based on a number of cases too small to present

( ) Based on less than 20 cases

Attempted suicides, though rare among the elderly, serve as an important indicator of suicide risk. The low suicide attempt rate in older people may be explained by their greater desire to die and their determination that the suicidal act be fatal. In this age group, unlike in young people, suicide attempts may be considered more as "failed" suicide rather than as a "cry for help" (60).

Thoughts about death have been reported in 15.9% of elderly persons (73), with highest rates in women and in individuals aged 85 years and older (63). Special attention should be addressed to this factor as a potential predictor of suicide in the elderly, because the vast majority of elderly suicide victims do not have a history of previous suicidal behavior, so early detection is difficult. Nevertheless, the identification of people at risk may be confounded by such factors such as anhedonia, being tired of life and wishing to die (63).

Suicidality among Arab and Jewish Israelis

In general, Islam forbids suicidal behavior (74), and suicide is considered illegal in Muslim countries (74). Data on suicidal behavior in Muslim countries are sparse, and much of the available research consists of descriptive studies. Since 1985, no Middle Eastern country other than Israel has provided data on suicide to the World Health Organization (wHO) (75).

Although underreporting of suicide may exist in countries where it is illegal, suicide rates indeed appear to be lower among Muslim countries than among individuals of other countries. This may also be the case in countries with populations belonging to different religions. These countries have an advantage for the comparative study of suicide rates because medical examiners and coroners are probably using similar criteria (75). In Israel, however, we need to consider the strong possibility that Arab society covers up, misclassifies or fails to report completed suicides.

The Arab sector in Israel is not a single homogeneous group. Levav and Aisenberg (71) found that Muslim Arabs had the lowest suicide rate of Jews, Druze and Christian Arabs. However, among teenagers, Kohn *et al.* (12) found that Christian Arabs had a lower rate of completed suicide than Muslim Arabs, while both groups had lower rates than Jews (75). This finding parallels the limited data from Jordan and Syria that suggest that Christian Arabs have a lower incidence of completed and attempted suicide than Muslim Arabs (74). According to 2000 to 2004 Ministry of Health figures, suicides numbered an average of 370 annually in the Jewish sector and 30 in the Arab sector. In the 15- to 24-year-olds, the suicide rate among Arab Israelis was 7.9 per 100,000 for men and none for women. The respective rates for Jewish Israelis, as mentioned before, were 12.8 per 100,000 and 2.1 per 100,000. Analysis by age revealed a rise in suicide in the past decade among Arab-Israeli adolescents, especially with regard to firearm-related suicides (75). The highest suicide rate in Arab Israelis was found among the 15- to 24-year-olds, whereas in the Jewish Israelis those 75 years or older had the highest rates. About a third of all suicides in the Arab-Israeli population were completed by adolescents compared to one-fifth in the Jewish/Druze population. Accordingly, professionals working with Arab-Israeli adolescents must be aware of this heightened risk and formulate appropriate preventive strategies (76).

Kohn *et al.* (12) had provided information on suicide rates among Jewish, Muslim Arab, Druze and Christian Arab-Israeli children (up to 14 years old) from 1979 through 1989. The authors noted an apparent increase in suicide during that time, especially among Muslim Israelis. In contrast to the pattern reported among adults (74), among children the rates of suicide combined with undetermined causes of death were statistically higher among non-Jews than Jews. However, no statistical differences were found between the various national/religious groups for suicides only (12). No recent studies are available assessing suicide in children. Even the Ministry of Health, which is Israel's official source of data on suicidality, does not publish such important information.

In contrast to findings for suicide (6.2 per 100,000 in Arab Israelis vs. 15.1 per 100,000 in Jewish Israelis), a comparison of national suicide attempts rates between Jews and Arabs is not available in the official Health Ministry publication (see reference 11). A limited study based on patients visiting the emergency room conducted in a general hospital in the Western Galilee, yielded higher suicide attempt rates among Arabs than among Jews (24.4 per 100,000 vs. 11.0 per 100,000, respectively) (48). A second important finding in this study was the significant inter-ethnic differences in gender, age and number of self-harm episodes. Specifically, among Jewish men, the rate of attempts rose markedly after age 40, while among their Arab counterparts, the distribution was even throughout all age groups. Among Jewish women, admissions for self harm rose gradually with age, whereas among Arab women, it peaked at age 20 to 29. These findings suggest that different ethnic groups may be characterized by differential risk patterns. Noteworthy, despite substantial differences in the Jewish and Arab sociodemographic and clinical profiles, the method, location and number of self-harm episodes were similar (48).

The interethnic crossover between suicide and attempted suicide in Arabs and Jews (48) suggests that among the former – more than among Jews – deliberate self harm is an expression of emotional distress rather than a wish to die (48). Furthermore, in Arab-Israeli women – who constitute a national minority in a patriarchal society (77) – deliberate self-harm may serve as a means to protest against oppression. At the same time, the typical midlife existential crisis could be responsible for the emergent age pattern of self harm among the Jewish-Israeli sub-population, as reported with regard to other Western urban populations (78, 79).

Suicidality in immigrants from the former Soviet Union and Ethiopia

Adjusting to a new culture and its accompanying stress of acculturation represents a challenge for immigrants (80). Dislocation, identity confusion, loss of social status and social networks, loneliness and rapid cultural change may all cause feelings of hopelessness and eventually lead to suicidal behavior (87) (see chapter 6).

For the years 2000–2007, the Ministry of Health reported higher suicide attempt rates for all age groups in immigrants from the former Soviet Union (FSU). The difference is especially evident in youths aged 15–24 (239.1 and 165 per 100,000 FSU-born females and males, respectively, compared with 194.8 and 118.2 Ethiopian-born females and males, respectively, and 162.2 and 79.9 Israeli-born females and males, respectively) (11).

Two surveys on suicidal ideation in FSU-born immigrants to Israel revealed different suicidal behavior patterns in both adolescents and adults compared to native-born Israelis.

In the first survey, a representative sample of 406 adolescents (aged 11 to 18) who had emigrated from the FSU during 1989 to 1993 was compared to 203 adolescents from Jewish high schools and the Jewish University in Moscow, in addition to 104 Israeli-born adolescents studying in Jerusalem high schools. The same door-to-door selection procedure and the same questionnaire were used for all three samples (81). The findings showed that approximately every tenth adolescent (10.9%) in the study group reported suicidal ideation during the six months preceding the survey. This rate was significantly higher than that of their peers living in the FSU, but not different from the rate in Israeli-born adolescents (8.7%). In addition, 95.4% (42/44) of these ideators had attempted suicide during the study period, compared to .5% (2/360) of those without suicidal ideation in the same period (81).

There were few gender differences in either suicidal ideation or attempts – although by age, rates of suicidal ideation in older adolescents were twice as higher than those in younger ones. The suicide ideators reported significantly higher levels of psychological distress and more behavioral problems than the non-ideators, and they had more immigration-based difficulties with language, physical health, personality characteristics and family problems. They also had less social support from the family (81).

The second national community survey of self-reported suicidal ideation and attempts compared a random group of recent immigrants from the FSU to Israel (N = 800) with a sample of Jews in the FSU (82). Almost all respondents had lived in Israel for less than five years. The same "door-to-door" selection procedure was used in both groups, with a 98.5% compliance rate. The FSU comparison group (N = 411) was matched for age and gender and did not differ significantly in sociodemographic characteristics (82). Analysis of the findings revealed a significantly higher one-month prevalence rate of suicide ideation in the immigrant sample (15.1%) than in their counterparts (6.6%). A total of 5.5% of the immigrants had ever made a suicide attempt compared to .5% of the controls. Risk factors for suicide ideation were younger age; living without a spouse; low level of social support; history of immigration from a country with a high suicide rate (Russia and the Baltic countries); and having lived in Israel for two or three years. The strongest risk factors were a higher level of psychological distress and symptoms such as depression, hostility and paranoid ideation, as well as low social support (82).

The Ministry of Health also reported a higher suicide rate in immigrants from the FSU than among Israeli-born Jews for all age groups, except for those 65 years and older. For example, during the years 2000–2004, the suicide rates in the FSU-born males aged 15 to 24 years were 2.6 higher than among non-immigrant Jews and others (including non-Arab Christians and those with no religious classification); 2.4 higher, for those aged 25–44; and 1.2 times higher, for those aged 45–64 (11). Between the years 1996 and 2004, the age-adjusted suicide rates ranged from 10.8 to 13.6 per 100,000 for FSU immigrants and 18.8 to 25.2 per 100,000 in FSU-born males. Suicide rates in FSU immigrants increased in younger age groups (15 to 44) with a larger increase in youths (from 10.8 in 1996–2000 to 13.5 per 100,000 in 2000–2004) (11) (table 4 and figure 2).

Table 4. Suicide rates per 100,000 for the population 15 year of age and older by immigrant status and by age group. Years 1996–2004 (11)

Age	2001–2004			1996–2000		
	Total	Men	Women	Total	Men	Women
Immigrants from the former USSR coming to Israel from 1990						
15–24	13.5	24.4	(2.2)	10.8	19.0	(2.3)
25–44	13.3	24.9	(2.8)	12.0	22.4	(2.8)
45–64	11.4	18.9	5.5	10.6	19.2	(3.6)
65+	12.9	21.3	7.7	13.3	22.7	7.6
Age-standardized rate	12.8	22.9	3.9	11.6	20.9	3.5
Immigrants from Ethiopia coming to Israel from 1980						
15–24	40.0	68.9	..	(20.6)	(34.9)	..
25–44	31.5	50.3	(14.0)	(20.6)	(29.8)	..
45–64	(25.9)	(41.8)	..	(42.7)	(65.6)	..
65+	..	..	..	(47.4)	(77.1)	(20.2)
Age standardized rate	30.8	50.0	(11.6)	29.5	46.1	(12.7)
Nonimmigrant Jews and others						
15–24	5.7	9.3	1.9	6.2	10.2	1.9
25–44	6.7	10.5	3.0	7.1	11.4	3.0
45–64	9.4	15.5	3.7	7.5	11.9	3.4
65+	12.6	21.6	5.6	16.5	25.7	9.4
Age standardized rate	7.8	12.8	3.2	8.2	13.1	3.7

( ) Based on less than 20 cases
..Number of cases too small to report
1996 Israeli population was set as standard population

Figure 2. Age-standardized suicide rates per 100,000 population 15 years
and older by Jewish males. Three year-average (11)

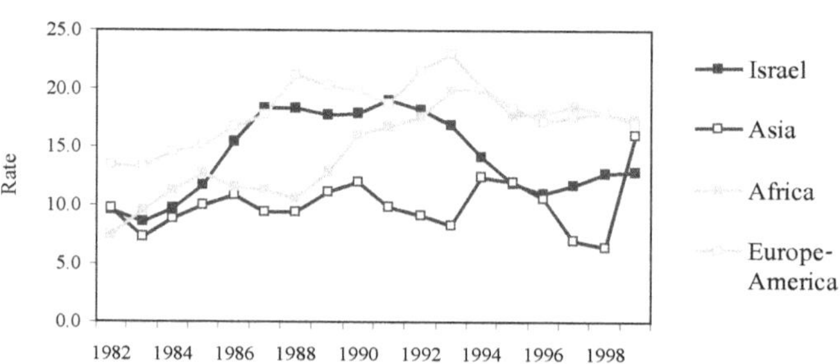

Compared to the immigrant population from the FSU, there are very few peer-reviewed studies on suicidal behavior (ideation or attempts) among Ethiopian immigrants to Israel. The newly released publication from the Ministry of Health points to lower rates compared to FSU immigrants in all age groups and quite similar to the age-adjusted rates of non-immigrant group of Jews and others (11). Regarding completed suicides, the Ministry (11) reported a strikingly higher number than in the general population in Israel (8, 46, 80–84). For instance, in 1984, the suicide rate was 25 per 100,000 among Ethiopian immigrants and six per 100,000 nationally; in 1986, the rate was sevenfold higher in the immigrant group. One decade later, this difference persists (85). In the newly released data from the Ministry, the latest data show an alarming increase: Suicide rates in Ethiopian males aged 15–44 was 59.1 per 100,000 during 2000–2004, compared to 32.4 per 100,000 during the years 1996–2000. Young Ethiopian males aged 15–24 had 7.4 time higher suicide rates compared to non-immigrant Jews and others, and 2.8 times higher rates when compared to FSU immigrants (table 4). The proportion of rates in the ages 25–44 years old people was 4.8 and 2.0, respectively.

Also, in Ethiopian males, the percentage of suicides from the total suicidal acts (attempted and completed suicides) is much higher (43%) compared to both FSU immigrants (21%) and non-immigrant Jews and others (17%).

In a small study, Arieli *et al.* (86) performed a "psychological autopsy" of Ethiopian suicide victims that provided information on the characteristics of suicide in this high-risk group. The authors interviewed the relatives and close friends of 44 of the total 49 Ethiopian immigrants who had attempted suicide from January 1983 to September 1992. They also examined detailed reports on the suicides as well as medical summaries of treatments in mental health clinics, whenever available. They found that the male: female ratio was twice that for suicide victims from the general community. The proportion of suicides was highest in the 20 to 39 age group. Only two suicide methods were used –hanging and jumping off high places. The distribution of these methods between men and women was the same (85).

Stress resulting from the immigration process itself may not fully explain the difference in suicidal tendency between immigrants in Israel from the FSU and Ethiopia. It is possible that certain psychiatric disorders among Ethiopian-born Israelis are under diagnosed because local psychiatrists are unaware of the culture-dependent presentations of mental symptoms, leading to insufficient treatment (85). Others proposed that the heightened risk among Ethiopian immigrants is associated with the different role of the head of the household in their country of origin in contrast to Israel and the distress experienced by married Ethiopian men following the loss of dominance in the home. Both situations may ultimately lead to depression and suicide. Also, as a result of the emigration to Israel, Ethiopian women lost the protection from community leaders that kept them safe from domestic violence in Ethiopia (86), thus leaving them more helpless and vulnerable.

❧ From epidemiology to mental health action

The unique ethnic and religious blend of the Israeli society demands research of societal cross-sections in order to formulate a comprehensive picture of suicidality in Israel.

This chapter summarized some of the research conducted over the past 20 years in Israel. This includes a focus on specific high-risk groups such as immigrants from the former Soviet Union and Ethiopia, Holocaust survivors and young army recruits, as well as research of specific high-risk age and gender subgroups across a religious and ethnic divide.

Despite advances in the research on suicidality in Israel, much remains unknown regarding specific risk and protective factors in various subpopulations. Future studies identifying these factors can help professionals formulate more effective and targeted intervention programs.

Centers in the US and many European countries have adopted several promising empirically-based prevention strategies, some of which are used in suicide-prevention programs. These include a battery of actions – establishing updated and detailed epidemiological database on suicide and attempted suicide; mental health and suicide-awareness campaigns; school-based skills training; prevention programs for students; screening for at-risk youths; education of primary-care physicians about depression and suicide; education by the public media; and lethal-means restriction (87).

To face this public health challenge – and in accordance with the Helsinki Declaration of 2005 adopted by the Ministerial Conference of the World Health Organization European Regional Office (88) – a national committee of experts in the field of suicidal behavior and relevant stakeholders has been established by the Ministry of Health. Its task is to formulate, implement and evaluate a preventive program for all age groups along the life cycle.

❧ References

1. Pfeffer CR. *The suicidal child*. New York: Guilford Press, 1986.
2. *Webster's New Collegiate Dictionary*, eighth edition. Springfield, MA: G&C Merriam Co., 1979.
3. Kaplan HL, Sadock BJ, Grebb JA. *Kaplan and Sadock's synopsis of psychiatry: behavioral sciences clinical psychiatry*, seventh edition. Baltimore, MD: Williams & Wilkins, 1994.
4. Schmidtke A, Bille-Brahe U, De Leo D, *et al*. The WHO/EURO multicentre study on suicidal behavior. In: Schmidtke A, Bille-Brahe U, De Leo D, *et al*., eds. *Suicidal behavior in Europe*. Gottingen, Germany: Hogrefe & Huber, 2004.
5. Maris R. The relationship of nonfatal attempts to completed suicides, In: Maris RW, Berman AL, Maltsberger JT, *et al*., eds. *Assessment and prediction of suicide*. New York: Guilford Press, 1992.
6. Apter A, Horesh N, Gothelf D, *et al*. Relationship between self- disclosure and serious suicidal behavior. *Comprehensive Psychiatry* 2001; 42: 70–75.
7. Moscicki EK. Identification of suicide risk factors using epidemiologic studies. *Psychiatry Clinics of North America* 1997; 20: 499–517.
8. Lubin G, Glasser S, Boyko V, *et al*. Epidemiology of suicide in Israel: a nationwide population study. *Social Psychiatry and Psychiatric Epidemiology* 2001; 36: 123–127.
9. Holinger P, Offer D. *Suicide and homicide among adolescents*. New York: Guilford Press, 1994.
10. Kellerman AL, Rivara FP, Somes G, *et al*. Suicide in the home in relation to gun ownership. *New England Journal of Medicine* 1992; 327: 467–472.
11. Haklai Z, Aburbeh M, Stein N. *Suicidality in Israel*. Jerusalem: Information and Computer Services. Health Information Department. Ministry of Health, State of Israel, 2008.
12. Kohn R, Levav I, Chang B, *et al*. Epidemiology of youth suicide in Israel. *Journal of the American Academy of Child and Adolescent Psychiatry* 1997; 36: 1537–1542.

13. Vijayakumar L, Nagaraj K, Pirkis J, *et al.* Suicide in developing countries. I. Frequency, distribution, and association with socio-economic indicators. *Crisis* 2003; 26: 104–111.

14. World Health Organization. *International classification of diseases – Tenth edition (ICD-10).* Version for 2007 [online]. 2007 [cited November 5, 2007]. Available from URL: http://www.who.int/classifications/apps/icd/icd10online/.

15. Ministry of Health. *Suicidality in Israel* (Hebrew) [online]. 2007 [cited November 5, 2007]. Available from URL: http://www.health.gov.il/pages/default.asp?maincat=2&catId=396&PageId=2707.

16. Levinson D, Haklai Z, Stein N, *et al.* Suicide attempts in Israel: age by gender analysis of a National Emergency Departments Database. *Suicide and Life-Threatening Behavior* 2006; 36: 97–102.

17. Levinson D, Haklai Z, Stein N, *et al.* Suicide ideation, planning and attempts: Results from the Israel National Health Survey. *Israel Journal of Psychiatry and Related Sciences* 2007; 44: 136–143.

18. Kposowa AJ. Marital status and suicide in the National Longitudinal Mortality Study. *Journal of Epidemiology and Community Health* 2000; 54: 254–261.

19. Wasserman D. A stress-vulnerability model and the development of the suicidal process. In: Wasserman D, ed. *Suicide: an unnecessary death.* London: Martin Dunitz, 2001.

20. Gould M, Greenberg T, Velting D, *et al.* Youth suicide risk and preventive interventions: a review of the past 10 years. *Journal of the American Academy of Child and Adolescent Psychiatry* 2003; 42: 386–405.

21. Anderson RN. Deaths: leading causes for 2000. *National Vital Statistics Report* 2002; 50: 16.

22. World Health Organization. Suicide rates and absolute numbers of suicide by country [online]. 2002 [cited August 1, 2002]. Available from URL: http://www.who.int/mental_health.

23. Centers for Disease Control and Prevention (CDC). Rates of homicide, suicide, and firearm-related death among children – 26 industrialized countries. *Mortality and Morbidity Weekly Report* 1997; 46: 101–105.

24. Williams M. *Suicide and attempted suicide: understanding the cry of pain.* London: Penguin Books, 2001.

25. Canetto SS, Sakinofsky I. The gender paradox in suicide. *Suicide and Life Threatening Behavior* 1998; 28: 1–23.

26. Brent DA. The aftercare of adolescents with deliberate self harm. *Journal of Child Psychology and Psychiatry* 1997; 38: 277–286.

27. Brent DA, Kolko DJ, Wartella ME, *et al.* Adolescent psychiatric inpatients' risk of suicide attempt at 6-month follow-up. *Journal of the American Academy of Child and Adolescent Psychiatry* 1993; 32: 95–105.

28. Shaffer D, Gould MS, Fisher P, *et al.* Psychiatric diagnosis in child and adolescent suicide. *Archives of General Psychiatry* 1996; 53: 339–348.

29. Beautrais A. Risk factors for suicide and attempted suicide among young people. *Australian and New Zealand Journal of Psychiatry* 2000; 34: 420–436.

30. Heikkinen M, Aro H, Lonnqvist J. Recent life events, social support and suicide. *Acta Psychiatrica Scandinavica* 1994; (suppl. 377): 65–72.

31. Kienhorst CWM, de Wilde EJ, Diekstra RFW, *et al.* Differences between adolescent suicide attempters and depressed adolescents. *Acta Psychiatrica Scandinavica* 1992: 85: 222–228.

32. Beck AT, Brown G, Berchick RJ, *et al.* Relationship between hopelessness and ultimate suicide: a replication with psychiatric outpatients. *American Journal of Psychiatry* 1990; 147: 190–195.

33. Neuringer C, Lettieri DJ. Cognition, attitudes and affect in suicidal individuals. *Suicide and Life Threatening Behavior* 1971; 1: 106–124.

34. Linehan M, Camper P, Chiles J, *et al.* Interpersonal problem-solving and parasuicide. *Cognitive Therapy Research* 1987; 11: 1–12.

35. Evans J, Platts H, Liebenau A. Impulsiveness and deliberate self-harm: a comparison of "first-timers" and "repeaters". *Acta Psychiatrica Scandinavica* 1996; 93: 378–380.

36. Pearce CM, Martin G. Locus of control as an indicator of risk for suicidal behavior among adolescents. *Acta Psychiatrica Scandinavica* 1993; 88: 409–414.

37. Apter A, Gothelf D, Orbach I, *et al.* Correlation of suicidal and violent behavior in different diagnostic categories in hospitalized adolescent patients. *Journal of the American Academy of Child and Adolescent Psychiatry* 1995; 34: 912–918.

38. Kerfoot M, Dyer E, Harrington V, *et al.* Correlates and short-term course of self-poisoning in adolescents. *British Journal of Psychiatry* 1996; 168: 38–42.

39. Herrington R, Saleem Y. Cognitive behavioral therapy after deliberate self-harm in adolescence. In: King R, Apter A, eds. *Adolescent suicide.* Cambridge: Cambridge University Press, 2003.

40. Brent DA, Perper JA, Moritz G, *et al.* Psychiatric risk factors of adolescent suicide: a case control study. *Journal of the American Academy of Child and Adolescent Psychiatry* 1993; 32: 521–529.

41. Brent DA, Perper JA, Goldstein CE, *et al.* Risk factors for adolescent suicide: a comparison of adolescent suicide victims with suicidal inpatients. *Archives of General Psychiatry* 1988; 45: 581–588.

42. Lewinsohn PM, Rohde P, Seeley JR. Adolescent suicidal ideation and attempts: prevalence, risk factors, and clinical implications. *Clinical Psychology: Science and Practice* 1996; 3: 25–46.

43. Reinherz HZ, Giaconia RM, Silverman AB, *et al.* Early psychosocial risks for adolescent suicidal ideation and attempts. *Journal of the American Academy of Child and Adolescent Psychiatry* 1995; 34: 599–611.

44. Gould MS, King R, Greenwald S, *et al.* Psychopathology associated with suicidal ideation and attempts among children and adolescents. *Journal of the American Academy of Child and Adolescent Psychiatry* 1998; 37: 915–923.

45. Fergusson DM, Woodward LJ, Horwood LJ. Risk factors and life processes associated with the onset of suicidal behaviour during adolescence and early adulthood. *Psychological Medicine* 2000; 30: 23–39.

46. Fergusson DM, Lynskey MT. Suicide attempts and suicidal ideation in a birth cohort of 16-year-old New Zealanders. *Journal of the American Academy of Child and Adolescent Psychiatry* 1995; 34: 1308–1317.

47. Farbstein I, Dycian A, Gothelf D, *et al.* A follow-up study of adolescent attempted suicide in Israel. *Journal of the American Academy of Child and Adolescent Psychiatry* 2002; 41: 1342–1349.

48. Ashkar K, Giloni C, Grinshpoon A, *et al.* Suicidal attempts admitted to a general hospital in the Western Galilee: an inter-ethnic comparison study. *Israel Journal of Psychiatry and Related Sciences* 2006; 43: 137–145.

49. Iancu I, Laufer N, Dannon PN, *et al.* A general hospital study of attempted suicide in adolescence: age and methods of attempt. *Israel Journal of Psychiatry and Related Sciences* 1997; 34: 228–234.

50. Gofin R, Avitzour M, Haklai Z, *et al.* Intentional injuries among the young: presentation to emergency rooms, hospitalization, and death in Israel. *Journal of Adolescent Health* 2000; 27: 434–442.

51. Lifshitz M, Gavrilov V. Deliberate self-poisoning in adolescents. *Israel Medical Association Journal* 2002; 4: 252–254.

52. Marttunen M, Henriksson M, Pelkonen S, *et al.* Suicide among military conscripts in Finland: a psychological autopsy study. *Military Medicine* 1997; 162: 14–18.

53. Schoderus M, Lonnqvist JK, Aro HM. Trends in suicide rates among military conscripts. *Acta Psychiatrica Scandinavica* 1992; 86: 233–235.

54. Gal R. *A portrait of the Israeli soldier.* Westport, CT: Greenwood Press, 1986.

55. Caldwell CB, Gottesman H. Schizophrenia – a high risk factor for suicide: clues to risk reduction. *Suicide and Life Threatening Behavior* 1992; 22: 479–493.

56. Murphy GH, Wetzel RD. The lifetime risk of suicide in alcoholism. *Archives of General Psychiatry* 1990; 47: 383–392.

57. Simpson SG, Jamison KR. The risk of suicide in patients with bipolar disorder. *Journal of Clinical Psychiatry* 1999; 60: 53–56.

58. Bleich A, Chen E, Levy A. Conflictual areas in the interaction between the Israeli adolescent and compulsory military service: a possible source of crisis situations. *Israel Journal of Psychiatry and Related Sciences* 1986; 23: 29–37.

59. Every two weeks a soldier commits suicide (Hebrew). NRG *Ma'ariv* [online]. 2007 [cited November 3, 2007]. Available from URL: http://www.nrg.co.il/online/43/art1/052/775.html (Hebrew).

60. Path-to-Life. Summary of meeting of the lobby for the struggle against suicidality in Israel [online]. 2007 [cited November 2, 2007]. Available from URL: http://path-to-life.org/index.php?cookie_lang=he&page_type=1&page_data[id]=4081& (Hebrew)

61. Bodner E, Ben-Artzi E, Kaplan Z. Soldiers who kill themselves: contribution of dispositional and situational factors. *Archives of Suicide Research* 2006; 10: 29–43.

62. Apter A, Bleich A, King RA, *et al.* Death without warning? A clinical postmortem study of suicide in 43 Israeli adolescent males. *Archives of General Psychiatry* 1993; 50: 138–142.

63. De Leo D, Meneghel G. The elderly and suicide. In: Wasserman D, ed. *Suicide: an unnecessary death.* London: Martin Dunitz, 2001.

64. Achte K. Suicidal tendencies in the elderly. *Suicide and Life Threatening Behavior* 1988; 18: 55–65.

65. Moscicki EK. Epidemiology of suicide. *International Psychogeriatrics* 1995; 7: 137–148.

66. Osgood NJ. Suicide in the elderly: etiology and assessment. *International Review of Psychiatry* 1992; 4: 217–223.

67. Ron R. Depression and suicide among community elderly. *Journal of Gerontological Social Work* 2002; 38: 53–71.

68. Perry CM, Johnson CL. Families and support networks among African American oldest-old. *International Journal of Aging and Human Development* 1994; 38: 41–50.

69. Ziv-Beyman S. Aged widows and married women: a multidimensional comparison. *Survey Review of Gerontology* 1996/7; 101: 20–23.

70. Baxter D, Appleby L. Case register study of suicide risk in mental disorders. *British Journal of Psychiatry* 1999; 175: 322–326.

71. Levav I, Aisenberg E. The epidemiology of suicide in Israel: international and intranational comparisons. *Suicide and Life Threatening Behavior* 1989; 19: 184–200.

72. Barak Y, Aizenberg D, Szor H, *et al.* Increased suicidal risk amongst aging Holocaust survivors. *General Hospital Psychiatry* 2003; 2 (Suppl 1): S151.

73. Scocco P, Meneghel G, Dello Buono M, *et al.* Death ideation and its correlates: survey of an over 65-year-old population. *Journal of Nervous and Mental Disease* 2001; 198: 210–218.

74. Chaleby KS. Issues in forensic psychiatry in Islamic jurisprudence. *Bulletin of the American Academy of Psychiatry and Law* 1996; 24: 117–124.

75. Lester D. Islam and suicide. *Archives of Suicide Research* 2006; 10: 77–97.

76. Morad M, Merrick E, Schwarz A, *et al.* Suicide behavior among Arab adolescents. In: Merrick J, Zalsman G, *et al. Suicidal behavior in adolescence: an international perspective.* London: Freund Publishing House, 2005.

77. Elnekave E, Gross R. The healthcare experiences of Arab Israeli women in a reformed healthcare system. *Health Policy* 2004; 69: 101–116.

78. Dudley MJ, Kelk NJ, Florio TM, *et al.* Suicide among young Australians, 1964–1993: an interstate comparison of metropolitan and rural trends. *Medical Journal of Australia* 1998; 169: 77–80.

79. Qin P, Nordentoft M. Suicide risk in relation to psychiatric hospitalization: evidence based on longitudinal registers. *Archives of General Psychiatry* 2005; 62: 427–432.

80. Cosik A. Acculturation strategies, coping process and acculturative stress. *Scandinavian Journal of Psychology* 2004; 45: 269–278.

81. Ponizovsky A, Ritsner M, Modai I. Suicide ideation and suicide attempts among adolescent immigrants from the former Soviet Union to Israel. *Journal of the American Academy of Child and Adolescent Psychiatry* 1999; 38: 1433–1441.

82. Ponizovsky A, Ritsner M. Suicide ideation among recent immigrants to Israel from the former Soviet Union: an epidemiological survey of prevalence and risk factors. *Suicide and Life Threatening Behavior* 1999; 29: 376–392.

82. Ratzoni G, Apter A, Blumensohn R, *et al.* Psychopathology and management of hospitalized Ethiopian immigrant adolescents in Israel. *Journal of Adolescence* 1988; 11: 231–236.

83. Arieli A, Gilat I, Aycheh S. Suicide by Ethiopian immigrants in Israel. *Harefuah* 1994; 123: 45–70 (Hebrew).

84. Nachman R, Yanai O, Goldin I, *et al.* Suicide in Israel: 1985–1997. *Journal of Psychiatry and Neurosciences* 2002; 27: 423–428.

85. Shoval G, Schoen G, Vardi N, *et al.* Suicide in Ethiopian immigrants in Israel: a case for study of the genetic-environmental relation in suicide. *Archives of Suicide Research* 2007; 11: 1–7.

86. Arieli A, Gilat I, Aycheh S. Suicide among Ethiopian Jews: a survey conducted by means of a psychological autopsy. *Journal of Nervous and Mental Disease* 1996; 184: 317–319.

87. Mann JJ, Apter A, Bertolote JM, *et al.* Suicide prevention strategies: a systemic review. *Journal of the American Medical Association* 2005; 294: 2064–2074.

88. World Health Organization, European Regional Office. Ministerial Conference. Facing the challenges, building solutions. Helsinki, January 2005.

SECTION III

Epidemiology Applied to the
Mental Health Services

Chapter 17

THE EPIDEMIOLOGY OF MENTAL HEALTH PROBLEMS
IN PRIMARY HEALTHCARE IN ISRAEL

Galit Geulayov, Joshua Lipsitz, Raz Gross

A high prevalence of mental health problems has been reported by general population surveys (1–4). According to the World Health Organization (WHO), about 450 million people affected with mental or behavioral disorders worldwide, and further increase is likely (5). Importantly, mental health problems have a considerable impact on the individual's physical and social wellbeing and are a significant contributor to the economic burden on society (6). Research shows that mental health problems are associated with increased physical morbidity (7, 8); mortality (7, 9, 10); cause significant disability; and impair quality of life (11).

Mental health problems result also in significant work loss (12) and are often associated with increased healthcare utilization and expenditure (13, 14). Moreover, persons with mental health problems frequently become victims of stigma and discrimination (5). Nevertheless, despite the substantial burden resulting from mental health problems, well-established diagnostic criteria and the existence of effective treatment options (15), many persons with mental health problems may remain untreated for many years. Data from the Israel National Health Survey (INHS), for example, showed that only about one-third of the persons with a mood (32.0%) or anxiety (36.0%) disorder contacted a healthcare provider for their mental health disorder in the year of illness onset – while the median treatment lag for any mood or anxiety disorder is 16 years (16).

Mental health problems are prevalent in primary care settings. A cross-cultural study conducted by the WHO at 14 sites (17) demonstrated that a substantial proportion – about 24.0% – of all patients in these settings had a mental disorder. The most common diagnoses in primary care settings are depression, anxiety and substance abuse disorders (5). A large proportion of people suffering from mental health problems do not turn to mental health services but rather to primary care practitioners (1, 18). In the INHS (19), findings showed that 7.5% of the respondents sought some form of assistance for mental health problems during a 12-month period, 59% of whom consulted some general health professionals. These professionals may have a pivotal role in providing mental healthcare services.

This chapter reviews Israeli studies carried out on psychiatric conditions in primary healthcare, including prevalence and risk factors for psychiatric morbidity. The chapter concludes with a discussion of issues related to relevant interventions in primary care.

§ The epidemiology of mental health disorders

Several methods are used to ascertain psychiatric disorders. In clinical settings, diagnosis of psychiatric conditions is typically made relying on a clinical interview and assessment. By contrast, research studies ascertain mental health disorders using structured or semi-structured diagnostic interviews, such as the Composite International Diagnostic Interview (CIDI) (20). Alternatively, self-report instruments such as the Center for Epidemiologic Studies Depression questionnaire (CES-D) (21); the Beck Depression Inventory (BDI) (22); the General Health Questionnaire (GHQ) (23); and the Patient Health Questionnaire (PHQ) (24) are used. A disorder or a condition is typically identified if a pre-determined cutoff score is met.

§ Depression

Depression has been the most widely studied mental health disorder in primary care settings worldwide, including in Israel. Depression refers to a wide range of mental health problems characterized by the absence of a positive affect (a loss of interest and enjoyment in ordinary things and experiences), low mood and a range of associated emotional, cognitive, physiological and behavioral symptoms (11). According to the *DSM-IV*, there are two main types of depressive disorders-major depressive disorder (MDD) and dysthymic disorder. To meet the diagnostic criteria of a major depressive episode, the person needs to experience depressed mood or loss of interest or pleasure and additional four symptoms (table 1), most of the day almost every day, for at least two weeks (25). Dysthymic disorder allows for more fluctuation in mood and requires fewer symptoms, but duration must be two years.

Table 1. Diagnostic symptoms of mental health disorders in primary care settings (Adapted from the DSM-IV) (25)

Disorder/ condition	Symptoms∞	Notes

Depression	A. Depressed mood
	B. Markedly diminished interest or pleasure
	  1. Significant weight or appetite change
	  2. Insomnia or hypersomnia
	  3. Psychomotor agitation or retardation
	  4. Fatigue or loss of energy
	  5. Feelings of worthlessness or excessive or inappropriate guilt
	  6. Diminished ability to think or concentrate, or indecisiveness
	  7. Recurrent thoughts of death or suicide
		MDD: 5 symptoms present for most of the day almost every day of which at least one is A or B
		
		mD*: 2 symptoms present for most of the day almost every day of which at least one is A or B

Anxiety disorders		

Table 1. Diagnostic symptoms of mental health disorders in primary care settings (Adapted from the DSM-IV) (25) (cont.)

Disorder/ condition	Symptoms∞	Notes

GAD	A. Excessive anxiety and worry occurring for at least 6 months
	B. The person finds it difficult to control the worry
	C. Anxiety or worry are associated with 3 or more of the following:
	  1. Restlessness or feeling keyed-up or on edge
	  2. Being easily fatigued or worn-out
	  3. Concentration problems
	  4. Irritability
	  5. Muscles tension
	  6. Sleep disturbance
	D. Anxiety or worry cause significant distress or impairment
	E. The disturbance is not due to the direct physiological effects of substance or a general medical condition and does not occur exclusively during another disorder	

Panic attacks	1. Palpitations, pounding heart, or accelerated heart rate 2. Sweating 3. Trembling or shaking 4. Sensations of shortness of breath or smothering 5. Feeling of choking 6. Chest pain or discomfort 7. Nausea or abdominal distress 8. Feeling dizzy, unsteady, lightheaded, or faint 9. Derealization (feelings of unreality) or depersonalization (being detached from oneself) 10. Fear of losing control or going crazy 11. Fear of dying 12. Paresthesias (numbness or tingling sensations) 13. Chills or hot flushes	A discrete period of intense fear or discomfort, in which four (or more) symptoms developed abruptly and reached a peak within 10 minutes

PTSD	A. Exposure to a traumatic event in which:
	  1. The person experienced, witnessed, or was confronted with an event or events that involved actual or threatened death or serious injury, or a threat to the physical integrity of self or others
	  2. The person's response involved intense fear, helplessness, or horror.
	B. The traumatic event is persistently re-experienced in ways of:
	  1. Recurrent and intrusive distressing recollections of the event, including images, thoughts, or perceptions
	  2. Recurrent distressing dreams of the event
	  3. Acting or feeling as if the traumatic event were recurring (includes a sense of reliving the experience, illusions, hallucinations, and dissociative flashback episodes, including those that occur on awakening or when intoxicated)
	  4. Intense psychological distress at exposure to internal or external cues that symbolize or resemble an aspect of the traumatic event
	  5. Physiological reactivity on exposure to internal or external cues that symbolize or resemble an aspect of the traumatic event
	C. Persistent avoidance of stimuli associated with the trauma and numbing of general responsiveness (not present before the trauma), as indicated by:
	  1. Efforts to avoid thoughts, feelings, or conversations associated with the trauma
	  2. Efforts to avoid activities, places, or people that arouse recollections of the trauma
	  3. Inability to recall an important aspect of the trauma
	  4. Markedly diminished interest or participation in significant activities
	  5. Difficulty falling or staying asleep
	  6. Irritability or outbursts of anger
	  7. Difficulty concentrating
		1 and 2 in A and at least 1 in B and at least 3 in C and at least 2 in D and E and F

Table 1. Diagnostic symptoms of mental health disorders in primary care settings (Adapted from the DSM-IV) (25) (cont.)

Disorder/ condition	Symptoms∞	Notes
	8. Hyper vigilance 9. Exaggerated startle response 10. Duration of the disturbance: symptoms in B, C, and D > 1 month 11. The disturbance causes clinically significant distress or impairment in social, occupational, or other important areas of functioning.	
Somatoform disorders		

Somatization	A. A history of many physical complaints beginning before the age of 30 years.
	B. Each of the following criteria must have been met:
	  1. 4 pain symptoms related to at least four different sites or functions (e.g., head, abdomen, back, joints, extremities, chest, rectum, during menstruation, during sexual intercourse, or during urination)
	  2. 2 gastrointestinal symptoms other than pain (e.g., nausea, bloating, vomiting other than during pregnancy, diarrhea, or intolerance of several different foods)
	  3. 1 sexual or reproductive symptom other than pain (e.g., sexual indifference, erectile or ejaculatory dysfunction, irregular menses, excessive menstrual bleeding, vomiting throughout pregnancy)
	  4. 1 pseudo neurological symptom not limited to pain (*conversion* symptoms such as impaired coordination or balance, paralysis or localized weakness, difficulty swallowing or lump in throat, *aphonia*, urinary retention, hallucinations, loss of touch or pain sensation, double vision, blindness, deafness, seizures; *dissociative* symptoms such as amnesia; or loss of consciousness other than fainting)
	C. Either (1) or (2):
	  1. Each symptom in criterion B cannot be fully explained by a general condition or the direct effect of a substance
	  2. The impairment cased is in excess of would be expected by an existing medical condition.
	D. Symptoms are not intentionally produced.	

Hypochondriasis	A. Preoccupation with fears of having, or the idea that one has, a serious disease based on the person's misinterpretation of bodily symptoms. B. The preoccupation persists despite appropriate medical evaluation and reassurance. C. The belief in Criterion A is not of delusional intensity (as in Delusional Disorder, Somatic Type) and is not restricted to a circumscribed concern about appearance (as in Body Dysmorphic Disorder). D. The preoccupation causes clinically significant distress or impairment in social, occupational, or other important areas of functioning. E. The duration of the disturbance is at least 6 months. F. The preoccupation is not better accounted for by Generalized Anxiety Disorder, Obsessive-Compulsive Disorder, Panic Disorder, a Major Depressive Episode, Separation Anxiety, or another Somatoform Disorder. Specify if: With poor insight: if, for most of the time during the current episode, the person does not recognize that the concern about having a serious illness is excessive or unreasonable.	
Pain disorder	Pain in one or more anatomical sites is the predominant focus of the clinical presentation and is of sufficient severity to warrant clinical attention. The pain causes clinically significant distress or impairment in social, occupational, or other important areas of functioning. Psychological factors are judged to have an important role in the onset, severity, exacerbation, or maintenance of the pain. The symptom or deficit is not intentionally produced or feigned (as in Factitious Disorder or Malingering).	

Table 1. Diagnostic symptoms of mental health disorders in primary care settings (Adapted from the DSM-IV) (25) (cont.)

Disorder/ condition	Symptoms∞	Notes
	The pain is not better accounted for by a Mood, Anxiety, or Psychotic Disorder and does not meet criteria for Dyspareunia. *Code as follows:* 307.80 Pain Disorder Associated With Psychological Factors: psychological factors are judged to have the major role in the onset, severity, exacerbation, or maintenance of the pain. (If a general medical condition is present, it does not have a major role in the onset, severity, exacerbation, or maintenance of the pain.) This type of Pain Disorder is not diagnosed if criteria are also met for Somatization Disorder. *Specify if:* Acute: duration of less than 6 months Chronic: duration of 6 months or longer 307.89 Pain Disorder Associated With Both Psychological Factors and a General Medical Condition: both psychological factors and a general medical condition are judged to have important roles in the onset, severity, exacerbation, or maintenance of the pain. The associated general medical condition or anatomical site of the pain (see below) is coded on Axis III. *Specify if:* Acute: duration of less than 6 months Chronic: duration of 6 months or longer Note: The following is not considered to be a mental disorder and is included here to facilitate differential diagnosis.	

* *Not included in DSM-IV as a diagnosis but in the appendix*

∞*Adapted from the DSM-IV*

Major Depressive Disorder (MDD); Minor Depression (MD); Generalized Anxiety Disorder (GAD); Post Traumatic Stress Disorder (PTSD)

Seven studies provide information about the prevalence of depressive disorders in Israeli primary care. The time frame for prevalence estimates varies across studies, with four of seven studies using point prevalence. Kafman *et al.* (6) identified 1.6% of 551 primary care patients, aged 18–90, as MDD positive. Using the same self-report instrument, the Inventory to Diagnose Depression (IDD) (26), however, Froom *et al.* (27) found that 3.4% of their sample of 207 kibbutz members (age ≥ 17) met criteria for MDD. This considerable difference is not readily explained. The two samples were similar in terms of age, however the proportion of women was slightly higher in the latter, 63.0%, as compared to the former study, 54.0%, which might account for some of the difference since women tend to show higher rates of depressive morbidity than do men (28). In another study, Simon *et al.* (14) studied 3613 primary care patients from rural practices in the south, and reported a prevalence of 4.5% for depressive disorder (i.e., MDD) using the CIDI. Shvartzman *et al.* (29) showed that the point prevalence of MDD in 2509 patients recruited from urban primary care clinics in the south was as high as 5.9%. In these two studies (14, 29), depression was assessed using a diagnostic interview as opposed to self-administered assessment tools as utilized by Kafman *et al.* (6) and Froom *et al.* (27).

These findings are surprising, because self-rated screening instruments usually produce more false positives and thus tend to yield higher prevalence rates of mental health disorders compared with diagnostic interviews (30, 31). None of the studies cited above described in detail the method used for sample selection, except for Shvartzman *et al.* who used a random sample. Indeed, the prevalence rate reported by Shvartzman *et al.* is consistent with that of studies from other countries (32). The relatively low prevalence rate reported in the studies cited above (6, 14, 27) could be accounted for by some selection bias.

Using the CIDI-SF (short form) diagnostic interview (33), Cwikel *et al.* (30) assessed the one-year prevalence rates of depressive disorders and subclinical conditions in a group of 976 patients aged 25 to 75 who were recruited from primary care clinics throughout Israel. The studies reported that 20.6% had a clinical diagnosis of depression (i.e., scored 4 to 7 on the CIDI-SF) during the year preceding the interview. A single Israeli study (34) that assessed the lifetime prevalence of dysthymic disorder in primary care using chart review found a .9% prevalence rate. However, this was part of a multinational study, and data specific to the local site were not reported.

Subclinical depression

Researchers have also studied mental health problems based on sub-threshold (sub-syndromal) diagnosis. The terms "minor depression" and "significant depressive symptoms" represent conditions characterized by the presence of depressive symptoms that may not fulfill the criteria for a depressive disorder. Nevertheless, these conditions are associated with significant disability (35), morbidity (36), and mortality (37) and may impose a significant economic burden (38). They also represent a significant predictor of later onset of MDD (35). Seven of 10 studies assessed subclinical depressive morbidity; all but one studied point prevalence.

The lowest prevalence rate of minor depression in primary care settings was 1.1%, as reported by Kafman *et al.* (6). Similarly, Shvartzman *et al.* (29) detected 1.6% with minor depression, yet Froom *et al.* (27) found a prevalence rate of 5.4% for minor depression in a group of kibbutz members, some of whom (approximately 30.0%) were recruited from the primary-care clinic. Differences could be explained by the use of different thresholds for clinical depression. Interestingly, the study by Froom *et al.* had a fairly high rate of minor depression and a low rate of major depression, while the inverse was found by Shvartzman *et al.* (29).

Current prevalence rates of clinically significant depressive symptoms also varied considerably across studies. Reis et al. (39) identified 7.0% of 238 primary-care patients recruited from 28 family practices throughout Israel. The authors found significant depressive symptoms using a three-item depression screening tool, while Shvartzman et al. found that 14.3% had significant depressive symptoms (29).

In another study, Biderman *et al.* (40) showed that 16.8% of their sample of persons over age 60 had elevated depressive symptoms scores. Herrman *et al.* (38) found that 24.0% of the sample studied had clinically significant depressive symptoms, while Cwikel *et al.* (30) used a diagnostic interview and reported a one-year prevalence rate of 4.8% for sub-threshold depression (i.e., CIDI-SF score=3) in 976 primary care patients aged 25–75 years. This considerable variability in findings probably reflects variability in the methods employed in these studies.

No two studies used the same instrument for assessing depressive symptomatology. Studies varied also with respect to methods of sampling (random vs. convenience samples), sample size (from N = 238 to N = 3613) and the sociodemographic characteristics of the population studied (such as age and gender). Notably, in a majority of the published studies, no adequate reference was found to the evaluation of the psychometric properties of the Hebrew version of the instruments used. In some of these papers, the authors cited another reference from which it was possible to extract information on the psychometric properties of the Hebrew version (table 2), but in other cases it was not possible to do so.

Table 2. Instruments used to assess mental health problems in primary care in Israel

Authors (Year)	Methods				Disorder/ condition	Instrument	Method of administration	Criteria for caseness	Prevalence rates	Validity/ reliability/ sensitivity/ Specificity tests of Hebrew version
	Sample	Sampling method	N	Age						
Depression										
Froom et al. (1995) (27)	Kibbutz members, some from PC 36.8% males	Not specified	207	≥17	Major depressive disorder (MDD) Minor depression (mD)	Inventory to Diagnose Depression (IDD)	SR	DSM algorithm: MDD=anhedonia or dysphoria + 4 other symptoms mD=anhedonia or dysphoria + 2 other symptoms	Current MDD: 3.4% mD: 5.4%	In Zimmerman et al. (1986): Agreement: 80% Kappa: .62
Reis et al. (1999) (39)	PC 49% males	Not specified	238	>21	Depressive symptoms	A 3-item depression screening tool	SR	N/A	Current 7%	N/S
Munitz et al. (2000) (34)	PC patient files 24.5% males	Consecutive	200	Mean (±SD) 54.3 (±16.9)	Depressive disorder (DDIS) Diagnosable depression (DD)	ICD-10 depressive symptoms checklist	Medical file examination	DDIS: diagnosis of depression in medical file DD: sufficient symptoms in file for a diagnosis of depression	3 months DDIS: N/A for the Israeli subsample DD: 4.4%	N/R
Biderman et al. (2002) (40)	PC patients 41% males	Not specified	283	age≥60	Depressive symptoms (DS)	Geriatric Depressive Scale (GDS)	SR	GDS≥7	Current 16.8%	In Cwikel et al (1989): Sensitivity: 72% Specificity: 57%
Herrman et al. (2002) (38)	PC patients 46% males	Not specified	3613	18–75	Depressive symptoms (DS)	Center for Epidemiologic Studies Depression Instrument (CES-D)	SR	CES-D≥16	Current 24%	N/S
Simon et al. (2002) (14)	PC patients 46% males	Not specified	3613	18–75	Depressive disorder	Composite International Diagnostic Interview (CIDI)	N/A	DSM-IV criterion for MDD	Current 4.5%	N/S

Table 2. Instruments used to assess mental health problems in primary care in Israel (cont.)

Authors (Year)	Methods				Disorder/ condition	Instrument	Method of administration	Criteria for caseness	Prevalence rates	Validity/ reliability/ sensitivity/ Specificity tests of Hebrew version
	Sample	Sampling method	N	Age						
Kafman *et al.* (2003) (6)	PC patients 46% males	Not specified	551	18–90	Major depressive disorder (MDD) Minor depression (mD)	Inventory to Diagnose Depression (IDD)	SR	Based on DSM algorithm: MDD = anhedonia, dysphoria + 4 other symptoms mD = anhedonia or dysphoria + 2 other symptoms	Current MDD: 1.6% mD: 1.1%	In Zimmerman *et al.* (1986): Agreement: 80% *Kappa*: .62
Shvartzman *et al.* (2005) (29)	PC patients 39.3% males	Random	2507	age 21–65	Major depressive disorder (MDD) Minor depression (mD) Depressive symptoms (DS)	Mini International Neuropsychiatric Interview (MINI)	Telephone interview	N/A	Current MDD: 5.9% mD: 1.6% DS: 14.3%	Refer to Sperber *et al.* (1994)
Heymann *et al.* (2007) (46)	Military PC enlisted males	Consecutive cases with a psychiatric diagnosis and matched controls	285	N/S	Depressive disorder	Medical file examination	N/R	Diagnosis in medical file	3 years Depression: 20% Anxiety: 25% Somatoform: 6%	N/R
Cwikel *et al.* (2008) (30)	PC patients 34.8% males	Consecutive	976	25–75	1. Depressive disorder 2. Sub-threshold depression	Composite International Diagnostic Interview (CIDI) CIDI-SF (short form) Symptom Checklist-90 (SCL-90)	SR	Depressive disorder: CIDI-SF score 4–7 Sub-threshold depression: CIDI-SF score 3	1-Year Disorder: 20.6% Sub-threshold: 4.8%	N/S

Table 2. Instruments used to assess mental health problems in primary care in Israel (cont.)

Authors (Year)	Methods				Disorder/ condition	Instrument	Method of administration	Criteria for caseness	Prevalence rates	Validity/ reliability/ sensitivity/ Specificity tests of Hebrew version
	Sample	Sampling method	N	Age						
Postpartum depression										
Glasser et al. (2000) (43)	Prenatal care clinic	Random	288	17–43	Postpartum depression (PPD)	The Edinburgh Postnatal Depression Scale (EPDS)	SR	EPDS≥10 at 6 weeks postpartum	Current 22.6%	N/S
Eilat-Tsanani et al. (2006) (44)	Delivery ward in Emek medical center	Consecutive	574	≥18	Postpartum depression (PPD)	The Edinburgh Postnatal Depression Scale (EPDS)	Telephone interview	EPDS≥13 at 2 months postpartum	Current 9.9%	N/S
Anxiety										
Heymann et al. (2007) (46)	Military PC enlisted males	Consecutive cases with a psychiatric diagnosis and matched controls	285	N/S	Anxiety disorders	Medical file examination	N/R	Diagnosis in medical file	3 years Any anxiety disorder: 25%	N/R
Cwikel et al. (2008) (30)	PC patients 34.8% males	Consecutive	976	25–75	Disorders: Generalized anxiety disorder (GAD) Panic attacks (PA) Obsessive compulsive disorder (OCD) Sub-threshold conditions: Panic attack	Composite International Diagnostic Interview (CIDI) CIDI-SF (short form) Symptom Checklist-90 (SCL-90)	SR	Disorders: GAD: N/A PA: CIDI-SF score 3–6 OCD: CIDI-SF score 3 Sub-threshold conditions: Panic attacks: CIDI-SF score 2	1-year disorders: GAD: 11.2% PA: 7.4% OCD: 3.9% Sub-threshold: Panic attacks: 4.4%	N/S

Table 2. Instruments used to assess mental health problems in primary care in Israel (cont.)

Authors (Year)	Methods				Disorder/ condition	Instrument	Method of administration	Criteria for caseness	Prevalence rates	Validity/ reliability/ sensitivity/ Specificity tests of Hebrew version
	Sample	Sampling method	N	Age						
Post-traumatic stress disorder										
Taubman-Ben-Ari et al. (2001) (47)	PC patients 40% males	Random	2975		Post-traumatic stress disorder (PTSD)	14-item PTSD scale	SR	Based on DSM-III: A traumatic event+1 or more symptoms relating to persistent re-experiencing the event+1 or more relating to avoidance of reminding situations+2 relating to increased arousal .	Current 9%	Test-retest: 82% Concurrent validity: Intrusion sub-scale r=.62; Avoidance sub-scale r=.40 Agreement: 75%
Cwikel et al. (2008) (30)	PC patients 34.8% males	Consecutive	976	25–75	Post-traumatic stress disorder (PTSD)	PTSD checklist	SR	N/S	1-Year 2.8%	N/S
Somatomoform disorder/related conditions										
Cwikel et al. (2008) (30)	PC patients 34.8% males	Consecutive	976	25–75	Disorders: Hypochondriasis Somatization Sub-threshold conditions: Hypochondriasis	Composite International Diagnostic Interview (CIDI) CIDI-SF (short form) Symptom Checklist-90 (SCL-90)	SR		1-Year Disorders: Hypochondriasis: 1.3% Somatization: 11.8% Sub-threshold: Hypochondriasis: .8%	N/S

Table 2. Instruments used to assess mental health problems in primary care in Israel (cont.)

Authors (Year)	Methods				Disorder/ condition	Instrument	Method of administration	Criteria for caseness	Prevalence rates	Validity/ reliability/ sensitivity/ Specificity tests of Hebrew version
	Sample	Sampling method	N	Age						
Eating disorders										
Cwikel et al. (2008) (30)	PC patients 34.8% males	Consecutive	976		Eating Disorder (ED)	Disordered eating behavior	SR	ED: N/A	1-Year ED: 15%	N/S
Emotional distress										
Shiber et al. (1990) (61)	PC patients	Not specified	776	≥18	Emotional distress	General Health Questionnaire (GHQ)	SR	GHQ≥5	Current 69%	N/S
Maoz et al. (1991) (60)	Military PC clinics 81% males	Random	182	Mean (±SD) 22.6 (±N/S)	Psychological distress	General Health Questionnaire (GHQ)	SR	GHQ≥5	Current 42%	N/S
Yagur et al. (2002) (58)	PC patients 55.2% males	Not specified	125	18–82	Psychological distress	Items related to depression and anxiety from BSI and PERI	SR	Score>2: clinically significant distress	Current 10.4%	Cronbach's = .92
Rabinowitz et al. (2005) (59)	PC patients 40% males	Not specified	2975	≥18	Psychological distress	General Health Questionnaire (GHQ)	SR	GHQ≥5	Current 38.2%	N/A

Abbreviations: NS – Not specified; NR – Not relevant; PC – Primary care; SR – Self report; MDD – Major depressive disorder;

BSI – Brief Symptom Inventory; PERI – Psychiatric Epidemiology Research Interview-Demoralization Scale

Risk factors

Many potential risk factors have been studied in relation to depression.

Gender: Israeli studies generally support the finding that women are more vulnerable to depression. Female gender has been associated with clinically significant depressive symptoms (34, 39), depressive disorder (30), minor depression (29) or diagnosable depression (sufficient depressive symptoms in the medical file suggestive of a depressive episode) (34). However, other studies found that depression was not associated with gender when compared to depressive symptoms (15), to no depression (6) nor to severity of depressive symptoms (41).

Age: There are no consistent findings regarding age as a risk factor for depressive morbidity. One study (6) found that the mean age of individuals with major or minor depression was significantly higher than that of people with no depressive morbidity, whereas another study (14) reported that depression was more prevalent in those younger than 65 years. Other reports found no association between age and clinically significant depressive symptoms (15, 29, 38, 40, 41) or depressive disorder (15, 29, 41).

Marital status: Studies conducted outside Israel reported that being married or cohabiting is protective with respect to depressive morbidity (28), while studies conducted in Israel did not demonstrate such an association. In one study (38, 41) severe depressive symptoms were more frequent in unmarried individuals. In another study (6), a higher rate of minor depression and MDD was found in married and widowed (vs. single) persons, while in other reports, marital status was unrelated to a clinically significant depression score (29, 40) or MDD (15, 29).

Socioeconomic status (SES): Studies seem to confirm that lower educational attainment represents a risk factor for depression. Findings showed that the number of years of schooling was inversely associated with depressive symptom scores (29, 38, 41) and MDD (15, 29) – although two studies reported no association between years of education and depressive symptoms scores (40) or MDD (6).

Regarding employment and income, there was some indication that unemployment and low income were associated with depression. One study (29) reported a higher proportion of depressive disorders (i.e., MDD) and depressive symptoms among the unemployed, while another study (30) found that depression was more prevalent among those not working full time. In a third study (15), there was no association between indices of employment and depression. Regarding income, Cwikel *et al.* (30) found that depression was more prevalent among individuals classified by the authors as having insufficient income.

Other factors studied in relation to depressive morbidity in primary healthcare in local studies include ethnicity, immigration status and religiosity. One Israeli study reported that depressive morbidity was associated with being a member of an ethnic minority group (34). In another study, depressive morbidity was associated with being an immigrant living in Israel for more than 10 years prior to the survey and with being secular (29).

In conclusion, consistent with reports from other countries (29), Israeli data showed that certain subgroups within the Israeli population identified in primary care settings are at a higher risk for developing depression. More specifically, it appears that female gender, low educational attainment and income and indices of unemployment are associated with depression and depressive symptoms in the primary-care populations.

℘ Postpartum depression

The term postpartum depression (PPD) refers to non-psychotic depression that occurs shortly after childbirth (see chapter 11). PPD is clinically no different from non-childbirth-related depressive episode, and the symptoms must meet the same diagnostic criteria. However, the symptoms should occur within four to six weeks after childbirth, although epidemiological studies show that vulnerability to symptoms may occur for a significantly longer period (42).

Two Israeli studies have been carried out on PPD (43, 44). Glasser *et al.* (43) conducted a prospective study in three prenatal care clinics in central Israel. The authors surveyed a random sample of 288 Israeli women, aged 17 to 43. Using the Edinburgh Postnatal Depression Scale (EPDS) (45), a self-administered questionnaire used to screen for symptoms of PPD, they found that 22.6% of women had PPD at six weeks post delivery.

However, Eilat-Tsanani *et al.* reported a much lower rate of PPD as assessed by the EPDS (44). The investigators studied a group of 574 women aged 18 and over in a northern town in Israel. Their study included a random sample of Arab and Jewish Israelis living in rural and urban communities. The rate of reported postnatal depression at two months after childbirth was 9.9%. Although this study was not conducted in primary healthcare settings but in a hospital, it is included here for the purpose of comparison. One way to explain the inconsistency in findings is the different EPDS cutoff scores used by the two studies to classify individuals as depressed. While Eilat-Tsanani *et al.* (44) considered those with an EPDS ≥ 13 to have PPD, Glasser *et al.* (43) used a cutoff score of 10 and above. Indeed, the former reported a significantly lower prevalence. When Glasser *et al.* used the EPDS≥13 cutoff-point, they found that 13% had PPD (S. Glasser, personal communication, October 2008). Furthermore, assessment during different time-frames might explain some of the differences in the findings. Glasser *et al.* (43) measured PPD at six weeks while Eilat-Tsanani *et al.* (44) assessed PPD at two months after childbirth. Studies conducted in other countries also reported great variation as a function of the time frame used to assess PPD (42).

Risk Factors

Several risk factors for postpartum depression have been assessed in the Israeli population. These include sociodemographic factors, psychosocial variables, pregnancy-related and health-related factors. Results show that Arab women are more vulnerable to postpartum depression than Jewish women in Israel and that new immigrants are at a higher risk compared to Israeli-born women (44). Similarly, being a homemaker was associated with PPD as compared to being employed at some job outside the home (44). Glasser *et al.* (43) identified marital disharmony and lack of social support as major risk factors for developing PPD. Furthermore, certain indices of health were identified as risk factors for PPD. Prolonged infant health problems (43), unplanned pregnancy, experiencing the course of pregnancy as "hard" and rating one's health as "not good" compared to "good" or "very good" (44), were all predictors of PPD. A further important point emerging from these two studies is the finding that past mental illness renders women vulnerable to PPD. More specifically, past diagnosis of depression (44), depressive symptoms during pregnancy and a history of emotional problems (43) were all predictors of PPD.

℘ · Anxiety disorders

Anxiety disorders refer to a group of disorders where the primary feature is abnormal or inappropriate anxiety (table 1). This group includes generalized anxiety disorder (GAD), panic disorder (PD), obsessive-compulsive disorder (OCD), post-traumatic stress disorder (PTSD) and different specific phobias. Limited research has been carried out on anxiety disorders in primary care in Israel.

Cwikel *et al.* (30) assessed anxiety in 976 patients, aged 25–75 years, recruited from primary care practices throughout Israel in face-to-face interviews using the CIDI structured questionnaire. They found that the prevalence rate of anxiety disorders during one year was 11.2%, for GAD; 7.4%, for panic attack; and 3.9% for OCD – i.e., a total of 18.7% had some form of anxiety disorder during one-year. In another study, Heymann *et al.* (46) assessed the prevalence of anxiety disorders in a military primary-care clinic. The investigators reviewed the medical files of 285 enlisted soldiers, 25.0% of whom had developed some form of anxiety disorder during their three years of military service. The sample selected for the study included 155 consecutive cases (i.e., soldiers with some mental health problem) and 130 matched controls.

Findings regarding PTSD in primary care were not consistent. Taubman-Ben-Ari *et al.* (47) studied PTSD in a random sample of 2,975 Israeli primary care attendees. They reported a PTSD point prevalence rate of 9%. However, Cwikel *et al.* (30) found that only 2.8% of their sample of 976 patients aged 25–75 years had PTSD during the past year. The conflicting findings may be explained in part by different methodologies (see table 2 for detailed methods). In contrast, studies conducted in other countries found that PTSD is rather prevalent in primary care. For example, Liebschutz *et al.* (48) reported a one-year prevalence of 26.0% in an urban primary care sample in the US, while Stein *et al.* (49) found that 11.8% met criteria for partial or full PTSD among 368 primary-care patients. Magruder *et al.* (50) reported that 11.5% of 746 randomly selected primary-care patients met criteria for PTSD. Neria *et al.* (51) estimated current prevalence rates for PTSD related to the terror attacks on the US on September 11, 2001. These ranged from 4.7% to 10.2%, depending on the criteria used for classification, in a sample of 930 adults at a New York City general medical clinic. The findings cited above seem to be more consistent with the results obtained by Taubman-Ben-Ari *et al.* in Israel (47).

Risk Factors

Even less is known about risk factors for anxiety disorders. Cwikel *et al.* (30) found that female gender was a risk factor for panic disorder, but surprisingly not for GAD or PTSD. Gender was unrelated to any sub-threshold anxiety conditions. Furthermore, years of education, lower income and not working full time were all associated with GAD, while only lower income was associated with panic attacks. More research is clearly needed to determine the prevalence of anxiety disorders and subclinical conditions as well as their correlates in primary care in Israel.

❧ Somatoform disorders and somatization

Somatoform disorder is the umbrella term used to describe a group of conditions characterized by the presence of physical symptoms causing significant distress or disability without evidence of a clear physiologic cause. The *Diagnostic and Statistical Manual of Mental Disorders – Fourth Edition (DSM-IV)* classifies somatoform disorders into six separate psychiatric disorders: *somatization disorder*; hypochondriasis; pain disorder; undifferentiated somatoform disorder; conversion disorder; and body dysmorphic disorder. This section will focus on the first three disorders.

Individuals with somatization disorder report symptoms affecting multiple organ systems or physical functions, including pain, gastrointestinal distress, sexual problems and symptoms that mimic neurological disorders (table 1). Hypochondriasis refers to excessive concern and fears of having a physical disease or injury. Individuals experiencing the disorder tend to over-react to minor physical symptoms or sensations.

The primary feature of pain disorder is physical pain that causes significant distress or disability or leads an individual to seek medical attention. Pain may be medically unexplained or it may be associated with an identifiable medical condition but far more severe than the condition would warrant. Limited research has been performed on somatoform disorders in primary-care settings in Israel. Cwikel *et al.* (30) studied the one-year prevalence rate of mental health disorders and subclinical conditions in 976 patients aged 25 to 75 years who had been recruited from primary care practices throughout Israel. They reported that 1.3% had hypochondriasis and 11.8% somatization disorder during one year. The authors identified five risk factors for somatization disorder – a lower level of education, lower income, unemployment and being 45 to 64 years old. Similarly, separated, divorced or widowed persons had higher prevalence of somatization compared to the married and single.

Somatic complaints that do not fulfill criteria for a disorder are a common problem in primary care (52). The term somatization has been broadly defined as the presentation of one or more medically unexplained somatic symptoms that do not fulfill DSM-IV criteria for somatization disorder or other somatoform disorder (53). Research into somatization in primary care is important for several reasons. First, somatization is common in primary care (54). Barsky *et al.* (55), for example, found that the point prevalence of somatization in primary care in the US was as high as 20.5%. However, only one study assessed the prevalence of sub-threshold somatoform conditions among Israeli primary care patients. Cwikel *et al.* (30) found that the one-year prevalence of sub-threshold hypochondriasis was .8%, a rate considerably lower than that reported in other countries. Second, patients with somatic symptoms experience significant distress and disability. Third, somatic symptoms are often the only presentation of emotional distress during the primary care visit and may be the key to identification (46). Furthermore, somatization may lead to multiple, and sometimes potentially hazardous and often costly unnecessary medical tests. Indeed, studies from countries other than Israel have shown that high level of medically unexplained somatic symptoms leads to increased healthcare utilization (55, 56).

§ Other mental disorders

Other mental health disorders and subclinical conditions commonly seen in primary-care settings include eating disorders and substance abuse and dependence, as well as psychological distress. Eating disorders are characterized by disturbances in eating behavior. Disorders in this category include mostly anorexia nervosa and bulimia nervosa. In the single study which assessed the prevalence of eating disorders in primary care, Cwikel *et al.* (30) found a one-year prevalence of 15.0% in 976 patients, aged 25–75 years, recruited from primary care practices throughout Israel. This rate is high and is comparable to that of depressive disorders reported in the same study, 20.6%, yet no further research on eating disorders in primary care settings has been reported. There has also been no research into substance abuse disorders within the Israeli primary care context.

❧ Emotional distress

This term refers to a nonspecific measure of psychopathology that usually includes, among others, symptoms of anxiety and depression (57). We identified four recent studies in primary care settings in Israel. The different studies show significant variation in findings. Yagur *et al.* (58) assessed emotional distress measured by a composite of items extracted from other standard instruments, in a sample of 125 consecutive patients aged 18 to 82 years recruited from a Jerusalem primary care clinic during the *Al-Aksa Intifada* (insurrection, in Arabic). They reported a 10.4% prevalence rate of psychological distress. The other three studies of emotional distress (59–61) used the same instrument i.e., the General Health Questionnaire (GHQ) (23) and the same cut-off score (GHQ ≥ 5) to screen for caseness. They did, however, produce inconsistent findings.

Rabinowitz *et al.* studied a sample of 2975 primary care patients, aged 18 or over. Their study showed that 38.2% of primary care users experience psychological distress at time of assessment (59). A slightly higher prevalence rate of 42.0% was reported by Maoz *et al.* (60), who used a random sample of 182 military primary care patients. Shiber *et al.* (61), that studied a sample of 776 patients aged 18 or over who had been drawn from primary care clinics in southern Israel, reported a much higher prevalence rate (69.0%) of emotional distress. However, as acknowledged by the investigators in a later publication (62), this rate is excessive and probably a reflection of the GHQ's high sensitivity. The prevalence rates reported by Maoz *et al.* (60) and Rabinowitz *et al.* (59) – 32.8% and 42.0% respectively – were more consistent with findings from studies conducted in other countries (63).

Risk factors

Rabinowitz *et al.* (59) found that distress was more prevalent in women and in older individuals, while in the Maoz *et al.*'s study (60) soldiers enlisted for military service were more likely to show psychological distress as compared to career soldiers; combat soldiers suffered from psychological distress at a lower rate than did soldiers serving in technical, maintenance and administrative positions. Nevertheless, more data are needed before we can draw any conclusion regarding risk factors for psychological distress in the Israeli primary care population.

❧ The impact of mental health problems in primary healthcare

Much of the Israeli literature on the impact of mental health problems tends to focus on the impact of depression. In general, studies seem to support the widely reported association between depression and disability, as well as an impaired quality of life. For example, studies reported that severity of depressive symptoms was associated with poor self-reported physical functioning (38), functional status, cognitive functioning and slow walking speed in elderly patients (40). Furthermore, functional impairment was found most severe in patients with MDD and least severe in individuals with no depression, while individuals with minor depression experienced intermediate level of functional impairment (27). In another study, having significant depressive symptoms was associated with chronic lower back pain (39).Consistent with findings from international studies (64), severity of depressive symptoms was inversely related to self-perceived physical health (41) and to satisfaction with health status (38, 41); it was positively associated with self-perceived poor health (14). Inverse relationship was also reported between depressive symptoms score and overall quality of life (38, 41). Like depression, psychological distress was inversely related to self-rated health (59).

Studies on the economic impact of depression focused on the association between depressive disorders or symptoms on the one hand and measures of health services utilization, healthcare expenditure, costs due to work disability, work loss days and lost productivity on the other. Use of health services was positively associated with a higher depressive symptom score (38) and having been diagnosed with depression (34). Moreover, mental and general medical costs were 40% higher for patients with clinical depression, compared to individuals with depressive symptoms (15). Similarly, individuals with MDD had significantly higher rates of health service utilization and costs compared to persons with either minor depression, depressive symptoms or no depression (29). Regarding indices of work-related productivity, depressed persons were slightly more likely to be absent from work compared to patients without depression (29); clinical depression was only slightly more costly in terms of work disability compared to depressive symptoms without a clinical diagnosis (15). The above suggests that depression has a significant impact on healthcare resource consumption and expenditure and that a clinical diagnosis may lead to greater consumption of resources (15) relative to that incurred by subclinical cases.

Other mental health problems were also related to resource consumption. PPD was associated with multiple visits to the pediatrician and to a family physician during two months after childbirth (44). In another study, psychological distress – a subclinical condition – was associated with more frequent visits to primary care physicians (59), with higher care-seeking behavior and higher prescription of sedative or hypnotic drugs (65).

﴾ From epidemiology to mental health action

Studies carried out in Israel showed the high prevalence rates of mental health conditions in primary care and their associated sociodemographic and clinical characteristics. However, transforming these findings into everyday clinical practice is a complex task. In the next section, we will try to elucidate some of the issues pertinent to implementation of interventions, including common barriers to implementation at different levels of the healthcare delivery system. We will also suggest ways in which these interventions can contribute to quality of healthcare and health outcomes.

Detection and adequacy of treatment

Identification of patients with mental health problems is clearly the first step towards effective management (46). Israeli studies show, however, that a large proportion of patients suffering from mental health problems are not detected in primary care settings. Froom *et al.* (27) found that for over a third of the patients in primary care clinics, MDD was previously undetected. Munitz *et al.* (34) reported that 22.0% of the patients they studied were correctly diagnosed by their physician with depression. Maoz *et al.* (60) found that 42.0% of their sample reported psychological distress; however, only 13.0% of these self-reported cases were identified by their treating physicians as such. Similarly, Shiber *et al.* (61) found that while 69.0% of their sample was found to be probable cases of psychological distress, the general practitioner assessed only 31% of the initial sample as cases, i.e., over half were not recognized. Similar findings emerge from studies carried out in other countries (66, 67). To address the problem of underdetection and misdiagnosis, there is a strong need to develop the use of effective methods for detecting common mental health disorders in primary care. This entails validation of screening instruments, education and training of primary healthcare practitioners and systematic evaluation and dissemination of research findings.

Israeli studies show that even among identified patients, many receive suboptimal treatment for their disorder. In fact, only a small proportion received appropriate care. From the Longitudinal Investigation of Depression Outcomes (LIDO) study, which aimed to address patterns of depression treatment and the association between treatment and clinical outcomes in primary care, it appears that a relative minority, 17.0%, of the sample was treated for depression during a nine-month follow-up. Moreover, only 10.0% of patients received potentially effective treatment (defined as the lowest effective dose) (68).

Many factors might account for underdetection and undertreatment of mental health problems. These fall into three main categories – patient, provider, and health care-related factors (69). Likelihood of detection is decreased when patients present with somatic rather than emotional complaints (70–72). Psychological distress expressed through somatic symptoms accounts for a significant proportion of psychiatric morbidity in primary care (60). In a United Kingdom study, Goldberg and Huxley (73) found that while 25.0% of the primary care patients had a mental health condition, only 7.8% presented with clear psychological symptoms. The others presented with various somatic, stress-related symptoms. Furthermore, patients may be concerned about stigma associated with mental health diagnosis and treatment, or hold beliefs that prevent them from seeking professional mental health help. One Israeli study found that patient-related barriers to treatment of depression included concern about medication costs and side effects; embarrassment about treatment; a belief that seeking treatment could compromise job opportunities; inconvenient treatment facilities; and discouragement by family or friends (68). More research is needed in order to elucidate patient-related barriers to recognition and treatment of mental health problems in the primary care system.

From the healthcare provider's perspective, barriers may include competing demands and time constraints (74); inadequate knowledge about diagnosis and treatment options (75); lack of psychological orientation (76); and inadequate insight into different cultural manifestations of mental disorders (77). In an Israeli study of provider-related factors, Shiber *et al.* found that factors such as clinician's specialization in family medicine, their interest in emotional health and belief in its importance; good communication; low patient load; and familiarity with the patients all predicted better identification of emotional distress (61).

Rabinowitz *et al.* (78) studied the characteristics of primary care clinicians who tended to treat depressive disorders by themselves. They devoted more time to continuing medical education; specialize in family medicine; conduct more home visits and more medical procedures; and perceived themselves as the first contact for psychosocial issues.

Furthermore, Goldfracht *et al.* (79) identified barriers to depression and anxiety care by primary care physicians. According to their study, 85.0% of primary care physicians ranked time constraints as the main barrier; 60.0%, indicated insufficient knowledge regarding diagnosis and treatment as barriers to care; 63.0%, cited lack of means to treat the disorders; and 69.0%, reported that shortage of expert support was a barrier. Additionally, 43.0% and 37.0% cited difficulty in speaking about mental health issues and a lack of personal interest in treating as a barrier. While factors such as knowledge and skills may be modifiable through education and training, others (e.g., lack of time, lack of expert support) may depend more on the healthcare system.

Healthcare system factors are a significant contributor to quality of mental healthcare in primary care. Important barriers to care may include, among others, the lack of a systematic method for detecting and managing patients with mental health problems (80), inadequate continuity of care (81) and insufficient resource allocation for mental health care. To the best of our knowledge, this issue of factors related to the healthcare system has not been addressed by Israeli researchers.

Very little is known about mental health outcomes in Israeli primary care. Existing studies focused on measuring outcomes unrelated to any specific intervention effort. Evidence seems to suggest that primary care patients with mental health conditions show poor outcomes (14, 60, 82). Remission and recovery have been reported in two papers based on a single multinational study (LIDO) including Israel as a site. The sample employed included 161 patients with major depression who were followed for up to 12 months, 17.0% of whom received treatment for depression during the follow-up period. Simon et al. (14) reported that 36% of the patients had persistent clinical depression at nine months. Full remission of depression following treatment was achieved by a little more than a third of the sample. Patients achieving complete remission at follow-up were younger, had more years of schooling, were more often employed at baseline, had fewer medical conditions and were less likely to have dysthymic disorder or anxiety (82). Maoz *et al.* (60) identified 42% of soldiers attending military primary care clinics with significant psychological distress at baseline. In a follow-up assessment at one year of those soldiers who were psychologically distressed at baseline, 48% had persistently high score of psychological distress. Further research is needed on outcomes of patients with mental health problems in primary care and the effect of specific interventions on outcomes.

Challenges and opportunities for mental health treatment in primary care

Under Israeli law, all citizens and *de jure* residents are medically insured. Medical services are delivered primarily by four public health funds (HMO-like organizations) except for mental health services, which until now have been delivered mainly by the Ministry of Health. However, mental health care is facing a major reform effort, including a proposed shift in responsibility for the provision of mental health services from the Ministry of Health to the four public HMOs. When responsibility for mental health services shift from the ministry to public insurers, the role of the primary care physician as a "gatekeeper" and guide is likely to become even more prominent.

In the four health funds, visits to hospital-based specialists usually require prior authorization, either from a primary care provider or a community-based specialist. However, access to some areas in community-based specialized care is controlled by the general practitioners (GP) in some of the health funds. For example, the largest one, *Clalit* Health Services, the GP plays more of a gatekeeper role; members have free access to specialists in six areas such as dermatology, gynecology or ophthalmology – but access to other specialists requires a referral from a primary care provider. In other health funds, members usually have free access to all fund-affiliated community-based specialists without prior authorization from a primary care provider (83).

As a gatekeeper for specialized mental health care, the primary care provider is facing several challenges in the treatment process. According to the model described Goldberg and Huxley (73), there are a number of filters in the process of getting to the specialized mental health care level (84). In the first place, a patient must recognize that he has a problem and seek help. Next, the GP needs to identify the exact problem. Finally, the GP has to treat or refer the patient to specialized care. In this model, it is essential for the GP to have the knowledge and skills to identify the mental health symptoms and well structured specialized services to allow further referral for psychiatric care.

Studies show, however, that a large proportion of patients with mental health symptoms seek help in primary care, and that *de facto* primary care physicians treat more than 50.0% of patients with mental health problems (85). Indeed, the INHS (19) found that the majority (59%) of those who sought help for their mental health symptoms chose to consult a general health-care professional. Hence, primary care physicians have a central role in detecting and treating mental health problems.

Israel's population is highly heterogeneous in terms of its cultural makeup, beliefs, mother tongues and customs (86). Primary care physicians are expected to respond to the needs of a diverse population. Culture may affect detection and treatment of mental health conditions. For example, patients from different cultural backgrounds may have different interpretations of the terms used in screening instruments, which might decrease the validity of the instrument. Furthermore, according to Kerr and Kerr (85), social norms may contribute to the implicit prohibition of use of certain self-descriptive terms, depending on the patient's gender. Men, for example, may not perceive themselves or be perceived as depressed if their gender role prohibits them from using conventional terms to describe emotional problems. These social norms and structure may exert their effect differently in different cultures, interfering with proper diagnosis. One way to overcome some of these difficulties may be through the validation of culturally-sensitive screening tools in mental health.

Somatic complaints such as headaches, change in appetite, and chronic pain may co-occur with psychological symptoms in many mental health conditions, such as depression. Primary care practitioners are more likely to miss a mental health disorder when somatic symptoms are the patient's major complaint. Cultural factors may influence the somatic manifestations of mental health problems. There is a need to address all these factors in future research to improve the understanding and practice in managing mental health problems in the Israeli primary care system.

A key issue in the present discussion is the quality of caregiver-patient relationship. Caregiver-patient relationship has inspired a large volume of research in recent years, and it is largely recognized that the quality of communication between the patient and the healthcare provider is related to outcomes of care. In one Israeli study, Gross *et al.* (65) assessed patients' satisfaction with physician discussion of emotional distress issues. The authors concluded that patients who reported discussing emotional distress with their primary care physician were significantly more satisfied with care. Studies conducted elsewhere have shown that satisfaction with care is associated with better health outcomes and improved adherence to medical recommendation (87, 88).

Comorbidities

Many primary care patients suffering from a mental health condition are also coping with a chronic medical disorder. In fact, studies from other countries consistently show that the prevalence of mental health problems is higher among patients with general medical disorder relative to those with no physical condition (89). For example, the prevalence of depression in patients with diabetes is twice as high as in persons without diabetes (90). Similar pattern has been observed with respect to other chronic medical disorders such as cardiovascular disease (91).

Furthermore, overlap between different mental health problems in primary care is common. For example, Barsky *et al.* (55) found that 20.5% of their sample had a diagnosis of somatoform disorder. Of those with a somatoform disorder, about a third had comorbid major depression. An additional one-sixth had sub-threshold depression and 18.8% had comorbid panic disorder. Similarly, Jackson *et al.* (66) found that 29.0% of their primary care sample had a depressive or anxiety disorder, with 34.0% of these having more than one disorder. Co-occurrence of mental health problems presents a complex challenge for primary care clinicians and might require additional skills and resources that the primary care clinician may not have readily available. Unfortunately, research-based information on this issue is still lacking in Israel.

Treatment options

Many options are available to treat mental health problems that are commonly encountered in primary care. Full discussion of treatment options for mental health problems is beyond the scope of the present chapter. However, as evidence emerging from well-designed studies carried out in Europe and the US indicate (11, 92), some of these options show promising results in improving outcomes and reducing healthcare expenditure for psychiatric problems in primary care. These include well-tolerated pharmacological treatments (92) and psychological interventions (93). The most suitable method of treatment depends on multiple factors (including the disorder itself), the patient's preferences and the availability of specific treatment options. Studies in the Israeli primary care facilities are needed to determine the effect of different treatment options.

❧ Conclusions

Psychiatric disorders are common in primary healthcare settings, but reported prevalence rates vary considerably across the Israeli studies. Regarding mental health disorders, studies showed that the point prevalence rates ranged from 1.6% to 5.9% for major depression and 9.9% to 20.6% for postpartum depression, while the one-year prevalence of depressive disorders was as high as 20.6%. Similarly, the one-year prevalence of any anxiety disorder was 22.5% and 13.1% for somatoform disorders. Prevalence of sub-threshold psychiatric conditions in the Israeli primary care population was 1.1% to 5.4% for minor depression; 7% to 24% for depressive symptoms; and 10.4% to 69.0% for psychological distress.

One important gap in the literature concerns the scope of psychiatric problems addressed in Israeli primary healthcare research. The majority of studies addressed depressive disorders and conditions despite the fact that other psychiatric conditions show prevalence rates comparable to those of depression. For example, the prevalence rates of anxiety or eating disorders are similar to that of depressive disorders yet very little research effort has been put forward to investigate these disorders. Future research should address the wider spectrum of psychiatric disorders commonly encountered in primary care, including anxiety disorders, eating disorders, substance abuse and somatization. Significantly more research effort is needed to determine prevalence rates, improve detection process of psychiatric morbidity and evaluate treatment outcomes following the implementation of different treatment modalities.

Selected sociodemographic and clinical characteristics such as female gender, lower income, low educational attainment and a history of psychiatric morbidity were identified as risk factors for psychopathology. In a system of limited health resources and competing demands, it might be useful to adopt a targeted approach in which screening efforts focus on subgroups within the population identified as high risk – for example, patients with past mental illness (43, 44) or a chronic medical condition.

Israeli studies show that only a small proportion of patients affected by mental health disorders are detected in primary care, despite the finding that well above 50.0% of them seek help for a psychiatric problem in primary care. Our review indicates that potentially effective treatment options are offered to a very small fraction of patients affected. Identification and treatment of mental health problems in primary care is a complex task and likely to involve multiple factors, including health policy, structure of the health services, cultural factors and other variables pertaining to health provider training and attitudes (78). As data on such factors are scarce, more research is clearly essential. Furthermore, there is a strong need to develop empirically based treatment guidelines for mental health problems in primary care. To accomplish that, treatment initiatives should be put forward by the four health funds, followed by systematic assessment of outcomes.

❧ References

1. Regier DA, Narrow WE, Rae DS, *et al*. The *de facto* US mental and addictive disorders service system. Epidemiologic catchment area prospective 1-year prevalence rates of disorders and services. *Archives of General Psychiatry* 1993; 50: 85–94.

2. Jenkins R, Lewis G, Bebbington P, *et al*. The National Psychiatric Morbidity Surveys of Great Britain – initial findings from the household survey. *Psychological Medicine* 1997; 27: 7 5–789.

3. Bijl RV, Ravelli A. Psychiatric morbidity, service use, and need for care in the general population: results of The Netherlands Mental Health Survey and Incidence Study. *American Journal of Public Health* 2000; 90: 602–607.

4. Kessler RC, Berglund P, Demler O, *et al*. The epidemiology of major depressive disorder: results from the National Comorbidity Survey Replication (NCS-R). *Journal of the American Medical Association* 2003; 18: 289: 3095–3105.

5. World Health Organization. *The world health report 2001. Mental health: new understanding, new hope.* Geneva: World Health Organization 9online]. 2001 [cited July 9, 2008]. Available from URL: www.who.int/whr/2001/en/.

6. Kafman M, Alon N, Hermoni D. Screening for depression in primary care clinics in Israel – how wide is the gap? *Harefuah* 2003; 142: 815–819 (Hebrew).

7. Ustun TB. The global burden of mental disorders. *American Journal of Public Health* 1999; 89: 1315–1318.

8. Wells KB, Sturm R, Sherbourne CD, *et al*. *Caring for depression*. Cambridge, MA: Harvard University Press, 1996.

9. Penninx BW, Geerlings SW, Deeg DJ, *et al*. Minor and major depression and the risk of death in older persons. *Archives of General Psychiatry* 1999; 56: 889–895.

10. Wulsin LR, Vaillant GE, Wells VE. A systematic review of the mortality of depression. *Psychosomatic Medicine* 1999; 6: 6–17.

11. National Institute for Clinical Excellence, NICE. *Depression: management of depression in primary and secondary care.* National Collaborating Centre for Mental Health Commissioned by the National Institute for Clinical Excellence [cited June 1, 2008]; Available from URL: http://www.nice.org.uk/CG023.

12. Broadhead WE, Blazer DG, George LK, *et al*. Depression, disability days, and days lost from work in a prospective epidemiologic survey. *Journal of the American Medical Association* 1990; 264: 2524–2528.

13. Simon G, Ormel J, VonKorff M, *et al*. Health care costs associated with depressive and anxiety disorders in primary care. *American Journal of Psychiatry* 1995; 152: 352–357.

14. Simon GE, Chisholm D, Treglia M, *et al*. Course of depression, health services costs, and work productivity in an international primary care study. *General Hospital Psychiatry* 2002; 24: 328–335.

15. Chisholm D, Diehr P, Knapp M, *et al*. Depression status, medical comorbidity and resource costs: evidence from an international study of major depression in primary care (LIDO). *British Journal of Psychiatry* 2003; 183: 121–131.

16. Wang PS, Angermeyer M, Borges G, *et al*. Delay and failure in treatment seeking after first onset of mental disorders in the World Health Organization's World Mental Health Survey Initiative. *World Psychiatry* 2007; 6: 177–185.

17. Goldberg DP, Lecrubier Y. Form and frequency of mental disorders across centres. In: Üstün TB, Sartorius N, eds. *Mental illness in general healthcare: an international study.* Chichester: Wiley & Sons on behalf of WHO, 1995.

18. Parslow RA, Jorm AF. Who uses mental health services in Australia? An analysis of data from the National Survey of Mental Health and Wellbeing. *Australian and New Zealand Journal of Psychiatry* 2000; 34: 997–1008.

19. Levinson D, Levav I, Bin Nun G, *et al*. Israel National Health Survey: new data for planners, clinicians, researchers and the public at large. *Israel Journal of Psychiatry and Related Sciences* 2007; 44: 79–80.

20. Robins LN, Wing J, Wittchen HU, *et al*. The Composite International Diagnostic Interview. an epidemiologic instrument suitable for use in conjunction with different diagnostic systems and in different cultures. *Archives of General Psychiatry* 1988; 45: 1069–1077.

21. Radloff LS. The CES-D scale: a self-report depression scale for research in the general population. *Applied Psychological Measures* 1977; 1: 385–401.

22. Beck A, Steer R, Brown G. *Manual for Beck Depression Inventory II* (BDI-II). San Antonio, TX: Psychology Corporation, 1996.

23. Goldberg DP. *The detection of psychiatric illness by questionnaire.* London: Oxford University Press, 1972.

24. Spitzer RL, Kroenke K, Williams JB. Validation and utility of a self-report version of PRIME-MD: the PHQ primary care study. Primary care evaluation of mental disorders. Patient health questionnaire. *Journal of the American Medical Association* 1999; 10; 282: 1737-1744.

25. American Psychiatric Association. *Diagnostic and statistical manual of mental disorders – Fourth edition (DSM-IV).* Washington, DC: American, Psychiatric Association, 1994.

26. Zimmerman M, Coryell W. The validity of a self-report questionnaire for diagnosing major depressive disorder. *Archives of General Psychiatry* 1988; 45: 738-740.

27. Froom J, Aoyama H, Hermoni D, *et al.* Depressive disorders in three primary care populations: United States, Israel, Japan. *Family Practice* 1995; 12: 274-278.

28. Fryers T, Brugha T, Morgan Z, *et al.* Prevalence of psychiatric disorder in Europe: the potential and reality of meta-analysis. *Social Psychiatry and Psychiatric Epidemiology* 2004; 39: 899-905.

29. Shvartzman P, Weiner Z, Vardy D, *et al.* Health services utilization by depressive patients identified by the MINI questionnaire in a primary care setting. *Scandinavian Journal of Primary Health Care* 2005; 23: 18-25.

30. Cwikel J, Zilber N, Feinson M, *et al.* Prevalence and risk factors of threshold and sub-threshold psychiatric disorders in primary care. *Social Psychiatry and Psychiatric Epidemiology* 2008; 43: 184-191.

31. Katon W, Schulberg H. Epidemiology of depression in primary care. *General Hospital Psychiatry* 1992; 14: 237-247.

32. Williams JW, Jr., Noel PH, Cordes JA, *et al.* Is this patient clinically depressed? *Journal of the American Medical Association* 2002; 287: 1160-1170.

33. Kessler RC, Andrews G, Mroczek D, *et al.* The World Health Organization Composite International Diagnostic Interview shortform (CIDI-SF). *International Journal of Methods in Psychiatric Research* 1998; 7: 171-185.

34. Munitz H, Valevski A, Weizman A, *et al.* Recognition and treatment of depression in primary care settings in six different countries: a retrospective file analysis by WHO. *European Journal of Psychiatry* 2000; 14: 85-93.

35. Rollman BL, Reynolds CF third. Minor and subsyndromal depression: functional disability worth treating. *Journal of the American Geriatrics Society* 1999; 47: 757-758.

36. Chwastiak L, Ehde DM, Gibbons LE, *et al.* Depressive symptoms and severity of illness in multiple sclerosis: epidemiologic study of a large community sample. *American Journal of Psychiatry* 2002; 159: 1862-1868.

37. Lesperance F, Frasure-Smith N, Talajic M, *et al.* Five-year risk of cardiac mortality in relation to initial severity and one-year changes in depression symptoms after myocardial infarction. *Circulation* 2002; 105: 1049-1053.

38. Herrman H, Patrick DL, Diehr P, *et al.* Longitudinal investigation of depression outcomes in primary care in six countries: the LIDO study. Functional status, health service use and treatment of people with depressive symptoms. *Psychological Medicine* 2002; 32: 889-902.

39. Reis S, Hermoni D, Borkan JM, *et al.* A new look at low back complaints in primary care: a RAMBAM Israeli Family Practice Research Network study. *Journal of Family Practice* 1999; 48: 299-303.

40. Biderman A, Cwikel J, Fried AV, *et al.* Depression and falls among community dwelling elderly people: a search for common risk factors. *Journal of Epidemiology and Community Health* 2002; 56: 631-636.

41. Bech P, Lucas R, Amir M, *et al.* Association between clinically depressed subgroups, type of treatment and patient retention in the LIDO study. *Psychological Medicine* 2003; 33: 1051-1059.

42. Leahy-Warren P, McCarthy G. Postnatal depression: prevalence, mothers' perspectives, and treatments. *Archives of Psychiatric Nursing* 2007; 21: 91-100.

43. Glasser S, Barell v, Boyko v, *et al.* Postpartum depression in an Israeli cohort: demographic, psychosocial and medical risk factors. *Journal of Psychosomatic Obstetrics and Gynaecology* 2000; 21: 99-108.

44. Eilat-Tsanani S, Merom A, Romano S, *et al.* The effect of postpartum depression on women's consultations with physicians. *Israel Medical Association Journal* 2006; 8: 406-410.

45. Cox JL, Holden JM, Sagovsky R. Detection of postnatal depression. Development of the 10-item Edinburgh Postnatal Depression Scale. *British Journal of Psychiatry* 1987; 150: 782-786.

46. Heymann AD, Shilo Y, Tirosh A, *et al.* Differences between soldiers, with and without emotional distress, in number of primary care medical visits and type of presenting complaints. *Israel Medical Association Journal* 2007; 9: 90-93.

47. Taubman-Ben-Ari O, Rabinowitz J, *et al.* Post-traumatic stress disorder in primary-care settings: prevalence and physicians' detection. *Psychological Medicine* 2001; 31: 555-560.

48. Liebschutz J, Saitz R, Brower v, *et al.* PTSD in urban primary care: high prevalence and low physician recognition. *Journal of General Internal Medicine* 2007; 22: 719-726.

49. Stein MB, McQuaid JR, Pedrelli P, *et al.* Posttraumatic stress disorder in the primary care medical setting. *General Hospital Psychiatry* 2000; 22: 261-269.

50. Magruder KM, Frueh BC, Knapp RG, *et al.* Prevalence of posttraumatic stress disorder in Veterans Affairs primary care clinics. *General Hospital Psychiatry* 2005; 27: 169-179.

51. Neria Y, Gross R, Olfson M, *et al.* Posttraumatic stress disorder in primary care one year after the 9/11 attacks. *General Hospital Psychiatry* 2006; 28: 213-222.

52. Weiss R, Fogelman Y, Yaphe J. Somatization in response to undiagnosed obsessive compulsive disorder in a family. *BMC Family Practice* 2003; 20: 4:1.

53. Ritsner M, Ponizovsky A, Kurs R, *et al.* Somatization in an immigrant population in Israel: a community survey of prevalence, risk factors, and help-seeking behavior. *American Journal of Psychiatry* 2000; 157: 385-392.

54. Dickinson WP, Dickinson LM, deGruy FV, *et al*. The somatization in primary care study: a tale of three diagnoses. *General Hospital Psychiatry* 2003; 25: 1–7.

55. Barsky AJ, Orav EJ, Bates DW. Somatization increases medical utilization and costs independent of psychiatric and medical co-morbidity. *Archives of General Psychiatry* 2005; 62: 903–910.

56. Sheehan B, Bass C, Briggs R, *et al*. Somatization among older primary care attenders. *Psychological Medicine* 2003; 33: 867–877.

57. United States Preventive Services Task Force, *et al*. (USPSTF). *Guide to clinical preventive services – Third edition*. Screening for depression. Periodic updates 2003; 1: 121–145.

58. Yagur A, Grinshpoon A, Ponizovsky A. Primary care clinic attenders under war stress. *Israel Medical Association Journal* 2002; 4: 568–572.

59. Rabinowitz J, Shayevitz D, Hornik T, *et al*. Primary care physicians' detection of psychological distress among elderly patients. *American Journal of Geriatric Psychiatry* 2005; 13: 773–780.

60. Maoz B, Mark M, Rabinowitz S, *et al*. Measuring psychological stress in primary care military medical clinics. *Israel Journal of Psychiatry and Related Sciences* 1991; 28: 19–24.

61. Shiber A, Maoz B, Antonovsky A, *et al*. Detection of emotional problems in the primary care clinic. *Family Practice* 1990; 7: 195–200.

62. Benjamin J, Maoz B, Shiber A, *et al*. Prevalence of psychiatric disorders in three primary-care clinics in Beersheba, Israel. Concurrent assessment by the General Health Questionnaire, general practitioners, and Research Diagnostic Criteria. *General Hospital Psychiatry* 1992; 14: 307–314.

63. Boardman AP. The General Health Questionnaire and the detection of emotional disorder by general practitioners. A replication study. *British Journal of Psychiatry* 1987; 151: 373–381.

64. Paykel ES, Brugha T, Fryers T. Size and burden of depressive disorders in Europe. *European Neuropsychopharmacology* 2005; 15: 411–423.

65. Gross R, Brammli-Greenberg S, Tabenkin H, *et al*. Primary care physicians' discussion of emotional distress and patient satisfaction. *International Journal of Psychiatry in Medicine* 2007; 37: 331–345.

66. Jackson JL, Passamonti M, Kroenke K. Outcome and impact of mental disorders in primary care at 5 years. *Psychosomatic Medicine* 2007; 69: 270–276.

67. Gonzales JJ, Magruder KM, Keith SJ. Mental disorders in primary care services: an update. *Public Health Reports* 1994; 109: 251–258.

68. Simon GE, Fleck M, Lucas R, *et al*. Prevalence and predictors of depression treatment in an international primary care study. *American Journal of Psychiatry* 2004; 161: 1626–1634.

69. Cepoiu M, McCusker J, Cole MG, *et al*. Recognition of depression by non-psychiatric physicians – a systematic literature review and meta-analysis. *Journal of General Internal Medicine* 2008; 23: 25–36.

70. Wittchen HU, Lieb R, Wunderlich U, *et al*. Comorbidity in primary care: presentation and consequences. *Journal of Clinical Psychiatry* 1999; 60 Suppl 7:29–36; discussion 7–8.

71. Jackson JL, O'Malley PG, Kroenke K. Clinical predictors of mental disorders among medical outpatients. Validation of the "S4" model. *Psychosomatics* 1998; 39: 431–436.

72. O'Connor DW, Rosewarne R, Bruce A. Depression in primary care. 1: elderly patients' disclosure of depressive symptoms to their doctors. *International Psychogeriatrics* 2001; 13: 359–365.

73. Goldberg D, Huxley P. *Mental illness in the community: the pathway to psychiatric care*. London: Tavistock Publications, 1980.

74. Goldman LS, Nielsen NH, Champion HC. Awareness, diagnosis, and treatment of depression. *Journal of General Internal Medicine* 1999; 14: 569–580.

75. Davidson JR, Meltzer-Brody SE. The underrecognition and undertreatment of depression: what is the breadth and depth of the problem? *Journal of Clinical Psychiatry* 1999; 60 (Suppl 7): 4–9; discussion 10–11.

76. Cooper LA, Brown C, Vu HT, *et al*. Primary care patients' opinions regarding the importance of various aspects of care for depression. *General Hospital Psychiatry* 2000; 22: 163–173.

77. Kirmayer LJ. Cultural variations in the clinical presentation of depression and anxiety: implications for diagnosis and treatment. *Journal of Clinical Psychiatry* 2001; 62 (Suppl 13): 22–28; discussion 9–30.

78. Rabinowitz J, Feldman D, Gross R, *et al*. Which primary care physicians treat depression? *Psychiatric Services* 1998; 49: 100–102.

79. Goldfracht M, Shalit C, Peled O, *et al*. Attitudes of Israeli primary care physicians towards mental health care. *Israel Journal of Psychiatry and Related Sciences* 2007; 44: 225–229.

80. McCall L, Clarke DM, Rowley G. A questionnaire to measure general practitioners' attitudes to their role in the management of patients with depression and anxiety. *Australian Family Physician* 2002; 31: 299–303.

81. Docherty JP. Barriers to the diagnosis of depression in primary care. *Journal of Clinical Psychiatry* 1997; 58 (Suppl 1): 5–10.

82. De Almeida Fleck MP, Simon G, Herrman H, *et al*. Major depression and its correlates in primary care settings in six countries: 9-month follow-up study. *British Journal of Psychiatry* 2005; 186: 41–47.

83. Rosen MP, Siewert B, Sands DZ, *et al*. Value of abdominal CT in the emergency department for patients with abdominal pain. *European Radiology* 2003; 13: 418–424.

84. Oiesvold T, Sandlund M, Hansson L, *et al*. Factors associated with referral to psychiatric care by general practitioners compared with self-referrals. *Psychological Medicine* 1998; 28: 427–436.

85. Kerr LK, Kerr LD, Jr. Screening tools for depression in primary care: the effects of culture, gender, and somatic symptoms on the detection of depression. *Western Journal of Medicine* 2001; 175: 349–352.

86. Geulayov G, Lipsitz J, Sabar R, *et al*. Depression in primary care in Israel. *Israel Medical Association Journal* 2007; 9: 571–578.

87. Vermeire E, Hearnshaw H, Van Royen P, *et al*. Patient adherence to treatment: three decades of research. A comprehensive review. *Journal of Clinical Pharmacology and Therapeutics* 2001; 26: 331–342.

88. Vermeire E, Wens J, Van Royen P, *et al.* Interventions for improving adherence to treatment recommendations in people with type 2 diabetes mellitus. Cochrane Database System Review 2005 (2):CD 003638.

89. Gill D, Hatcher S. A systematic review of the treatment of depression with antidepressant drugs in patients who also have a physical illness. *Journal of Psychosomatic Research* 1999; 47: 131–143.

90. Talbot F, Nouwen A. A review of the relationship between depression and diabetes in adults: is there a link? *Diabetes Care* 2000; 23: 1556–1562.

91. Burg MM, Benedetto MC, Rosenberg R, *et al.* Presurgical depression predicts medical morbidity 6 months after coronary artery bypass graft surgery. *Psychosomatic Medicine* 2003; 65: 111–118.

92. Mann JJ. The medical management of depression. *New England Journal of Medicine* 2005; 353: 1819–1834.

93. DeRubeis RJ, Gelfand LA, Tang TZ, *et al.* Medications versus cognitive behavior therapy for severely depressed outpatients: mega-analysis of four randomized comparisons. *American Journal of Psychiatry* 1999; 156: 1007–1013.

Acknowledgement: Saralee Glasser, MA, provided helpful comments.

Chapter 18

PSYCHOPHARMACOEPIDEMIOLOGY IN PRACTICE

Hanan Munitz

Pharmacoepidemiology is the study of the utilization and effects of drugs in populations, and its methodology is derived from both, pharmacology and epidemiology. In addition to the classical subdivision of descriptive and analytical epidemiology, pharmacoepidemiology has an additional field of application called pharmacovigilance (1).

This chapter deals with the field of psychopharmacological epidemiology, which refers to the use of psychotropic medications in the population, mainly for psychiatric care. One of the principal obstacles in the study of the use of psychopharmacological agents is the non-specificity in the use of these drugs. For example, certain antidepressants are used to treat pain disorders, as well as for anxiety syndromes. In fact, most psychiatric medications are used to treat several different mental health disorders, e.g., antipsychotics are used for the treatment of schizophrenia, organic psychosis and mania, while antiepileptic drugs are used for seizure disorders and as mood stabilizers.

There is a single publication in Israel that describes drug utilization over a period of a year (2). One interesting finding in this publication is that psychotropic drug use in Israel has been similar to that in other European countries. Another equally interesting finding was that many patients do not receive proper drug treatment; a mere 20.0% received psychotropic medication. In Israel, like everywhere else, we encounter the paradox that people who need psychotropic medications do not take them, while they are prescribed to people who do not need them.

There are several factors contributing to the overall pattern of drug utilization: the epidemiology of the disorders; policy; marketing; availability; costs; and results of the conflict between "renovism" and conservatism.

❧ Psychotropic drug utilization

The reported results on the epidemiology of mental health disorders in Israel differ only slightly from those in other Western countries, though at the lower range of service utilization (2).

Under the National Health Insurance Law of 1994, there is a nationally agreed "basket" of health technologies. However, the patient is required to participate in the cost through out-of-pocket copayments. Drugs that are not included in the health basket but approved by the Health Ministry may be purchased in private pharmacies, and the patient pays the entire cost.

There are four Health Maintenance Organizations (HMOs) in Israel, but private practice is quite common. Naturally, drugs included in the health basket have a marketing advantage and are used more frequently than those not included. It should be pointed out that once a drug is included in the health basket there is no efficient way to eliminate it.

A public committee appointed by the government meets over several months at the end of each calendar year to study the hundreds of new medical technologies proposed for inclusion in the new basket and make recommendations to the Ministries of Health and Finance. New drugs are added annually.

Psychotropic drugs must compete with other drugs to be included in the health basket. Indeed, since there has been a tendency to prefer lifesaving drugs to medications that improve patients' quality of life, psychiatric drugs are at a disadvantage. As a result, their chances of being introduced into the health basket are reduced.

Marketing

Marketing in Israel is similar to most other countries. Marketing proves to be important in the introduction of new medications, tending to favor newer drugs at the expense of older drugs. Marketing influences clinical decision-making and, in a paradoxical way, it creates a conflict between the physician who believes in new medications and the general health system. The latter operates under both financial constraints and the assumption that rationing is an absolute necessity.

Availability

Availability should be viewed as a complex concept. The general concept deals with the ease of obtaining medication. It is influenced by varied factors, such as costs, bureaucratic difficulties and stigma. For example, people suffering from schizophrenia often experience financial hardships, and these may contribute to their tendency to opt for less-costly drugs. In addition, bureaucracy can be a hindrance in drug prescription. Finally, stigma and fear of medication bear a strong influence on the readiness to use psychotropic drugs (3).

The "renovism" – "conservatism" conflict

Today, there are currently strong forces, such as pharmaceutical companies and professional bodies, pushing for the utilization of new and more expensive medications. However, there are also forces causing the patient to prefer older and well-known medications. This may be due to the fear of changing habits and/or it is based on the often realistic belief that old medications are just as useful as the new ones. The same conflict is faced by the physician, who knows very well what present medications have achieved, but does not know for sure if the new drug is better or may cause harm. It may thus be safe to assume that the physician will tend to use new drugs in newly recruited medication users and be more conservative with the elderly population. If this were true, we should expect an age gradient in the relative use of old and new medications.

In this chapter, the *Clalit* Health Services (CHS) database is used to examine the pattern of psychotropic drug utilization. CHS is the largest health fund or HMO in the country with

3,841,000 members in 2007; that is about 55% of the population. CHS has its own network of local pharmacies and purchases its medication independently. This means that, although the following findings do not portray the full use of medication in all the population, they do show suggestive trends.

The use of antipsychotic medications

The following table reflects the use of anti-psychotic drugs according to the division between typical and atypical drugs and age.

Table 1. Use of typical and atypical antipsychotic medication (%) in the CHS-insured population by age group

Age group	Typical antipsychotics		Atypical antipsychotics		Total
	n	%	n	%	n
0–14	1938	63.8	1098	36.2	3036
15–24	4747	61.6	2961	38.4	7708
25–44	15,785	65.4	8337	34.6	24,122
45–64	25,514	78.4	7041	21.6	32,555
65+	30,007	89.6	3493	10.4	33,500
Total N	77,991	77.3	22,880		100,871
%				22.7	100.0

From table 1 it appears that only 22.7% of the CHS members who received antipsychotic medications were treated with the new atypicals. This is a lower rate than that found in most Western countries (4). However, when age is taken into account, two distinct groups emerge: In people younger than 45, the proportion reaches nearly 40%, a percentage similar to the use in those countries. This age-related pattern of use may be explained by the fact that the elderly are treated for dementia-associated psychopathology, coupled by the possible reluctance of physicians and patients to switch medication.

Table 2. The use of antipsychotic medications (%) in the CHS-insured population by age group

Age group	%
0–14	.3
15–24	1.3
25–44	2.0
45–64	4.1
65 and above	6.8
Total	2.6

Of the insured population, 2.6% received an antipsychotic drug in 2007. This rate is similar to that in France (4). It can be seen that the use of antipsychotics is age dependent, 65.5% of the insured that are being prescribed are aged 45 and over. It seems that the majority of antipsychotic medications are prescribed for other diagnosis than schizophrenia.

Clozapine

Of a total of 100,871 patients in 2007 receiving antipsychotic medication, only 2.3% received clozapine. In view of the fact that it is the drug of choice for resistant schizophrenia, this is a surprisingly low rate.

The use of antidepressant medications

Seven percent of the study population received an antidepressant medication in 2007. Table 3 shows the penetration of the new antidepressant medications. Similarly to the anti-psychotics, the penetration of new drugs is more pronounced in the younger age group with the exception of the very young. It is possible that this latter finding reflects the use of tricyclic drugs in the treatment of enuresis in this age group.

Table 3. The use of old and new antidepressant medications (%) in the CHS-insured population by age group

Age group	Old antidepressants n	New antidepressants n	Total n	% Old antidepressants	% New antidepressants
0–14	1087	1453	2540	42.8	57.2
15–24	1906	9363	11,269	16.9	83.1
25–44	8349	39,345	47,694	47.4	82.6
45–64	23,532	64,318	87,850	26.7	73.3
65+	34,385	85,426	119,811	28.7	71.3
Total N	69,259	199,905	269,164	25.7	74.3

The use of anti depressant medications varies according to age. Table 4 shows that the use of antidepressants seems to increase with age, with a third of the aged insured population receiving such a medication. Of all antidepressants, 77.2% are prescribed to people over the age of 45.

Table 4. The use of antidepressant medications (%) in the CHS-insured population by age group

Age group	%
0–14	.3
15–24	1.6
25–34	3.2
35–44	6.6
45–54	9.8
55–64	12.2
65–74	17.9
75–84	29.7
85 and above	33.9
Total	7.0

The use of anxiolytic medications

One of the unusual features in the health basket is the inclusion of two old "natural" anxiolytic products: valerian and calmanervin. Tables 5 and 6 depict the relative use of modern and natural anxiolytics and by age.

Table 5. The use of modern and natural anxiolytic medications (%) in the CHS-insured population by age group

Age group	Modern anxiolytics n	%	Natural anxiolytics n	%	Total n	%
0–14	12,014	1.2	2016	.2	14,030	1.4
15–24	5746	1.0	3216	.6	8962	1.6
25–34	18,142	3.1	5028	.9	23,170	4.0

Table 5. The use of modern and natural anxiolytic medications (%) in the CHS-insured population by age group (cont.)

Age group	Modern anxiolytics		Natural anxiolytics		Total	
	n	%	n	%	n	%
35–44	13,147	3.3	5905	1.5	19,052	4.8
45–54	29,666	7.1	10,558	2.5	40,224	9.6
55–64	45,131	12.2	12,498	3.4	57,629	15.6
65–74	51,446	20.8	13,314	5.4	69,760	26.2
75–84	62,335	33.7	14,977	8.1	77,312	41.8
85+	24,362	38.4	5588	8.9	29,950	47.3
Total N	261,989	6.8	73,190	1.9	335,179	8.7

Table 6. The use of modern and natural anxiolytics (%) in the CHS-insured population by age group

Age group	Modern anxiolytics	Natural anxiolytics
	%	%
0–14	85.6	14.4
15–24	64.1	35.9
25–34	78.3	21.7
35–44	69.0	31.0
45–54	73.8	26.2
55–64	78.3	21.7
65–74	73.7	26.3
75–84	80.6	19.4
85 and above	81.3	18.7
Total	78.2	21.8

Overall, these results suggest that old habits die hard. About one in five patients uses an old-fashioned preparation; this use also exists in the younger age group. A possible reason is that the old-fashioned drugs can be accessed without a prescription, whereas a prescription is needed for other anxiolytics. Of the insured population, 6.9% use modern anxiolytics and 1.9%, old-fashioned ones.

The use of hypnotic medications

Table 7. The use of hypnotic medications (%) in the CSH-insured population by age group

Age group	n	Rate %
0–14	321	–
15–24	1952	.3
25–34	5280	.9
35–44	8021	2.0
45–54	18,625	4.5
55–64	31,197	8.4
65–74	40,770	16.4
75–84	55,300	29.9
85 and above	25,421	40.4
Total N	186,887	14.9

The use of these drugs is obviously age related, and its use in the elderly seems to reach an epidemic quality. Taking into account the increased risk of falls and confusion in the elderly using hypnotic medications, proper interventions should be considered seriously to improve this present reality.

The use of Ritalin

Table 8. The use of Ritalin (%) in the CHS-insured population by age group

Age group	n	Rate %
0–14	26,612	2.7
15–24	8977	1.6
25–34	1686	.3
35–44	627	.2
45–54	503	.1
55–64	164	–
65–74	39	–
75–84	23	–
85 and above	–	–
Total N	38,631	

It seems that the use of Ritalin in the CHS insured population is lower than reported in the literature (5). In my opinion, the health providers should seek better ways of reaching the needed and adopt a less defensive attitude regarding the use of this effective drug.

The use of lithium

Table 9. The use of lithium by age group in the CHS-insured population

Age group	n
0–14	24
15–24	321
25–34	632
35–44	646
45–54	946
55–64	843
65–74	499
75–84	267
85+	53
Total N	4231

The rate of use of lithium in the population is a meager .1%. It is the only mood stabilizer analyzed, as it was impossible to evaluate how much of the other mood stabilizers available were prescribed due to psychiatric diagnosis or to other medical conditions.

Total psychopharmacological use

In 2007, 11.8% of CHS members used at least one psychotropic (not including hypnotics). If the hypnotics were added, then the figure would reach 14.3%.

The average number of drugs taken by an average patient is 1.7. This shows that polypharmacy is common. Obviously, this does not reflect the usual recommendation of good medical practice

§ From epidemiology to mental health action

Based on the CHS-insured population, it is safe to assume that the use of psychotropic drugs in Israel is higher than that reported previously (2) and rather similar to studies conducted in other countries (6–9).

This study also showed that such use is usually age-related, and it appears not to follow known disease epidemiology or good medical practice. It is thus incumbent upon the responsible parties to elucidate the reasons for this pattern of use. More generally, what this chapter has shown is the continuous need to monitor the use of psychotropic medication in the population.

§ References

1. Storm BL, Kimmel SE, eds. *Textbook of pharmacoepidemiology,* Fourth edition. Sussex: Wiley and Sons, 2006.
2. Grinshpoon A, Marom E, Weizman A, *et al.* Psychotropic drug use in Israel: results from the national health survey. Primary care comparison. *Journal of Clinical Psychiatry* 2007; 9: 356–363.
3. Freedman DX, Stahl M. Policy implications of new psychiatric drugs. *Health Affairs* 1992; 11: 157–163.
4. Underwood BR. Dominance of second generation antipsychotics: time for reflection? *Psychological Bulletin* 2007; 31: 233.
5. Teeter – Ellison A, Pottick KJ, Zito J, *et al. Identification and treatment of* ADHD: *a lifespan perspective.* Washington, DC: SAMHSA National Mental Health Information Center, 2002.
6. Lecadet J, Vidal P, Baris B, *et al.* Psychotropic medications prescriptions and use in metropolitan France. *Revue Médicale de l'Assurance Maladie* 2003; 34: 75–84 (French).
7. Linden M, Bar T, Helmchen H. Prevalence and appropriateness of psychotropic drug use in old age: results from the Berlin aging study (BASE). *International Psychogeriatrics* 2004; 16: 461–480.
8. Angermeyer AJ, Bruaerts BS, Brugh R, *et al.* Psychotropic drug utilization in Europe: results from the European study of the epidemiology of mental disorders ESEMED project. *Acta Psychiatrica Scandinavica* (suppl.) 2004; 420: 55–64.
9. Thiels C. Utilization of psychotropic medication. *British Journal of Psychiatry* 2005; 186: 167–168.

Chapter 19

THE EPIDEMIOLOGY OF TREATED MENTAL AND BEHAVIORAL DISORDERS IN ISRAEL

Yaacov Lerner and Daphna Levinson

Mental health care in Israel has entered a period of transition in a major reform currently being implemented in the system. The main targets of the reform are the proper allocation of resources to enable the shift from inpatient to community-based care, and the inclusion of mental health care as a component of the health insurance coverage.

To fully understand the magnitude of the proposed changes, it is necessary to first review the development of the mental health services in last few decades – with an emphasis on recent years. This review is based on Ministry of Health databases and epidemiological and other studies that have been conducted. The mental health care system consists of a variety of interdependent components. For convenience, the findings will be presented in three sections – inpatient psychiatric care, ambulatory mental health services and rehabilitation services.

❧ Inpatient care

Historical overview

The mental health system in the state's early days consisted of a nationwide network of psychiatric hospitals using the buildings of vacant British army camps. This was perhaps the only possible and immediate response to the problems created by the large influx of new immigrants – many of them Holocaust survivors – suffering from mental disorders. How to provide immediate shelter and treatment facilities became an urgent policy issue (1).

The focus on hospital treatment was influenced by the prevailing medical model approach and the orientation towards curative medicine with an emphasis on acute states. Consequently, there was reluctance to deal with (or perhaps ignorance of) the need for rehabilitation and supportive care for people with chronic mental disorders. Most of the latter ultimately ended up in institutions that were similar to boarding houses. The increase in psychiatric hospital beds reached its peak in the late 1960s and early 1970s (2.4 beds per 1000 population). In the 1980s, bed rates gradually began to decline (table 1) following the community-oriented reorganization of the mental health services in the late 1970s that called for the delivery of comprehensive mental health services in geographically defined catchment areas or areas of service responsibility (2).

Table 1. Rates of psychiatric beds and inpatient days per 1000 population. Years 1958–1995 (55)

Year	Rate	Days
1958	2.1	734
1966	2.4	–
1970	2.4	915
1975	2.3	–
1980	2.2	712
1985	1.8	–
1990	1.5	495
1995	1.2	414

The monitoring and evaluation of inpatient services has been facilitated by the Psychiatric Case Register (PCR), established and maintained by the Ministry of Health since the early 1950s. All inpatient and day-care psychiatric facilities are required by law to report all admissions and discharges. The PCR cumulatively records basic demographic and psychiatric information for each admitted individual. Diagnoses are recorded for each episode at admission and discharge (3).

Trends in hospital stays

A comparison between the mental health systems of Israel and New York State, which was conducted in 1986 (see below), showed a similar residential rate – 1.9 per 1,000 population (4). The data were based on surveys covering all patients seen in public mental health services in both locations within the same week.

In Israel, inpatient care was provided mainly in psychiatric hospitals, while the general hospitals played a limited role. In contrast, the proportion of inpatients treated in NYS general hospitals reached 90%. The psychiatric bed rates in Israel continued to decrease (from 1.5 per 1000 population in 1990 to .9 in 2000). However, the proportion of psychiatric beds in Israeli general hospitals has remained low – about 5.0% of the total number of psychiatric beds in the first decade of the first century (5) compared to 20.0% in the US (6) and 10.0% to 28.0% across various European countries (7).

The limited number of psychiatric beds in general hospitals probably results from both organizational and historical reasons and budgetary constraints (4). The decline in bed rates has been accompanied by a parallel decrease in the length of inpatient stays. Levinson *et al.* (8) examined accumulated lengths of stay during seven years following first psychiatric admissions of patients admitted in the years 1960, 1970, 1980 and 1990. The results showed a decline in the accumulated lengths of stays, mainly of patients with schizophrenia and among those with long hospital stays (table 2).

Table 2. Average accumulated length of stay by four cohorts and diagnosis. Years 1960–1990 (8)

Length of stay, days	1960			1970			1980			1990		
	M	SD	n	M	SD	n	M	SD	n	M	SD	n
Schizophrenia[1]												
1–90[2]	53	23	33	54	22.2	115	51	23	162	42	24	189
91–365	196	73.9	76	191	77.4	152	196	74.4	211	186	73.7	197
366–730	540	110.5	30	502	110.5	37	508	101.1	63	482	94.3	65
731+[3]	1807	591.2	45	1695	647.2	66	1297	495.6	59	1473	610.3	57
Affective disorders[4]												
1–90[5]	53	22	44	39	24	86	42	21	102	44	25	117
91–365	193	75	28	191	71	52	177	73	74	180	78	92
366–730	517	130	9	488	113	9	456	94	24	480	95	17
731+	1849	679	7	1675	822	4	1726	592	6	1139	260	5

1 *Overall difference between cohorts* $F_{(3,1272)} = 8.59, p < .0000$
2 $F_{(3,414)} = 6.03, p < .0005$
3 $F_{(3,180)} = 5.08, p < .0021$
4 *Overall difference between cohorts* $F_{(3,660)} = 27.79, p < .0000$
5 $F_{(3,345)} = 3.68, p < .0124$

Trends in involuntary psychiatric hospitalization

The Israel Mental Health Act (MHA) was implemented in 1991. It replaced the previous MHA, which was adopted in 1955. Several authors examined the trends of involuntary hospitalization over the decade after the MHA's implementation (9–11), and all of them noted an increase in the proportion of involuntary admissions.

Bauer *et al.* (11) reported that the proportion of involuntary admissions among the total inpatient admissions per year rose significantly from 23.9% in 1991 to 38.1% in 2000. In parallel, annual involuntary admission rates per 100,000 population doubled over the follow-up period. They argued that this increase cannot be explained by implementation of the MHA, since this act aimed to reduce the number of compulsory admissions through the establishment of strict criteria, including involuntary examinations that ought to precede issuing state commitments to psychiatric institutions. According to the authors, one possible cause for this increase is the reduction of psychiatric inpatient beds during this decade. Bed unavailability might have delayed admissions, thus leading to the worsening of symptoms, poorer compliance with medication and more frequent episodes of violence. A similar claim has been mentioned in the literature by Wall *et al.* (12) in England.

Immigration and hospitalization

Since the establishment of the state in 1948, several million Jewish refugees and immigrants from all over the world arrived to its shores. Although there exists a vast amount of research literature on immigrants' mental health (13) (see chapter 6), only a few addressed the issue of hospitalization.

Popper and Horowitz (14) found that yearly psychiatric admission rates of new immigrants in 1990 to 1991 were 3.5 per 1000 compared with 2.5 per 1000 for the general population. They also found that while 6.0% of all patients who were admitted remained hospitalized for over a year, among immigrants the respective figure was 9.0%. Similar findings were reported by Shemesh *et al.* (15). These authors compared admission rates between immigrants and native-born Israelis in the years 1972–1980 and in 1990. In the 1970s, the admission rate for immigrants was 3.3 per 1000, while the rate for the local born was 2.0 per 1000. In 1990, the rates were 3.1 per 1000 vs. 2.0 per 1000, respectively. Clearly, the stress of transition and the lack of social support may have heightened the probability of psychiatric hospitalization. Indeed, 50.0% of admissions of new immigrants occurred within three months of their arrival (14). Another factor that may account for those results is that Jewish immigration is not restricted by medical criteria, thus formerly hospitalized psychiatric patients are granted permission to immigrate.

War and hospitalization

Israel has endured several wars and long periods of terrorist acts in between. Surprisingly, there are only a few studies related directly to the implications of war on psychiatric hospitalization After the Yom Kippur War, a rear unit for the treatment of soldiers with combat reactions was established based on psychodynamic and sociological theories. These indicated that it is essential to: (a) focus on the immediate experience of the soldier, (b) counteract strong regressive pulls, and (c) build on the support of the unit (16). In setting up such a unit instead of a hospital, the Israel Defense Forces hoped to preserve to the fullest the continued functioning of the soldier. The authors did not report controlled results – but based on observations they estimated that about 70% of the soldiers had improved considerably by the end of their service in the unit. After the first Gulf War, Knobler *et al.* (17) compared these psychiatric admissions to those at a major Jerusalem hospital during two parallel periods – one and two years before and one year after the war. Psychiatric hospitalizations did not decline, unlike during the previous Yom Kippur War of 1973 (18). A possible explanation is that unlike earlier wars, in the Gulf War, missiles were aimed at densely populated areas causing casualties among the civilian population. Most of the patients who were admitted had chronic psychiatric disorders in acute exacerbation. Another study on that war by Bleich *et al.* (19) examined civilians suffering from psychological symptoms who were admitted to the emergency rooms of general hospitals located in the area under attack. The authors stated that the uncertainty about the time, the target sites and type of warhead (conventional or chemical) was a source of many traumatic stress reactions at or near the missile attack sites. About 43.0% of the 773 casualties evacuated to hospitals were diagnosed as psychological casualties. When this chapter was written, there were still no such publications about the Second Lebanon War in 2006.

Levav *et al.* (20) examined the effects of escalation of terrorism in Jerusalem during the *Al-Aksa Intifada* (insurrection in Arabic) on the help-seeking behavior of the city's adult population. Regarding psychiatric admissions, there was no increase in first admissions but a short-term increase in readmissions to inpatient services (a possible effect of stress on a vulnerable group).

Correlates of psychiatric hospitalization

Several studies dealt with the correlates of psychiatric admissions and of length of stay. Lerner *et al.* (21) examined the longitudinal patterns of utilization of inpatient services. A nationwide random sample of patients admitted to psychiatric hospitals in 1980 was followed up until the end of 1984. Data were obtained from the Psychiatric Case Register. Two main contrasting patterns emerged. One consisted of a single short hospitalization for the entire four-year period.

This pattern was found among more than 50% of those patients for whom this hospitalization was the first of their lives. The second pattern characterized the patients who accumulated long periods of inpatient care – at least one year during the follow-up period (15.0% for patients on first admission and 34.0%, among patients with more that one admission). For the latter group, the main variables predicting a long cumulative stay were age (being 65 years old and over); marital status (being single); and hospitalization history (long duration and high frequency of previous hospitalizations) (22). Rabinowitz *et al.* (23) tried to identify predictors for revolving-door patients defined as "patients with four or more admissions with less than 2.5 years between consecutive admissions" based on data from the PCR. The main predictors were not being married at the time of first hospitalization, being unemployed and having a serious diagnosis such as schizophrenia. Not being married and employed remained significant predictors for a revolving door pattern, even after controlling for diagnosis of schizophrenia. They concluded that this may support the belief that social networks are important in reducing the revolving-door pattern. Berman and Zilber (24) found that predictors for a single brief psychiatric hospitalization over a follow-up of seven to eight years differ between hospitalized civilians and soldiers. For civilians, multivariate analysis revealed three main predictors – academic profession, diagnosis of neurosis and full military service (prior to hospitalization). For soldiers, the three main predictors were admission because of the risk for self harm, having been born in Israel and a need for remaining under observation. The study concluded that in civilian circumstances those individuals would have not been hospitalized.

The potential triggers for hospitalization of patients diagnosed with depression were explored in a cohort of inpatients in the Jerusalem area (25). Age over 60, immigration during the preceding five years and concomitant physical illness were the three most common potential triggers. The study limitation was the absence of a comparison group of depressed patients who were not hospitalized.

Resource allocation by the insurers according to the National Health Insurance Law of 1994 is primarily based on the age of the insured, which is a criterion less relevant for the establishment of eligibility for people with mental illness. Ginsberg *et al.* (26) examined PCR data to find gross predictors of the utilization of hospital-based psychiatric care. They found that the cumulative number of days of psychiatric hospital-based service use during the previous five years was a main predictor of future utilization. This study was done prior to the implementation of the Rehabilitation of the Mentally Disabled Act, and results of a study carried out today could well be different.

The impact of the socioeconomic status (SES) of the person's neighborhood of residence on psychiatric admissions had been studied by Rahav *et al.* (27) in Jerusalem. They found higher rates of psychiatric admission in areas of lower SES. Levinson *et al.* (28) examined the relationship between SES level of localities all over the country and psychiatric hospitalization measures. These authors found significant correlations between SES and admission rates, lengths of inpatient episodes and length of tenure in the community. Indeed, the higher the SES the lower the admission rates except for individuals in the lowest SES level, who may not be aware of the existing services and thus may not seek care in the health system.

§ Structural reform: 2000 to 2005

In the year 2000, based on the recommendations of a national committee (29) the Ministry of Health set a target of actively reducing the number of psychiatric beds between 2001 and 2005 to a bed ratio of .5/1000. The basic guiding concept was that only patients with active psychiatric symptoms should be hospitalized (30). This policy was greatly advanced following the passage of the Rehabilitation of the Mentally Disabled Act. This legislation made it possible for the Treasury to allocate an additional budget to the Ministry of Health for the transfer of patients with chronic and disabling conditions – from the hospital to sheltered housing projects if they were not in an active episode of the disorder. The purpose was to reduce the number of psychiatric beds. Indeed, a comparison of the number of patients hospitalized for over one year at the end of the 2000 to 2006 period (table 3) shows a significant drop in the number of those patients, specifically in the private hospitals (which admit only long-term stay inpatients and are characterized by poorer facilities and lower quality of care).

Table 3. Number of extended stay-patients (over one year) at the end of each year by hospital ownership. Years 2001–2007.

Year	Public hospitals	Private hospitals	Total
2001	1448	1079	2527
2002	1396	1021	2417
2003	1212	937	2149
2004	1061	844	1905
2005	1010	844	1854
2006	987	568	1555
2007	985	315	1300

Moreover, not only did the number of "old chronic patients" decreased, but there was also a decline in the yearly addition of the "new chronic patients." The percentage of yearly admissions who stayed over one year decreased from 4.0% to 2.6% (table 4).

Table 4. Psychiatric admissions extending over one year in public psychiatric hospitals (general hospitals excluded). Years 2000–2004.

Year	Number of admissions	Admissions extending over one year N	Admissions extending over one year %
2000	15,178	656	4.0
2001	14,884	511	3.4.
2002	15,397	451	2.9
2003	15,905	424	2.7
2004	16,527	429	2.6

Even most of these new patients with chronic disorders were discharged during the subsequent four years (figure 1).

Figure 1. Psychiatric admissions of patients staying over one year. Years 2000–2004

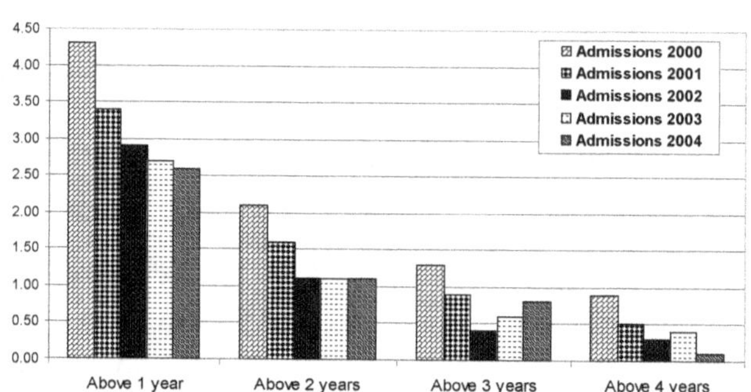

Children showed an even more dramatic decrease in the number of hospitalizations – from a peak of 6.0% in 2000 to an average of 1.0% in 2003 (31).

To cope with the rise in the absolute number of admissions due to population growth but without adding beds, it was agreed between the Ministries of Health and Finance that until the end of 2005, the mean duration of inpatient stay for active patients should drop to 32 days. During the same period, the percentage of readmissions within 30 days was targeted to drop to 12.0% and within 180 days to 36.0%, while the yearly admission rate was not to raise above 3.2/1000 (29). These aims were so far only partially achieved (table 5).

Table 5. Comparison between reform goals and achieved results. Years 2000–2006.
Mean days of inpatient stay of patients with active disorders.

Year		2000	2001	2002	2003	2004	2005	2006
Reform-goals	Adults	38.0	37.0	36.0	35.0	34.0	33.0	
	Children						60.0	
Results	Adults	37.6	38.1	36.0	36.6	36.7	33.3	32.3
	Children	52.6	55.3	55.7	56.5	59.2	56.1	54.4

Percentage of readmissions within 30 days from discharge.

Year	2000	2001	2002	2003	2004	2005	2006
Reform-goals	16.0	16.0	15.0	14.0	13.0	12.0	–
Results	16.5	16.0	15.6	17.0	16.7	17.0	17.9

Percentage of readmissions within 180 days from discharge.

Year	2000	2001	2002	2003	2004	2005	2006
Reform-goals	38.0	38.0	37.5	37.0	36.5	36.0	–
Results	39.0	39.5	39.2	39.8	40.1	40.8	41.1

Yearly admission rate per 1,000 population.

Year	2000	2001	2002	2003	2004	2005	2006
Reform-goals	≤ 3.2	≤ 3.2	≤ 3.2	≤ 3.2	≤ 3.2	≤ 3.2	
Results	2.9	2.8	2.8	2.8	2.8	2.9	3.0

The mean days of inpatient stay indeed decreased without a rise in the yearly admission rate. The more ambitious goal of lowering the percentage of early readmissions was not achieved, probably because of its partial dependence on significant improvements in community-based mental health services. The discharge of a large number of long-stay patients should enable the relocation of resources from inpatient stay to the community and thus to decrease the re-admission rates.

§ Ambulatory services

This section of the chapter provides an overview of the ambulatory services. It is based primarily on statistical reports published by the Ministry of Health and on two nationwide surveys conducted in 1986 and 2003. These two are described first. Next we describe the structure of the ambulatory mental health service system and patterns of service utilization. Finally, we discuss rehabilitation services.

§ Nationwide epidemiological surveys on mental health

Study I

The first nationwide survey of public mental health inpatient and outpatient facilities was conducted by the Ministry of Health during the last week of May 1986 (32, 33). The survey's outpatient component amassed information on the facilities' structural features, including number of staff slots and type of human resources, as well as information on the demographics, diagnostics and type of care provided to all 13,500 outpatients who came for treatment at those facilities during one typical week (a week containing neither holidays nor vacations) (32, 33). Survey questionnaires were completed by the professional staff for every patient visit, with a completion rate of 100%. The survey was carried out concomitantly with one in New York City that used the same methodology, with the purpose of comparing the two systems (32).

The survey painted a comprehensive picture of the content of care provided in the outpatient facilities, but issues relating to the prevalence of mental health disorders and the need for mental health care were left unanswered.

Study II

The Israel National Health Survey (INHS), also reviewed in many chapters of this book, was conducted in 2003 and 2004. It aimed specifically at providing estimates of prevalence of common mental disorders such as depression and anxiety and utilization levels of health and other services by adults with psychiatric problems (34). Both estimates are of major importance, especially due to the inclusion of mental health services in the mandatory "basket of services" that the four public health funds (Health Maintenance Organizations or HMOs) must provide to all their members (35).

The INHS followed the procedures established by the leading team from Harvard University and the World Health Organization (WHO) (36). The sample (34) was extracted from the National Population Register and comprised non-institutionalized legal residents aged 21 and over. It was designed to reflect a fixed distribution of respondents combining gender, age groups and population sectors (Arabs, immigrants (post-1990 immigrants from the former Soviet Union) and Jews and others (born in Israel, pre-1990 immigrants or post-1990 immigrants from countries other than the former Soviet Union).

Face-to-face interviews were conducted at the respondents' homes between May 2003 to April 2004 in Arabic, Hebrew or Russian. The survey was administered by professional interviewers using laptop computer interviews. Each interview took on average of 60 minutes, and the overall response rate was 73% (88%, among Arabs; 71%, among Jews), totaling close to 5000 interviews.

The survey provided a thorough description of the range of services used by the population for the treatment of mental health problems, as well as a detailed account of the dimensions of mental health vulnerability. This was aimed at estimating the needs for mental health care beyond the mere presence of a condition listed in the *Diagnostic and Statistical Manual of Mental Disorders – Fourth Edition* (DSM-IV).

The structure of the ambulatory mental health services

To better assess the epidemiological data presented here, we provide a quick overview of ambulatory mental health services. Mental disorders and mental health problems are treated by a variety of caregivers who work in diverse types of facilities and services (37). The specialty mental health sector is comprised of mental health professionals such as psychiatrists, psychologists, psychiatric nurses, psychiatric social workers and occupational therapists trained specifically to treat people with mental disorders. In 2007, there were 196 public mental health clinics (table 6); of them, 101 or 51.0% were owned and run by the Ministry of Health.

They are an integral part of mental health centers or linked to psychiatric hospitals and general hospitals. Of the other clinics, 38% were run by the HMOs and about 10.0% belonged to private or other public organizations About half of the clinics treat all age groups, while 18.0% of them only children or youth. In 2007, 67 urban localities (of the 226 in Israel) (38) had public mental health services. In most areas, the ratio was one clinic per about 35,000 population. Specialty mental health services were also provided privately by psychiatrists, psychologists and psychiatric social workers.

Table 6. Specialty mental health clinics by providers, target age group and district (56)

Ownership	Children and youth n	All age groups n	Adults only n	Total
Government & municipalities	21	37	43	101
Private and NGOs	2	5	0	7
Public hospitals	2	10	2	14
HMOs	10	34	30	74
Total	35	86	75	196

Age groups	Southern region	Haifa	Jerusalem	Central region	Northern region	Tel Aviv	Total
Children and youth	4	8	4	8	6	5	35
All age groups	9	13	14	22	12	16	86
Adults only	11	13	6	17	16	12	75
Total	24	34	24	47	34	33	196
(*) Population (thousands)	1021	864	870	1691	1203	1204	7117

(*) *Source: http://www.cbs.gov.il/shnaton58/download/st02_09x.xls*

Human resources

The number of staff posts in specialty mental health clinics run by the government and health funds (the largest of which, *Clalit*, was formerly run by the *Histadrut* – General Federation of Labor) was ascertained in the 1986 survey (33) and in the 1997 survey on professional resources in public mental health clinics (39). Then these clinics were almost the sole public providers of mental health care. The rates of psychiatrists and psychiatric nurses per 1000 population did not change much between the two surveys; in both periods there were about .04 posts of psychiatrists and about .02 posts of nurses per 1000. The rates of psychologists and social workers decreased between the two periods per 1000 population from .06 to .03 and from .035 to .025 respectively. The geographical distribution of human resources remained the same between the two periods, with the highest rates in the Tel Aviv district and the lowest in the north and south.

According to unpublished data from the Ministry of Health, in 2003 there were 777 full posts in all governmental and *Clalit* Health Services specialty mental health clinics. However, due to the emergence of new providers of mental health specialty services, it is not clear whether the rates per resident have changed since the 1997 survey.

Patterns of service use: Data from Study 1

The clinical disorders of the service users undergoing care in the public mental health specialty services were explored in the 1986 survey (33, 40). Service users belonged to two distinct groups, but almost equal in proportion. One group was comprised of service users affected by schizophrenia, paranoid states, affective disorders, organic conditions or functional impairment – which qualified them for disability pensions. The second group comprised of service users affected by neuroses, psychosomatic disorders, personality disorders, adjustment disorders, stress reactions, childhood disturbances or had no psychiatric diagnosis. None of the members in this group qualified for a disability pension.

The rate of patients with schizophrenia who used ambulatory services out of the total sample during that typical week in 1986 was 34.0%. Among new users –those who had their first contact during the month preceding that week – the proportion of users with schizophrenia was only 19.0%. This difference was explained by the policy of keeping patients with chronic disorders in treatment. The findings demonstrated clearly the difference between the prevalence of those seeking help in public mental health clinics and that of mental disorders in the community.

The 1986 survey revealed differences in the type of care both groups received. Individual ("talk") therapy was provided to 61.0% of the second group but to only 24.0% of the first group. Slightly over than half of the users (52.0%) in the first group received psychotropic medication (40). Users in the second group made more frequent visits to the clinic; more than half attended at least once a week. In contrast, 35.0% of users in the first group visited the clinic at least once a week.

This difference was related to the length of stay in ambulatory care. More than half of users in the first group had been in treatment for more than two years compared to only one-quarter in the second group. Findings also showed that in both groups, the longer the period of treatment the less frequent the visits are and that the majority of patients who have been under care for more than two years received medications.

The difference between these two groups of patients appeared also in two others studies done in 1986 in all of Jerusalem's outpatient clinics (41, 42). The two studies found treatment policy differences between clinics only in the treatment of neuroses and other less severe diagnostic categories (second group).

Clinics with greater psychotherapeutic orientation placed a larger percentage of newly referred patients after being registered on waiting lists or transferred them to other facilities. Clinics without this orientation had admitted most patients of this group to short-term treatment plans. Both types of clinics offered similar treatment to patients with schizophrenia or other psychotic disorders.

The 1986 survey showed a clear pattern in the use of ambulatory care resources: During a 12-month period, 50.0% of the adults made one to five visits, while another 12.0% visited more than 20 times. In other words, 8.0% of the adults made 26.0% of all visits, while 50.0% of the adults made only 9.0% of all visits (40). Using the formula developed by Laska *et al.* (43), an estimate for the yearly total number of public mental health service users was calculated from the data collected during one typical week (40). The estimate was 1.9 per 1000 population or about 2.0% per year.

Patterns of service use: Data from Study 11

The INHS (34) was conducted to estimate the mental health care needs of adults aged 21 and older residing in the community. This survey showed that in a given year, about 10.0% of the adult population had severe symptoms of mood or anxiety at a level that met DSM-IV criteria for mood or anxiety disorders (44). The survey also showed that in a given year, 10.3% of the adult population sought help for mental health-related problems (37). Table 7 presents those seeking help during one year by the type of provider and clinical severity.

Table 7. Use of services by diagnosed common mental disorders and severity level during the last twelve months (37)

| | n | Mental health professionals | | | | General health Professionals | | | Any prof. health services | Religious/ Spiritual | Any Prof. |
		Public clinic	Private practice	Non-health Services	Total	Doctor/ other health prof.	Medi-cations	Total			
Total N	4859	2.0 (.2)	2.1 (.2)	.5 (.1)	4.6 (.3)	1.6 (.2)	2.8 (.2)	4.4 (.3)	9.0 (.4)	1.3 (.2)	10.3 (.4)
AD	470	9.1 (1.4)	7.4 (1.3)	1.9 (.6)	18.6 (1.9)	5.9 (1.3)	5.5 (1.0)	11.4 (1.6)	30.1 (2.2)	4 (.9)	34.1 (2.3)
Severe	168	13.5 (2.7)	9.4 (2.3)	2.9 (1.3)	26.5 (3.5)	11.8 (2.9)	6.1 (1.8)	17.9 (3.3)	44.4 (4.1)	4.4 (1.7)	48.8 (4.1)
Moderate	166	8.5 (2.2)	8.3 (2.3)	1.8 (1.0)	18.6 (3.2)	3.4 (1.5)	5.1 (1.6)	8.5 (2.2)	27.1 (3.6)	6.4 (1.9)	33.5 (3.7)
Mild	136	3.9 (1.7)	3.5 (1.7)	.6 (.6)	8.0 (2.5)	1.1 (.8)	5.3 (1.9)	6.4 (2.0)	14.4 (3.1)	.6 (.6)	15 (3.1)
No AD	4389	1.2 (.2)	1.5 (.2)	.3 (.0)	3.1 (.3)	1.2 (.2)	2.5 (.2)	3.6 (.3)	6.7 (.4)	1.0 (.2)	7.7 (.4)

AD: *Any anxiety or depressive disorder; Prof.: Professional; Medications: psychotropic medications.*

Overall, 4.6% of the general population consulted a mental health professional; another 4.4% visited general or other physicians; and 1.3% visited only traditional "healers." About half of those consulting mental health professionals attended public mental health clinics (2.0%), while the other half sought private services. A negligible minority (.5%) discussed their problems with professionals at facilities outside of the healthcare sector (37).

Interestingly, the INHS showed the same annual rate of public mental health service use as noted in Study I. The 13 years that elapsed between the two surveys did not change the figure of 2.0% use of the public system (37, 40). However, the INHS showed that the public mental health facilities serve only 20.0% of the annual user population.

Respondents with mood or anxiety disorders (AD) had much higher consultation rates than users that did not meet any DSM-IV criteria, yet only half of the AD group (48.0%) had ever talked about their problem. In the 12 months preceding the date of the survey, only 34.1% of individuals with AD had any form of treatment; for 22.8% of them the treatment included psychotropic medication.

Consultation rates and utilization of psychotropic medication were related to the severity of the disorders (table 7). Among respondents with severe disorders, 48.8% had some type of consultation in the preceding 12 months, and 32.2% had used psychotropic medication. Individuals with moderate or mild levels of AD had lower rates of consultation (33.5% and 15.0%, respectively) and lower rates of psychotropic drug use (2.0% and 13.0%, respectively).

There were very few differences in the preferred type of treatment among individuals who sought any type of mental health treatment. The highest proportion of consultations among all respondents with a disorder was with mental health professionals (53.0% to 56.0%), with a slight preference for those in public settings, (25.0% to 28.0%).

Respondents with more severe disorders consulted with primary care doctors proportionally more often than those with less severe (moderate or mild) disorders (24.0%, 10.0% and 7.0% respectively) and used only psychotropic medication much less than the mild group (13.0% compared with 35.0%). Those with moderate disorders used religious/alternative counselors proportionally more often than the other groups (19.0% compared to 9.0% for severe and 4.0% for mild cases).

Treatment lag

The proportion of respondents who made treatment contact in the year the mood or anxiety disorders began ranged between 30.0% and 40.0%. The proportion was higher among respondents with panic or bipolar disorders (57.0% and 50.0% respectively). Within the first five years after onset, 50.0% to 60.0% of respondents with mood or anxiety disorders had contacted services regarding their disorder.

Except for panic and bipolar disorders, the median treatment-contact lag for anxiety disorders was three years, and six years for mood disorders. That is, 50.0% of respondents with mood disorders did not seek treatment within six years of the first manifestation of the disorder. A comparison of the median duration of the proportion of respondents making treatment contact within the first year showed that unless treatment contact is made within the first year, the likelihood of treatment diminishes steadily.

Number of visits in the preceding 12 months

The overall mean number of visits to mental health professionals in the past 12 months was 14, while the mean number of visits to GPs was only three. The mean and the median number of visits to both types of professional was the same for those with and without AD.

Predictors of utilization

The predictors of utilization of health services for mental or emotional problems among individuals with AD in the past 12 months showed that service utilization was significantly more prevalent in the 35-to 64-year-old group, but it was not related to level of education, level of income, gender or marital status.

Demand for ambulatory services under the new mental healthcare legislation

The relatively new legislation on mental health care (NLMH) (35) proposes to shift responsibility for mental health services to the four HMOs for all those who meet criteria for mental health disorders. The INHS (37) and other surveys have shown that the rate of use of mental health care in a population lags far behind the prevalence rate of psychiatric disorders (45–48). Yet, having an estimate for the population's prevalence of mental health disorders still leaves open the practical question of the annual numbers of the population that might demand dedicated mental health care.

The INHS (34), which focused on the prevalence of common mental disorders and the use of services for mental health problems, provided the opportunity to estimate the size of the population that is not only eligible for specialty mental health care but that will also demand ambulatory mental health specialty care from public providers.

Assuming no change in the patterns of service use observed in the survey, the analysis showed that 5.5% of the population was both eligible for care under the NLMH and likely to demand services (49). Uncertainty about the way the new legislation would change patterns of service use produced a modular estimate, depending on assumptions about who might be switching providers for financial reasons or the possibility of referring clients to public mental health providers. The estimates ranged between 1.2% – the size of the population legally eligible and using public mental health services at the time of the survey – to 5.5%, the highest limit of the estimate based on the assumption that those who "perceived the need to use" services would act on their need.

§ Rehabilitation services

Organized activities to promote rehabilitation of patients with chronic psychiatric disorders were launched in 1979 with a network of social clubs by *Enosh*, an NGO (50). It was followed by another NGO, *Eshet*, which in 1984 opened eight centers for sheltered employment and by psychiatric hospitals. *Eshet* opened 15 rehabilitation units for psychosocial and medical services for their outpatients with chronic psychiatric disorders.

In 1993, the Ministry of Health added a special rehabilitation component to its department of mental health services. Its specific goal was to develop services for long-term inpatients discharged after many years and enable them to reintegrate into the community.

The biggest boost to the rehabilitation programs followed the passage in the *Knesset* (Parliament) of the Rehabilitation of The Mentally Ill Law in July 2000 (50). It allocated special funds for rehabilitation and stipulated the procedures by which entitlement for services is determined and the rehabilitation needs are assessed.

The need to provide "baskets of services" to persons with mental illness set off a wave of initiatives for programs in housing, social activities, education, case management and employment (50).

The effects of the transfer from psychiatric hospitals to community-based hostels or other community housing projects were investigated in four different studies (19–22 and 51–54). The earliest study showed that about one-third of former inpatients were readmitted during their hostel residence and for shorter periods compared to equivalent pre-hostel periods (51). These results were repeated later (52, 53). One study found that following the closure of two long-stay psychiatric hospitals in 1997 and 2000, there was a lower readmission rate for those who were discharged into the community in the post-law period (after 2000) (52). Another study found that in 2000 and 2001, the re-hospitalization rate was significantly lower than in 1990 and 1991 for patients with schizophrenia who were hospitalized longer than six months, but not for short-stay patients with schizophrenia or for patients with affective disorders (53).

In another prospective evaluation (54) of a group discharged to hostels, patients were checked with a battery of tests two weeks before their resettlement and after six months of hostel residence. The results showed that psychopathological symptoms had declined and social interaction had increased. Hostel-based deinstitutionalization programs are a promising alternative for long-term psychiatric inpatients. Table 8 presents the increase in the number of users of rehabilitation services from the year 1999 and shows that the rate of registered users of any type of rehabilitation services increased from 1.15 to 2.62 per 1000 adults in just five years. The types of services in the highest demand were housing and the vocational services.

Table 8. Use of rehabilitation services by type. Years 1999–2005 (57)

Year	n	Rates per 1000 (18+)	Housing (*)	Vocational services (*)	Social and leisure (*)
1999	4708	1.15	1552	1968	2284
2000	5678	1.35	2117	2234	2399
2001	5914	1.37	2468	2091	3620
2002	8178	1.85	3824	3637	2743
2003	9744	2.17	4650	4422	3771
2004	11074	2.44	5491	5260	3605
2005	12213	2.62	6283	6053	3821

(*) Individuals enrolled here may also be counted under other types of services

§ Conclusions

The mental health system has changed considerably during Israel's first 60 years. The primarily inpatient care system became a diversified one of inpatient and outpatient care and rehabilitation modalities. The government is no longer the sole provider of services, and almost half of all ambulatory mental health care recipients are treated by primary care doctors.

All these transitions make possible the dual reform proposed by the Ministry of health. The reform's first component in the mental health system – the reduction of inpatient stay (cut in the number of inpatient beds, mainly of long-stay patients) – has almost been completed. Resources have been shifted to rehabilitation care with impressive results.

The second component – the inclusion of mental health care in the insurance coverage – can bring about the needed expansion of ambulatory services and specialty mental health services, and primary care doctors will increasingly care for the wide range of needs in the population.

❧ References

1. Aviram, U. Facilitating deinstitutionalization: a comparative analysis. *International Journal of Social Psychiatry* 1985; 27: 23–32.

2. Tramer L. A proposal for the reorganization of the mental health services system: a comprehensive integrated plan. *Public Health* 1975; 18: 1–12 (Hebrew).

3. Rahav M, Popper M, Nahon D. The psychiatric case register of Israel: initial results. *Israel Journal of Psychiatry and Related Sciences* 1981; 18: 251–267.

4. Siegel C, Handelsman M, Haugland G, *et al.* A comparison of the mental health systems of New York State and Israel. *Israel Journal of Psychiatry and Related Sciences* 1993; 30: 130–141.

5. Ministry of Health, Department of Information and Computation. *Psychiatric institutions in Israel, 2006*, vol. 1. Jerusalem: Ministry of Health, 2007.

6. Witkin MJ, Atay JE, Manderscheid RW. Highlights of organized mental health health services in 1994, In: Manderscheid RW, Henderson MJ, eds. *Mental health United States 1998.* DHHS Pub. No. (SMA) 99–3285. Washington, DC, 1998.

7. Levav I, Grisnshpoon A. Editorial: Beds in mental hospitals or beds in general hospitals, where should they be located? *Israel Journal of Psychiatry and Related Sciences* 2004; 41: 157–160.

8. Levinson D, Lerner Y, Lichtenberg P. Reduction in inpatient length of stay and changes in mental health care in Israel over four decades. *Israel Journal of Psychiatry and Related Sciences* 2003; 40: 240–247.

9. Bar-El Y, Durst R, Mazar Y, *et al.* Compulsory hospitalization in the light of the new legislation from the aspect of human rights. *Harefuah* 1999; 138: 15–20 (Hebrew).

10. Nahon D, Pugachova I, Yoffe R, *et al.* The impact of human rights advocacy, mental health legislation and psychiatric reform on the epidemiology of involuntary psychiatric hospitalizations. *Medicine and Law* 2006; 25: 283–295.

11. Bauer A, Rosca P, Grinshpoon A, *et al.* Trends in involuntary psychiatric hospitalization in Israel 1991–2000. *International Journal of Law in Psychiatry* 2007; 30: 60–70.

12. Wall S, Hotopf M, Wessely S. Trends in the use of the Mental Health Act: England, 1984–96. *British Medical Journal* 1999; 318: 1520–1521.

13. Lerner Y, Mirsky J, Barasch M. New beginning in an old land; refugee and immigrant mental health in Israel. In: Marsella AJ, Borneman T, Ekblad S, *et al.*, eds. *Amidst peril and pain.* Washington, DC: American Psychological Association, 2002.

14. Popper M, Horowitz R. *Psychiatric hospitalization of immigrants: 1990–1991. Statistical report 7.* Jerusalem: Ministry of Health, Mental Health Services, Department of Information and Evaluation, 1992 (Hebrew).

15. Shemesh AA, Horowitz R, Levinson D, *et al.* Psychiatric hospitalization of immigrants to Israel from the former USSR: assessment of demand in future waves if immigration. *Israel Journal of Psychiatry and Related Sciences* 1993; 30: 213–222.

16. Moses R, Bargal D, Calev J, *et al.* A rear unit for the treatment of combat reactions in the wake of the Yom Kippur War. *Psychiatry* 1976; 39: 153–162.

17. Knobler HY, Fainstein V, Maizel S, *et al.* Admissions to a psychiatric hospital during the Persian Gulf War. *Israel Journal of Medical Sciences* 1994; 30: 524–527.

18. Landau SF. Subjective social stress indicators and the level of reported psychopathology: the case of Israel. *American Journal of Community Psychology* 1990; 18:19–39.

19. Bleich A, Dycian A, Koslovsky M, *et al.* Psychiatric implications of missile attacks on a civilian population. Israeli lessons from the Persian Gulf War. *Journal of the American Medical Association* 1992; 268: 613–615.

20. Levav I, Novikov I, Grinshpoon A, *et al.* Health services utilization in Jerusalem under terrorism. *American Journal of Psychiatry* 2006; 163: 1355–1361.

21. Lerner Y, Popper M, Zilber N. Patterns and correlates of psychiatric hospitalization in a nationwide sample: I. Patterns of hospitalization with special reference to the "new chronic" patients. *Social Psychiatry and Psychiatric Epidemiology* 1989; 24: 121–126.

22. Zilber N, Popper M, Lerner Y. Patterns and correlates of psychiatric hospitalization in a nationwide sample II. Correlates of length of hospitalization and length of stay out of hospital. *Social Psychiatry and Psychiatric Epidemiology* 1990; 25: 144–148.

23. Rabinowitz J, Mark M, Popper M, *et al.* Predicting revolving-door patients in a 9-year national sample. *Social Psychiatry and Psychiatric Epidemiology* 1995; 30: 65–72.

24. Berman Ch, Zilber N. *Predictors of one-time psychiatric hospitalization. Society and Welfare* 1998; 18: 223–240 (Hebrew).

25. Lerer B, Shapira B, Bloch M, *et al.* Possible precipitants of psychiatric hospitalization in patients with major depression: results from the Jerusalem collaborative depression project. *Depression and Anxiety* 1999; 9: 156–162.

26. Ginsberg G, Lerner Y, Mark M, *et al.* Prior hospitalization and age as predictors of mental health resource utilization in Israel. *Social Science and Medicine* 1997; 44: 623–633.

27. Rahav M, Goodman AB, Popper M, *et al.* Distribution of treated mental illness in the neighborhoods of Jerusalem. *American Journal of Psychiatry* 1986; 143: 1249–1254.

28. Levinson D, Lachman M, Lerner Y. The SES setting of psychiatric hospitalization in Israel. *Social Psychiatry and Psychiatric Epidemiology* 2006; 41: 364–368.

29. Elizur A, Baruch Y, Lerner Y. The reform in mental health in Israel. In: Kop Y, ed. *The allocation of resources for social services 2004.* Jerusalem: Taub Center for Research of Social Policy in Israel, 2004.

30. Shani M. The Israeli reform of psychiatric hospitalization. *Israel Medical Association Journal* 2005; 7: 818–819.

31. Baruch Y, Kotler, M, Lerner Y, *et al.* Psychiatric admissions and hospitalization in Israel: an epidemiologic study of where we stand today and where we are going. *Israel Medical Association Journal* 2005; 7: 803–807.

32. Siegel C, Handelsman M, Haugland G, *et al.* A comparison of the mental health systems of New York State and Israel. *Israel Journal of Psychiatry and Related Sciences* 1993; 30: 130–141.

33. Feinson MC, LernerY, Levinson D, *et al.* Ambulatory mental health treatment under universal coverage: policy insights from Israel. *The Milbank Quarterly* 1997; 75: 235–260.

34. Levinson D, Paltiel A, Nir M, *et al.* The Israel National Health Survey: Issues and methods. *Israel Journal of Psychiatry and Related Sciences* 2007; 44: 85–93.

35. Haver E, Shani M, Kotler M, *et al.* Reform in mental health services – from whence and to where. *Harefuah* 2005; 144: 327–331 (Hebrew).

36. Kessler RC, Ustun TB. The World Mental Health (wmh) Survey Initiative Version of the World Health Organization (who) Composite International Diagnostic Interview (cidi). *International Journal of Methods in Psychiatry Research* 2004; 13: 93–121.

37. Levinson D, Lerner Y, Zilber N, *et al.* Twelve-month service utilization rates for mental health reasons: data from the Israel National Health Survey. *Israel Journal of Psychiatry and Related Sciences* 2007; 44: 114–125.

38. Central Bureau of Statistics. *Statistical abstracts of Israel 2007.* Localities and population (by district, sub-district and type of locality) Table 2.9 *http://www.cbs.gov.il/reader/shnatonhnew_site.htm.*

39. Levinson D. *Manpower in mental health clinics in Israel: a survey.* Jerusalem: Department of Information and Evaluation, Mental Health Services, Ministry of Health, 1998 (Hebrew).

40. Levinson D, Popper M, Lerner Y, *et al.* Patterns of ambulatory mental health services' utilization in Israel: analysis of data from a national survey (1986) and from a follow-up (1994). Jerusalem: Department of Information and Evaluation, Mental Health Services, Ministry of Health, and jdc – Israel Falk Institute for Mental Health and Behavioral Studies, 1996 (Hebrew).

41   Lerner Y, Zilber N, Barasch M, *et al.* Utilization patterns of community mental health services by newly referred patients. *Social Psychiatry and Psychiatric Epidemiology* 1993; 28: 17–22.

42. Lerner Y, Wittman L, Zilber N, *et al.* Long-term utilization of community mental health outpatient services in Jerusalem. *Social Psychiatry and Psychiatric Epidemiology* 1991; 26: 34–39.

43. Laska EM, Meisner M, Siegel C. Estimating the size of a population from a single sample. *Biometrics* 1988; 44: 461–472.

44. Levinson D, Zilber N, Lerner Y, *et al.* Prevalence of mood and anxiety disorders in the community: results from the Israel National Health Survey. *Israel Journal of Psychiatry and Related Sciences* 2007; 44: 94–103.

45. Wang PS, Aguilar-Gaxiola S, Alonso J, *et al.* Use of mental health services for anxiety, mood, and substance disorders in 17 countries in the who world mental health surveys. *The Lancet* 2007; 370: 841–850.

46. Bijl RV, de Graaf R, Hiripi E, *et al.* The prevalence of treated and untreated mental disorders in five countries. *Health Affairs* 2003; 22: 122–133.

47. Kessler RC, Demler O, Frank RG, *et al.* Prevalence and treatment of mental disorders, 1990 to 2003. *New England Journal of Medicine* 2005; 352: 2515–2523.

48. Alonso J, Codony M, Kovess v, *et al.* Population level of unmet need for mental healthcare in Europe. *British Journal of Psychiatry* 2007; 190: 299–306.

49. Levinson D, Lerner Y, Zilber N. Estimating the changes in demand for public mental health services following changes in eligibility: analysis of a national survey data. *The Journal of Mental Health Policy and Economics* (In press).

50. Shershevsky Y. Rehabilitation of the mentally ill in the community in Israel: processes and challenges. In: Aviram U, Ginath Y, eds. *Mental health services in Israel: trends and issues.* Tel Aviv: Tcherikover, 2006 (Hebrew).

51. Grinshpoon A, Shershevsky Y, Levinson D, *et al.* Should patients with chronic psychiatric disorders remain in hospital? Results from a service inquiry. *Israel Journal of Psychiatry and Related Sciences* 2003; 40: 268–273.

52. Grinshpoon A, Zilber N, Lerner Y, *et al.* Impact of a rehabilitation legislation on the survival in the community of long-term patients discharged from psychiatric hospitals in Israel. *Social Psychiatry and Psychiatric Epidemiology* 2006; 41: 87–94.

53. Grinshpoon A, Abramowitz MZ, Lerner Y, *et al.* Re-hospitalization of first-in-life admitted schizophrenic patients before and after rehabilitation legislation: a comparison of two national cohorts. *Social Psychiatry and Psychiatric Epidemiology* 2007; 42: 355–359.

54. Grinshpoon A, Naisberg Y, Weizman A. A six-month outcome of long-stay inpatients resettled in a hostel. *Psychiatric Rehabilitation Journal* 2006; 30: 89–95.

55. Ministry of Health. *Mental health in Israel. Statistical annual.* Jerusalem: Ministry of Health, 1996.

56. Ministry of Health. *Ambulatory services.* Jerusalem: Mental Health Services, Ministry of Health, 2007

57. Ministry of Health. *Mental health in Israel. Statistical annual.* Jerusalem: Ministry of Health, 2006.

Index[1]

---

1.   Numbers in italic refer to figures and tables.